AF676908

N. von Steinbüchel D. Y. von Cramon
E. Pöppel (Eds.)

# Neuropsychological Rehabilitation

With 12 Figures and 13 Tables

Springer-Verlag
Berlin Heidelberg New York
London Paris Tokyo
Hong Kong Barcelona
Budapest

Dr. rer. biol. hum. Dipl.-Psych. Nicole von Steinbüchel
Institut für Medizinische Psychologie
Goethestraße 31
W-8000 München 2
Federal Republic of Germany

Professor Dr. med. Dr. med. habil. Detlev Yves von Cramon
Städtisches Krankenhaus München-Bogenhausen
Abteilung für Neuropsychologie
Englschalkinger Straße 77
W-8000 München 81
Federal Republic of Germany

Professor Dr. phil. Ernst Pöppel
Institut für Medizinische Psychologie
Goethestraße 31
W-8000 München 2
Federal Republic of Germany

ISBN 3-540-54769-X Springer-Verlag Berlin Heidelberg New York
ISBN 0-387-54769-X Springer-Verlag New York Berlin Heidelberg

Library of Congress Cataloging-in-Publication Data.
Steinbüchel, N. von (Nicole), 1955– Neuropsychological rehabilitation / N. von Steinbüchel, D. Y. von Cramon, E. Pöppel. p. cm. Includes bibliographical references and index.
ISBN 3-540-54769-X (alk. paper). – ISBN 0-387-54769-X (alk. paper)
1. Brain damage – Patients – Rehabilitation – Congresses. 2. Clinical neuropsychology – Congresses. I. Cramon, Detlev von. II. Pöppel, Ernst. III. Title. [DNLM: 1. Brain Injuries – rehabilitation. 2. Cognition Disorders – rehabilitation. 3. Neuropsychology. WL 354 S819n]
RC387.5.S74 1992 616.8′043–dc20 DNLM/DLC for Library of Congress 92-2177 CIP

This work is subject to copyright. All rights are reserved, whether the whole or part of the material is concerned, specifically the rights of translation, reprinting, reuse of illustrations, recitation, broadcasting, reproduction on microfilm or in any other way, and storage in data banks. Duplication of this publication or parts thereof is permitted only under the provisions of the German Copyright Law of September 9, 1965, in its current version, and permission for use must always be obtained from Springer-Verlag. Violations are liable for prosecution under the German Copyright Law.

© Springer-Verlag Berlin Heidelberg 1992
Printed in the United States of America

The use of general descriptive names, registered names, trademarks, etc. in this publication does not imply, even in the absence of a specific statement, that such names are exempt from the relevant protective laws and regulations and therefore free for general use.

Product Liability: The publishers cannot guarantee the accuracy of any information about dosage and application contained in this book. In every individual case the user must check such information by consulting the relevant literature.

Typesetting: K+V Fotosatz GmbH, Beerfelden
26/3145-5 4 3 2 1 0 – Printed on acid-free paper

# Preface

The neuropsychological rehabilitation of patients with brain injuries presents a new challenge for medicine and psychology. In any society patients who have suffered a stroke or a traumatic brain lesion constitute a large group requiring special therapy; even nowadays only a small group of these patients obtain adequate rehabilitational support. Brain injuries may lead to loss or impairment of functions like language, sight, memory, attention, emotional control, or movement, and such impairments are usually accompanied by handicaps in the patient's daily life. Every attempt should be made to improve functional competence and the patient's capacity to cope with their disability and handicap.

In recent years, the aim of much research in the basic sciences has been to gain insight into the mechanisms of restitution of function, partly by trying to understand the pathophysiological mechanisms that are initiated by a traumatic event. However, in spite of this broad research initiative into recovery of function and the possibilities of cognitive remediation, our knowledge is still rather limited, with respect to both the neurobiological mechanisms that may underlie functional plasticity and the factors that may account for neuropsychological rehabilitation. In spite of these shortcomings, we would like to stress that progress can only be expected if an intense research effort is made to unite the concepts and results from the basic sciences with the practical demands of neuropsychological rehabilitation.

With this in mind, a meeting was held at which representatives from both fields came together to present ideas and results from their particular area of research. The papers from this conference are collected here; they are grouped around six major themes, each of which is followed by a critical evaluation prepared by invited discussants. The first section of the book, *basic hypotheses*, emphasizes theoretical issues and the neurobiological basis of neuropsychological rehabilitation. In particular, the concepts of local and global representations and plasticity of function are discussed with respect to recovery and rehabilitation. In the second section, different *concepts of rehabilitation* and their theoretical background, ranging from behavioral to psychoanalytically oriented approaches, are evaluated. As in any scientific field, *methodology* presents a complex problem. Some researchers prefer single case studies, whereas others believe that only classical group designs allow conclusions to be drawn about the efficacy of a treatment. The editors believe that the suitability of single case studies in allowing statements about therapeutic effects is often underestimated.

A particular methodological problem in *diagnostics* depends on the selection of the level at which a function is defined and measured. Before conducting a diagnostic survey, a decision has to be made whether one is interested in the specific functional impairment, or the patient's disability or handicap. Some researchers are of the opinion that precise knowledge of reduced basic functions is essential, whereas others believe that the patient's performance in activities of daily life should be of primary interest. In the following section on *various approaches to treatment*, a wide spectrum of therapeutic attempts is presented ranging from neuropharmacological to cognitive, psychotherapeutic, and social interventions. On a theoretical rather than an applied level, different treatment concepts are currently viewed as independent domains. We would strongly support a complementary attempt in which different therapeutic approaches can be integrated. In the final section the *treatment of functional deficits* is exemplified using the problems most often found in clinical practice such as those in speech and language, memory, attention, problem solving, and affect. It is reasonable to assume that each functional deficit requires a particular rehabilitational approach.

To improve the functional status and the quality of life of patients with a brain injury, different societies may adopt different strategies. We would like to mention here what seems to be reasonable for our country. As a first step, it appeared to be advisable to invite experts from different countries to hear how they approach the area of neuropsychological rehabilitation. On the basis of such expert knowledge, practical consequences may be envisaged. The Minister for Research and Technology provided funds for an international conference on the topic. This book contains the papers presented at this conference, which was held in October 1989. It is hoped that, on the basis of the knowledge and the opinions presented in this book, the problems of neuropsychological rehabilitation have been made more explicit, and practical solutions can be implemented. The editors would like to express their gratitude to the Minister for Research and Technology and the project managers, in particular Dr. Giesecke, Mr. Stumm, and Dr. Lehmann, for their strong support, the Carl Friedrich von Siemens-Stiftung in Munich, in particular Dr. Meier, for providing their excellent facilities for the conference, and Springer-Verlag, in particular Dr. Thiekötter and Mrs. Berger, for their interest and help in publishing this book, which will hopefully help to advance the important field of neuropsychological rehabilitation.

Munich

*Nicole von Steinbüchel-Rheinwall*
*Detlev Y. von Cramon-Taubadel*
*Ernst Pöppel*

# Contents

## Basic Hypotheses



## Controversial Concepts of Rehabilitation

## Methodology



## Diagnostics



## Various Approaches for Treatment

# List of Contributors

*Paul Bach-y-Rita,* M. D.
University of Wisconsin-Madison,
Department of Rehabilitation Medicine,
E3/348 Clinical Science Center, 600 Highland Avenue,
Madison, WI 53792, USA

*Anna Basso*, Ph. D.
Istituto di Clinical Neurologica, Università di Milano,
Via Francesco Sforza 35, 20122 Milan, Italy

*Leo Blomert*, Ph. D.
Anelt-Project, Sarphati-Park 67, 1073 CF Amsterdam,
The Netherlands

*Neil Brooks*, Ph. D.
University of Glasgow, Department of Psychological Medicine,
6 Whittinghame Gardens, Great Western Road,
Glasgow, G120AA, Scotland, UK

*Anne-Lise Christensen*, Ph. D.
Centre for Hjerneskade, Kobenhavns Universitet, Amager,
Njalsgade 88, 2300 Copenhagen S, Denmark

*Rudolf Cohen*, Ph. D.
Sozialwissenschaftliche Fakultät, Fachgruppe Psychologie,
Universität Konstanz, Postfach 5560, W-7750 Konstanz 1, FRG

*Detlev v. Cramon-Taubadel*, M. D.
Neuropsychologische Abteilung,
Städtisches Krankenhaus München-Bogenhausen,
Englschalkingerstr. 77, W-8000 Munich 81, FRG

*L. Fasotti*, Ph. D.
Institute for Rehabilitation Research, Zandbergsweg III,
6432 Hoensbroeck, The Netherlands

*Cesare Fieschi,* M. D.
Università degli Studi di Roma "La Sapienza",
Dipartimento di Scienze Neurologiche, III Clinica Neurologica,
Viale dell' Università 30, 00185 Rome, Italy

*Guido Gainotti,* M. D.
Università Cattolica del Sacro Cuore,
Facoltà di Medicina e Chirurgia "Agostino Gemelli",
Istituto di Clinica delle Mallatie Nervose e Mentali,
Largo Agostino Gemelli, 8, 00168 Rome, Italy

*David Howard,* Ph. D.
Psychology Department, Birkbeck College, Malet Street,
London WC1 E7HX, UK

*Walter Huber,* Ph. D.
Neurologische Klinik,
Rheinisch-Westfälische Technische Hochschule, Pauwelsstr. 30,
W-5100 Aachen, FRG

*Bryan Jennett,* M. D.
Department of Neurosurgery,
Institute of Neurological Sciences,
The Southern General Hospital, Glasgow G51 4TF,
Scotland, UK

*William Jenkins,* Ph. D.
Coleman Laboratory U-499, University of California,
Medical Center, San Francisco, CA 94143-0732, USA

*Andrew Kertesz,* M. D.
Department of Clinical Neurological Sciences,
St. Joseph's Hospital, London, Ontario N6A 4V2, Canada

*Muriel D. Lezak,* Ph. D.
School of Medicine, Dept. of Neurology,
Oregon Health Sciences University,
3181 S.W. Sam Jackson Park Road, L226,
Portland, Oregon 97201-3098, USA

*Norbert Mai,* Ph. D.
Entwicklungsgruppe klinische Neuropsychologie,
Dachauerstr. 164, W-8000 Munich 19, FRG

*Antony J. Marcel,* Ph. D.
MRC Applied Psychology Unit, 15 Chaucer Road,
Cambridge CB2 2EF, UK

*John Marshall,* Ph. D.
The Radcliffe Infirmary, Neuropsychology Unit,
Woodstock Road, Oxford OX2 HE, UK

*Gabriele Matthes-v. Cramon,* Dipl.-Psych.
Städtisches Krankenhaus München-Bogenhausen,
Englschalkingerstr. 77, W-8000 Munich 81, FRG

*Michael M. Merzenich,* Ph. D.
Coleman Laboratory U-499, University of California,
Medical Center, San Francisco, CA 94143-0732, USA

*Ernst Pöppel,* Ph. D.
Institut für Medizinische Psychologie,
Ludwig-Maximilians-Universität, Goethestr. 31,
W-8000 Munich 2, FRG

*George P. Prigatano,* Ph. D.
Barrow Neurological Institute,
St. Joseph's Hospital and Medical Center,
350 West Thomas Road, Phoenix, Arizona 85013-4496, USA

*Christian Rüger,* M. D.
Klinikum der Justus-Liebig-Universität,
Medizinisches Zentrum für Psychosomatische Medizin,
Klinik für Psychosomatik und Psychotherapie, Friedrichstr. 28,
W-6300 Gießen, FRG

*Viktor Shklovsky,* M. D.
Moskovskij Nauchno-Issledovatelskij, Institut Psichiatrii,
Vsesojuznyi Centr Patologii Rechi, Ul. Potesknaja 3,
107258 Moscow, Russia

*Donald G. Stein,* Ph. D.
The State University of New Jersey,
Rutgers Graduate School – Newark,
360 King Boulevard/401 Hill, Newark, New Jersey 07102, USA

*Nicole v. Steinbüchel-Rheinwall,* Ph. D.
Institut für Medizinische Psychologie,
Ludwig-Maximilians-Universität, Goethestr. 31,
W-8000 Munich 2, FRG

*Lance E. Trexler,* Ph. D.
The Center for Neuropsychological Rehabilitation, Inc.,
8925 North Meridian Street, Suite 100,
Indianapolis, Indiana 46260, USA

*Derick T. Wade*, M.D.
Rivermead Rehabilitation Centre, Abingdon Road,
Oxford OX1 4XD, UK

*Esther Wicab Bach-y-Rita*, Ph.D.
University of Wisconsin-Madison,
Department of Rehabilitation Medicine,
E3/348 Clinical Science Center, 600 Highland Avenue,
Madison, WI 53792, USA

*Klaus Willmes*, Ph.D.
Neurologische Klinik,
Rheinisch-Westfälische Technische Hochschule, Pauwelsstr. 30,
W-5100 Aachen, FRG

*Barbara Wilson,* Ph.D.
Medical Research Council (MRC), Applied Psychology Unit,
15 Chaucer Road, Cambridge CB2 2EF, UK

*Michael Wirsching*, M.D.
Klinikum der Justus-Liebig-Universität,
Medizinisches Zentrum für Psychosomatische Medizin,
Klinik für Psychosomatik und Psychotherapie, Friedrichstr. 28,
W-6300 Gießen, FRG

*Rodger Li Wood,* Ph.D.
St. George's House, 56 Billing Road, Northampton NN1 5DB,
UK

*Ed van Zomeren*, Ph.D.
Academisch Ziekenhuis Groningen, Oostersingel 59,
Postbus 30.001, 9700 RB Groningen, The Netherlands

# Basic Hypotheses

# Neuropsychological Rehabilitation from a Theoretical Point of View

*E. Pöppel and N. von Steinbüchel*

## Introduction

In neuropsychological rehabilitation of patients who have suffered a brain injury the mode of representation of function has to be taken into account. Rehabilitation of brain injured patients without neuropsychological foundation is of course possible, but taking neurobiological mechanisms into account seems a likely possibility to improve therapy.

If neuropsychology is to provide a basis for rehabilitation, the first step is to clarify how functions are represented in the brain and how lesions result in functional deficits. The theory about the mode of functional representation determines the selection of diagnostic procedures and therapeutic strategies. Many programs in neuropsychological rehabilitation are explicitly or implicitly based on the concept of a local representation of elementary functions. A local (or regional) representation of elementary functions is referred to here as modular or algorithmic representation; this terminology indicates that programs within neuronal assemblies or networks that are generally implemented in circumscribed brain areas and characterized by specific transmitter systems guarantee the availability of elementary psychological functions. This notion does not imply that a specific brain area necessarily represents only one function. It is conceivable that neurochemical differentiations allow the representation of different functions within one area; the information transfer between neurons which are located in one area can be distinguished by different transmitters, thus resulting in a spatially overlapping representation of functions within a circumscribed region.

Although a spatial segregation of functional representation has been repeatedly demonstrated, this representational mode of function has also been questioned. An alternative opinion on a more holistic representational mode is especially expressed by some researchers who work on the problem of restitution of function and rehabilitation. Several observations may indeed favor a representational mode not supporting a strict localizing principle (e.g., Marshall 1984; Meier et al. 1987; Stein 1988; Bach-y-Rita 1990). It could, however, also be the case that secondary factors mask a spatial localization of function. An additional source of controversy may be due to the fact that it often remains unclear what is meant by function. In principle, it appears possible that the localizing principle applies for one class of functions but not for another.

In what follows we want to describe a classification of elementary functions that can be used as a basis for their identification and perhaps their definition. In this classification, two classes of functions are distinguished (Saper and Plum 1985; Pöppel 1988; Berrol 1990), namely those that are responsible for the content of consciousness (the what of subjective experience) and those that have to be considered as the formal or logistical prerequisite of mental activity (the how). We hope that this distinction will help to settle certain disagreements about localization or non-localization of function. Furthermore, we believe that the different models formulated for neuropsychological rehabilitation can be discussed comprehensively within the general framework suggested by this classification. In addition, neurobiological mechanisms considered essential for restitution of functions can be referred to more precisely (e.g., von Monakow 1911; Teuber 1975; Gage et al. 1982; Marshall 1984; Diller 1987; Meier et al. 1987; Stein 1988).

## Localization of Function

In a critical evaluation of the localization principle, Damasio and Geschwind (1985) stressed that a large number of factors have to be considered if the correlations between structure and functions are to be discussed. Since Broca's observations (1865), circumscribed lesions of the brain have been used to investigate the relationship between structure and function. If the relationship between structure and function is evaluated at first sight it may appear unreasonable to assume an isomorphic mapping between a defined psychological event and a circumscribed area of the brain. It appears more sensible to look for the activity of an area within the framework of the neuronal activity of the entire central nervous system. The importance of evaluating the activity pattern of the brain in its entirety and not only in discrete regions has already been stressed by von Monakow (1911) and by Luria (1970), and it is certainly supported by observations using measurements of regional cerebral blood flow or glucose metabolism while a subject or patient is performing a certain task (e.g., Risberg 1986; Corbetta et al. 1990). However, although neuronal activity in several different brain areas characterizes specific mental acts like speaking or reading, it is also evident that circumscribed brain areas have to be functional to provide all the qualitative elements that characterize mental activity or phenomenal reality (Kertesz 1983).

To correlate the hypothetical relationship between structure and function the following factors have to be taken into account (Damasio and Geschwind 1985); some of the indicated factors may mask a close association between a defined function and a circumscribed area, i.e., a spatial localization of function:

*Mode of the Pathological Process.* For a correlational analysis, it is important to know whether the functional loss is due to stroke, trauma, tumor, infection, toxic, inflammatory, chronic degenerative processes, or other reasons.

*Size and Region of the Lesion.* If some kind of spatial organization for functional representation is suspected one has to know where the lesion is located. Furthermore the extent of the lesion is essential; paradoxically, quite often small lesions result in a greater functional loss than large lesions (Irle 1987).

*Speed of the Pathological Process.* Since the last century it has been known that slowly growing tumors result in a smaller functional deficit than sudden processes, like traumata. A similar conclusion on the importance of the time factor can be drawn from experiments on the serial lesion effect (Stein 1988).

*Time of the Diagnostic Evaluation.* It is very important how soon after a brain injury a diagnostic procedure is performed; this has already been pointed out by von Monakow (1911). It has, for instance, been noted that diagnostic analyses using computer tomography give different results immediately after the onset of a disease and sometime later (Damasio and Geschwind 1985).

*Instationary Observation Conditions.* Brain injury can cause changes of general nature that also can mask a close relationship between structure and function. For instance, it is wellknown that patients tire more easily after a brain lesion, their motivation is reduced, their capacity to concentrate is impaired, and the speed of basic mental processes is slowed down. If not controlled, these factors may increase the variance of measurements obtained with such patients and indicate a greater divergence in the relationship between structure and function than actually exists (Poppelreuter 1917; Pöppel et al. 1978).

## Content of Consciousness

With respect to functional representation we distinguish between two different classes of elementary functions. One domain comprises those functions which provide the content of mental activity or consciousness (the what); the other domain comprises those functions that determine the how, i.e., the necessary formal or logistical basis for the availability of what-functions. These two functional domains are usually not distinguished which may sometimes lead to unnecessary misunderstandings. Whereas the modular (in the special case local) representation may apply to what-functions, the neuronal algorithms for the logistical how-functions may be less well or not at all localized.

The content of consciousness is, for instance, determined by perception. When we perceive – an act which is characterized by an intentional relationship between subject and object – there is always something specific that is represented in consciousness. It has been shown for the visual system using neuroanatomical and neurophysiological techniques that elementary attributes of vision are represented according to the principal of segregation of functions (Zeki 1978), although in addition to the principle of segregation (or dissociation) a potential association of elementary functions has been demonstrated in neuropsychological investigations (e.g., Milner and Teuber 1968; Pöppel et al. 1978). An association can be expected if functions are represented by neuronal algorithms that share one area using different neurochemical markers or if the output of one area is needed as input in another area and the first area is affected by an injury. Experiments on perceptual completion suggest that one area codes visual information using one of two different neuronal algorithms, depending on whether stimuli are stationary or moving (Pöppel 1985a).

The fact that defined functions may be lost with interindividual constancy if circumscribed areas of the brain are destroyed supports the modular or algorithmic principle of perceptual representation rather convincingly. This mode of functional representation also applies to the other what-functions (e.g., Pöppel 1988), namely stimulus processing (association, learning and memory), stimulus evaluation (emotion), and stimulus response (action and reaction). The wellknown case of the patient H. M., who lost specific aspects of his memory systems following brain surgery because of a bilateral hippocampal ablation (Scoville and Milner 1957), is one example of the modular representation of the mnemonic processing functions. Because of the ablation, H. M. is no longer capable of storing new referential information although his short-term memory as well as recall mechanisms for information stored prior to the operation are still intact. Evaluation functions as represented by emotions are also characterized by a modular representation, as has been demonstrated by brain stimulation in neuroethological studies (Ploog 1980).

Irrespective of whether a circumscribed area may represent one or several functions, one has to ask the question according to which principle functions are represented within such areas. Of particular interest is whether topological principles are used for representation and, if so, what the variables are that define topological maps for functions for whom such a topological representation is not self-evident, like emotions or referential memory. For intramodular neuronal computations – and perhaps for intermodular ones also – neuronal oscillations that could be used for the binding of information between different neurons have recently been suggested (Gray et al. 1989; Pöppel et al. 1990, 1991). Although speculation concerning oscillations is interesting, knowledge of the neuronal mechanisms underlying elementary functions is still rather limited. Neuronal oscillations could also serve other purposes, like the creation of system states for the entire central nervous system (Pöppel 1970, 1985b; Pöppel et al. 1990). Obviously, the functional binding of the activities of different neurones is only one of the necessary basic operations in intramodular computations that is needed to provide functional availability on a macroscopic (i.e., behavioral or experiential) level.

Within this context, one should recall the principles of equipotentiality and mass action suggested by Lashley (1963). These principles may be quite important for a better understanding of restitution of function after brain injury. We propose the hypothesis that within one neuronal module the law of equipotentiality and mass action may apply to those neurones (or a partial set of neurones) that belong to the network subserving one defined function. After an incomplete injury within one neuronal module it is assumed that a set of equipotential neurones remains functional and that by improving their synaptic efficacy, functional improvement may be obtained.

The principle of equipotentiality does not preclude that the relationship between cellular function and an elementary psychological function on a macroscopic level can sometimes show long-term variation. That such relations are not absolutely fixed can be derived from observations on the neuronal plasticity in the motor system (Glees and Cole 1960), the somatosensory system (Wall and Egger 1971; Merzenich et al. 1983), and from considerations about the divergence of projection in the visual system that has been suggested as an underlying mechanism in the blindsight phenomenon (Pöppel et al. 1973) or the functional improvement of visual-field size after occipital lesions (Pöppel 1977; Zihl and von Cramon 1979). Because of morphological constraints (like a marked divergence and, thus, convergence of projection) limited functional reassignments due to a specific functional use or particular training appear feasible. A potential neuronal plasticity is of great importance for rehabilitation of function, although it could well be that functional plasticity is easier to obtain in the motor than in the sensory domain (Pöppel et al. 1987).

If one accepts a correlation between circumscribed brain areas or specific neuronal algorithms and defined elementary what-functions (although this relationship sometimes can be masked by secondary factors), if one assumes that, on the basis of different transmitter systems within one such area, different functions may be represented, and if one takes into account a potential long-term reassignment (or "plasticity") of function, it appears possible to unite several observations on restitution of function within one conceptual framework. To do so comprehensively, however, one has to distinguish between the what-functions that represent the content of consciousness and the how-functions that are responsible for the logistics of mental activity.

## Logistics of Mental Activity

It appears practical to differentiate between two different logistical functions i.e., activation and temporal coordination of functions. An increase or decrease of these functions after brain injury may lead to severe neuropsychological impairments, disabilities and handicaps. Without a minimal amount of activation, mental functions are not available in consciousness, or their subjective intensity is reduced as in patients in coma or those who go through different stages of reduced activation after a coma (von Cramon 1979; Saper and Plum 1985). This reduced activation after brain injury is an important problem which has to be dealt with extensively in the rehabilitation of function. Reduced activation can be reflected in a decrease in concentration, attention, and a marked fatiguability. Heightened activation can for instance be reflected in flight of ideas and disturbances of the problem-solving capacities.

Within the general area of activation, the mechanism of selective attention is of particular importance. New observations using positron-emission-tomography (PET scans) show that selective attention is controlled by a top-down mechanism (Corbetta et al. 1990). It has been demonstrated that focusing attention on particular attributes of an event results in higher activity within typical patterns of different brain areas; these patterns of enhanced activity vary according to the attentional foci. It appears possible that after a brain injury this top-down guidance of focusing and shifting attention may be disturbed, although elementary functions might be available.

Another domain of logistical functions is the temporal organization of elementary functions. Such temporal mechanisms are important to relate the neuronal activity of different elementary functions to each other and to temporally integrate information which is collected successively throughout time (Pöppel 1985b, 1989; Pöppel et al. 1991). As different what-functions are presumably represented in different areas or with particular neuronal algorithms within one area, one can assume the existence of a specific logistical mechanism which temporally organizes the various functions and relates them to one other; the different activities separated either spatially or algorithmically must be integrated somehow. If there is a disturbance in this temporal reference system, unified mental acts may no longer be possible (as suggested by the thought disorder observed in some schizophrenic patients).

An additional temporal integration mechanism has to be assumed that is available for the binding of successive information processed in different sensory channels like in the visual and auditory modality. This temporal integration mechanism must be responsible for linking discrete mental events. It has been demonstrated that an automatic binding mechanism is responsible for integrating successive information up to temporal intervals of approximately three seconds (Pöppel 1985b). In aphasic patients, this temporal integration mechanism appears to be disturbed. It is conceivable that in attentional problems after frontal lobe injuries this automatic process of binding discrete mental events has also suffered.

## Domains of Neuropsychological Rehabilitation

If one accepts the basic principles of the classificatory system presented here, i.e., that elementary functions are represented by special neuronal algorithms sometimes associated with circumscribed areas of the brain, that furthermore activation is necessary to guarantee the availability of these functions, and that particular programs have to provide the interaction between these modules, then the following potential disturbances can be predicted:

1. A lesion may result in a *partial* loss of a circumscribed area representing one or several particular functions.
2. A lesion may result in a *complete* loss of a circumscribed area representing one or several particular functions.
3. A lesion may result in a reduction of *activation* of all functional areas or a partial set of circumscribed areas representing a class of particular functions.
4. A lesion may result in a disturbance (or even interruption) of the *interaction* between the different circumscribed areas representing particular functions.

Obviously, various combinations of disturbances are also possible as is usually the case. A brain injury may result in a partial loss of one function, and (or) the complete loss of another function, and (or) a reduction of activation, and (or) problems in relating the remaining functions to each other. Using a combinatoric rule one can in principle predict 15 different pathological patterns after brain injury on the basis of the taxonomy of functions outlined here.

1/2 Partial loss of one function and complete loss of another function
1/3 Partial loss of one function and problems with activation
1/4 Partial loss of one function and problems in the interaction between this and the remaining functions
2/3 Complete loss of one function and problems with activation
2/4 Complete loss of one function and problems in the interaction in other remaining functions
3/4 Problems with activation and the interaction of different functions
1/2/3 Partial loss of one function, complete loss of another function, and problems with activation
1/2/4 Partial loss of one function, complete loss of another function, and problems in the interaction between remaining or partially spared functions
1/3/4 Partial loss of one function, problems with activation, and problems in the interaction between remaining or partially spared functions
2/3/4 Complete loss of one function, problems with activation, and problems in the interaction between remaining functions
1/2/3/4 Partial loss of one function, complete loss of another function, problems with activation, and problems in the interaction between remaining or partially spared functions.

To keep the argument simple, the relationship between pathological patterns and neuropsychological rehabilitation models as they have been described (e.g., Diller 1987) is indicated only for the discrete functional classes 1–4 mentioned above. The pathological patterns and neuropsychological rehabilitation models are:

– Partial lesions of circumscribed areas of the brain may result in a reduction of functional competence. In neuropsychological rehabilitation, such a pathological situation which leads to a lack of proper experience is referred to as the deficiency model. For therapeutic interventions this model suggests a structured training of the impaired functions.

- A lesion may result in a total loss of an area representing one or several functions, and it cannot be expected that the specific function can be saved or improved. In neuropsychological rehabilitation, this situation is referred to as the absence model, which is characterized by other therapeutical methods, like substitution of function.
- A lesion may disrupt or disturb the interaction between different circumscribed areas that represent separate functions. In rehabilitation research, such a situation is referred to as the interference model. The removal of the interference is the goal of different therapeutical interventions as for instance the isolation or suppression of interfering activities (Diller 1987).
- Apparently, in the different neuropsychological rehabilitation models reduced activation is not considered as an independent domain for functional rehabilitation. Based on the classification of functions presented above we would like to suggest, however, that four independent domains of rehabilitation have to be appreciated because qualitatively different neuronal algorithms are responsible for the availability of the what- and how-functions, i.e., activation of function should be treated as a separate entity. Thus, the four domains of rehabilitation are:
  1. *Restitution* of function after partial lesions of circumscribed areas or specific neuronal algorithms
  2. *Substitution* of function after complete lesions of circumscribed areas or defined neuronal algorithms
  3. *Activation* of function(s) after a pathological alteration of activation being too low or too high
  4. *Integration* of functions if the interaction between functional modules or their temporal relationship is deficient.

For these different therapeutical domains – restitution, substitution, activation and integration – different therapeutical strategies have to be envisaged. For restitution of function, specific functional training with varying complexity of the experiences might be useful. In substitution of function, the provision of alternative behavioral strategies to compensate for the complete functional loss may prove effective. For activation, psychopharmaca or behavioral modification could be appropriate. For integration of function, specific training programs or psychopharmaca might be useful.

As lesions usually effect several of the basic mechanisms in a concrete case, the different strategies have to be combined according to the patient's specific deficit pattern. Thus, in a rather simple case, only restitution or substitution of function may be sufficient, but in most cases a combination of strategies is probably advisable. The different therapeutic models propagated in neuropsychological rehabilitation are not mutually exclusive as alternative strategies but have to be looked upon as complementary.

Obviously, the decision to apply a specific rehabilitation program has to be based on detailed analyses of still intact, partially spared, or completely lost functions using appropriate diagnostic tools (e.g., Goldstein 1987). One has to emphasize that the selection of the kind of therapy depends on the level of diagnosis. If the brain injury is measured on the level of impairment, disability, or handicap (e.g., Wade, this book) different therapy strategies are indicated. On the level of the handicap for instance, activities of daily life, the ADL's (Brown et al. 1980) are assessed. For language therapy a measurement of ADL's, i.e., the patient's verbal communication in daily living, can have an implication for therapy. A training will not only deal with linguistic disturbances but with the patients capacity to get along in daily life situations of communication.

Complementary to the till now mentioned therapeutical interventions which are based on neurobiological and neuropsychological concepts the following considerations supported by the psychologically oriented systems theory have to be taken into account as well. Besides the neurological and neuropsychological consequences a brain injury also has to be understood as a traumatic interruption of the intra- and interpersonal system that provides the individual integrity and identity of a patient. Usually, a brain injury leads to great emotional disturbances, conflicts and quite often to personality changes. These personal alterations have to be dealt within appropriate counselling and individual and/or group therapy (Prigatano 1986, 1987; Ellis 1989). Besides the direct support that has to be provided by psychotherapeutic interventions the patient often has to develop an awareness of the disease at first in order to start a promising neuropsychological rehabilitation. A later aim of the therapeutical process is to prepare the patient to accept or better get used to the fact that particular functions might never again be available. The patient has to develop a new life style that is compatible with his abilities. Coping mechanisms and the patients acceptance of the chronic impairment have to develop. After brain injury, constant training and motivation is necessary to keep up a regained functional level. Such motivation can be one consequence of psychotherapy; it is most often also provided by family members or the patients' immediate social environment. Often the personal surrounding of the patient also requires psychotherapeutic counselling and support.

## Neurobiological Concepts of Rehabilitation

Recently, attention has been focused on which morphological or neurochemical mechanisms might be important for rehabilitation of function. We would like to relate the different therapeutic approaches indicated above (restitution, substitution, activation, and integration) to some of these neurobiological processes.

Restitution of function appears to be possible when a certain redundancy of functional representation is present. During development, such redundancy is well established (Changeux and Danchin 1976; Huttenlocher 1990); a surplus of synaptic contacts is available and only a partial set of these synaptic contacts are stabilized, i.e., selected for further neuronal processing (Edelman 1987). A potential structural basis for redundancy that remains potentially operative throughout life may be provided by a marked degree of divergence and convergence of projection in the afferent pathways. Possibly, the widely propagated strict topological representation of sensory maps onto cortical areas may well be overemphasized. Divergence of projection can be conceived of as a structural basis for potential recovery of perceptual functions after brain injury. After local lesions, adjacent areas within a functional module that have remained unaffected by the lesion may be activated to improve the partially lost functional competence. Enhanced functional competence may be possible because of an improvement of synaptic efficacy in the remaining tissue (Glees and Cole 1960; Pöppel 1977; Merzenich et al. 1983).

Another structural basis for restitution of function may be provided by the multiple representation of functions which is theoretically possible if such pluripotentiality of functional representation can actually be demonstrated. It is conceivable that different functions are represented in multiple areas in the brain (like in the two hemispheres) and that after an injury of one area the other area may jump in to take over the function on the behavioral level. This principle of vicarious representation could also imply that the output of a circumscribed area representing a function can be transiently suppressed. Some observations on speech representation in children suggest that, at least up to the end of maturation, speech functions may be represented in both hemispheres, although the dominant left hemisphere may provide a higher potential for the development of linguistic competence (Woods and Teuber 1973).

Another possibility of restitution can be seen in the principle of compensation of function. This means that within an area partially effected by a lesion, an internal reorganization of neuronal activity may occur to represent the function appropriately. Since throughout life a loss of neurons within every neuronal module is constantly occurring, a compensatory mechanism must always be in operation. From a theoretical point of view, it appears to be suggestive to link the neuronal mechanism responsible for compensation of function to the principles of equipotentiality and mass action mentioned above (Lashley 1963).

Restitution of function may also depend on the disappearance of a neuronal shock after brain injury. This phenomenon has been described as diaschisis by von Monakow (1911). Diaschisis implies that there is an imbalance between excitation and inhibition between different areas after a brain injury. The gradual disappearance of this imbalance results in the reinstatement of functional competence that has been masked transiently. Thus, the fading away of diaschisis does not represent an active restitutional process but a functional unmasking.

Such an imbalance between excitation and inhibition between different areas has been observed experimentally in the visual system of the cat (Sprague 1966) and it has been suggested for visual mechanisms in the human (Pöppel and Richards 1974; Singer et al. 1977). An injury in the occipital lobe will result in a contralateral blindness. It has been shown that such a blindness can be removed if the contralateral colliculus superior is ablated or when the tectal commissure is cut. Both experimental manipulations lead to restitution of function because the initial manipulation apparently resulted in an imbalance of excitation and inhibition between the colliculi and the cortical areas. Under normal circumstances each occipital lobe excites the ipsilateral colliculus superior, and both colliculi inhibit each other. After the ablation of one cortical area, the ipsilateral colliculus receives too much inhibition because the excitatory input is lacking. The second operation removes the inhibitory input and, thus, reinstates functional competence. Equivalent phenomena could be described in humans (Pöppel and Richards 1974). Furthermore, it has been suggested that the collicular system in the human participates in the control of selective visual attention (Singer et al. 1977). With respect to restitution of function, these observations indicate the importance of an equilibrium of excitation and inhibition between functionally related areas. Disturbances on this level may also lead to an impaired integration of functions that are represented in different areas (see below).

Substitution of function is required if restitution of function is no longer possible because of the complete loss of circumscribed areas normally representing a function. For substitution of function, brain areas have to be used that have remained unaffected or are partially spared after stroke, trauma, or whatever the pathological process has been. Substitution of function refers mainly to new behavioral strategies to replace the original function with a useful behavioral alternative. The acquisition of new strategies in behavioral organization after brain injuries play an important role in daily life activities. From a practical point of view, substitution of function may often be more useful than restitution of function if the functional resources of elementary functions after a lesion are too limited. Substitution of function also refers to providing technical help, like specific protheses that can be used to mimic the original behavior.

Neuronal mechanisms tapped in substitution of function if alternative behavioral strategies are implemented may be similar to those involved in the development of conditioned behavior. If a conditioned reflex is established previously unconnected functions represented in different regions of the brain or by different neuronal algorithms are linked to provide a new behavioral category. It has been demonstrated that the neuronal traces of a conditioned behavior are not limited to the peripheral level, but involve central areas as well. The basic idea of the installment of functional links between unlinked areas has to be considered as an interesting mechanism for substitution of function. It would be reasonable to use the rich material from this experimental paradigm to obtain a better understanding of substitution of function.

Activation of functions can probably be reached mainly by pharmacological means, but it may also be possible to provide higher activation if the environment within which a patient has to function is enriched, as is indicated by some animal experiments (Will et al. 1977). A reduction in activation may result in a deficiency of motivation, increased fatiguability, or a reduction in the speed of mental processes. Training procedures and other therapeutic interventions are probably more successful with an appropriate level of activation. Cope (1988) mentions several areas where psychopharmacologic interventions might be useful: Agonists of the katecholaminergic system can be useful in the control of coma, and they can be administered in patients with a reduced level of activation; antidepressants may help to overcome a personal crisis and establish the necessary attitude for a successful rehabilitation; cognitive problems like memory functions or attentional mechanisms might be improved; finally, the agitation of the patients may have to be controlled (Levine 1988), which is probably the most frequent indication for psychopharmacologic interventions: "as head injured patients get better they get worse".

From a neurobiological view point integration of functions after brain lesions appears to be the least developed field in neuropsychological rehabilitation. The reason for this fact can be seen in the obvious lack of a theoretical orientation in neuropsychological rehabilitation, which is characterized by an eclectic orientation rather than a principal neurobiological foundation. A specific aspect of this therapy appears to be that it is not a particular function or the potential competence of the patient that has to be trained but that within a certain ecological context (which is of course different for each patient) integrated mental activity as reflected in the patient's performance has to be improved by removing the detrimental interference (e.g., Diller 1987). At present the therapeutic methods suggested within the domain of the so-called interference model (that comes closest to the problem indicated here) seem to be rather removed from a neurobiological basis.

We shall discuss one specific aspect of aphasia research which emphasizes the problem one is confronted with in integration of function. An aphasic patient is usually treated with a linguistically oriented therapy (e.g., Poeck et al. 1977; Kertesz 1985). If his lexical competence has suffered, he has to relearn a vocabulary; if he is agrammatic, one attempts to improve his syntactic competence; if his speech does not make sense, his semantic competence is treated. In these cases, emphasis is put on specific aspects of language behavior, i.e., different linguistic competences are singled out, and one tries to improve these competences if they have been impaired by the injury.

There are, however, alternative approaches to the problem of aphasia after brain injury and potential improvement by neuropsychological rehabilitation (e.g., Blomert, this volume). The approach we would like to suggest, however, is neurobiologically orientated and is based on the observation that after brain injuries central neuronal processes are usually slowed down. A retardation of neuronal processes implies that an area with a partial lesion operates in a different time domain than other unaffected regions. These different temporal processes may put an extra burden on the integration of functions that are represented in different regions.

A slowing down of central temporal processing mechanisms can be demonstrated by measuring order thresholds (von Steinbüchel 1987). The order threshold can for instance be determined using click stimuli presented binaurally; the subject has to indicate which one of two stimuli comes first. In healthy subjects, the auditory order threshold is close to 30 ms; in patients with acquired speech defects this threshold is prolonged up to more than 100 ms. Thus, the brain-injured patient needs much more time to indicate the sequence of two discrete auditory events. This slowing down of central nervous processes as reflected in the prolonged order threshold might be directly reflected in problems of language understanding (von Steinbüchel and Pöppel 1991). Auditory information that determines speech sounds is characterized by rather strict temporal constraints; if a receiving organ is slowed down in its processing of information, normal speech may be too fast for the patient. In such a situation, an integration of sensory information with the semantic component or other aspects of language may become difficult or even impossible. Experimental evidence shows (von Steinbüchel 1987) that such patients have difficulties in discriminating voiced and unvoiced phonemes (like "da" vs "ta"). A training of temporal order threshold up to a normal level was paralleled by an improvement in the phonetic domain. We propose that functional training – in this case, specific temporal training – can constitute a prerequisite for the successful integration of function. Only if neuronal algorithms operate in the same time domain can one expect efficient integration.

## Restitution of Function as a Neurobiological Challenge

In recent neurobiological research, a number of specific neuronal mechanisms at the cellular level have been discussed with respect to restitution of function. In this context neuromorphological and neurochemical mechanisms should be distinguished (Marshall 1984). It is still an open question whether these mechanisms relate to functional rehabilitation at the behavioral level (and if so how).

At the morphological level, collateral and regenerative sprouting (Raisman 1969) have been proposed as potential candidates for rehabilitation. Furthermore, it has been indicated that inactive afferents can regain activity after a lesion; this would imply an improvement of synaptic efficacy dependent on specific training after a brain injury. Finally, the principle of retained collaterals (Cajal 1968) could prove useful for rehabilitation. The principle of reduced diaschisis as expressed by von Monakow (1911) has already been mentioned as well as the principle of vicarious representation. In addition, new functional commitments in case a lesion happens in early states of ontogeny appear to be possible (Schneider 1973; Frost and Metin 1985).

On the neurochemical level several mechanisms have also been suggested as potential candidates for rehabilitation. After a brain injury, an improvement of postsynaptic sensitivity is usually observed; this phenomenon has been called "law of denervation" (Cannon and Rosenblueth 1949). Another mechanism appears to be presynaptic hyperactivity after brain injury. Thus, there appears to be both a pre- and postsynaptic effect based on an endogenous mechanism meant to compensate for a functional disturbance following a brain injury.

Furthermore, it has been suggested (e.g., Stein 1988) that after lesions trophic factors in the area of the lesion may be stimulated, possibly overcoming the detrimental effects. At the same time, however, toxic substances may be emitted, resulting in secondary effects leading to functional suppression. Such adaptive and maladaptive processes, i.e., the trophic and toxic factors, may compete with each other after brain injuries. The experimenter must determine what can be done to minimize the toxic effects that may represent one aspect of secondary brain injury. Possibly, the effects of gangliosides may be seen within this context (Sabel et al. 1984).

The morphological mechanisms hitherto suggested as being critical for the restitution of function may play only a minor role because sprouting is observed only at the lesion site itself or in the immediate vicinity. Sprouting may even be maladaptive for restitution of function. Collateral and regenerative sprouting has been verified (e.g., Raisman 1969), but its full potential for restitution of function remains unclear.

More important than sprouting for the restitution of function may be that previously inactive afferents may be reactivated after an injury. Such a phenomenon has been suggested by the experiments of Glees and Cole (1960) or Wall and Egger (1971). If one assumes a significant degree of divergence of projection in afferent pathways, it is possible that after local injuries the reactivation of afferents due to an improvement of synaptic efficacy next to the lesion site could be one of the neurobiological mechanism essential in the restitution of function. The observations on visual-field enlargement after occipital lesions that have been described after the application of specific functional training (Pöppel et al. 1978; Zihl and von Cramon 1979) can be interpreted on such a neurobiological basis. A direct link between the functional alterations and the neurobiological bases remains to be definitely demonstrated, and the relationship between observed behavioral changes and cellular mechanisms present a major challenge for future research in neuropsychological rehabilitation.

## References

Bach-y-Rita P (1990) Brain plasticity as a basis for recovery of functions in humans. Neuropsychologia 28:547–554

Berrol S (1990) Issues in cognitive rehabilitation. Arch Neurol 47:219–220

Broca P (1865) Sur le siège de la faculté du langage articulé. Bull Soc Anthropol 337–393

Brown M, Diller L, Fordyce W, Jacobs D, Gordon W (1980) Rehabilitation indicators: their nature and uses for assessment. In: Bolton B, Cook DW (eds) Rehabilitation client assessment. University Park, Baltimore, pp 102–117

Cannon WB, Rosenblueth A (1949) The supersensitivity of denervated structures. MacMillan, New York

Cajal SY (1968) Degeneration and regeneration of the nervous system. Hafner, New York (Original 1928)

Changeux J-P, Danchin A (1976) Selective stabilization of developing synapses as a mechanism for the specification of neuronal networks. Nature 264:705–712

Cope DN (1988) Neuropharmacology and brain damage. In: Christensen A-L, Uzzell BP (eds) Neuropsychological rehabilitation. Kluwer, Boston, pp 19–38
Corbetta M, Miezin FM, Dobmeyer S, Shulman GL, Peterson SE (1990) Attentional modulation of neural processing of shape, color, and velocity in humans. Science 248:1556–1559
Damasio AR, Geschwind N (1985) Anatomical localization in clinical neuropsychology. In: Frederiks JAM (ed) Clinical neuropsychology. Elsevier, Amsterdam, pp 7–22 (Handbook of Clinical Neurology, vol 1/45)
Diller L (1987) Neuropsychological rehabilitation. In: Meier MJ, Benton AL, Diller L (eds) Neuropsychological rehabilitation. Churchill Livingstone, Edinburgh, pp 3–17
Edelman GM (1987) Neural darwinism. Basic, New York
Ellis DW (1989) Neuropsychotherapy. In: Ellis DW, Christensen A-L (eds) Neuropsychological treatment after brain injury. Kluwer, Boston, pp 241–270
Frost DO, Metin C (1985) Induction of functional retinal projections to the somatosensory system. Nature 317:162–164
Gage FH, Dunnett SB, Björklund A, Stenevi U (1982) Functional recovery following brain damage: conceptual frameworks and biological mechanisms. Scand J Psychol (Suppl) 1:112–120
Glees P, Cole J (1960) Recovery of skilled motor functions after small repeated lesions of motor cortex in macaque. J Neurophysiol 13:137–148
Goldstein G (1987) Neuropsychological assessment for rehabilitation: fixed batteries, automated systems, and non-psychometric methods. In: Meier MJ, Benton AL, Diller L (eds) Neuropsychological rehabilitation. Churchill Livingstone, Edinburgh, pp 18–40
Gray CM, König P, Engel AK, Singer W (1989) Oscillatory responses in cat visual cortex exhibit inter-columnar synchronization which reflects global stimulus properties. Nature 338:334–337
Huttenlocher PR (1990) Morphometric study of human cerebral cortex development. Neuropsychologia 28:517–527
Irle E (1987) Lesion size and recovery of function: some new perspectives. Brain Res Rev 12:307–320
Kertesz A (1983) Issues in localization. In: Kertesz A (ed) Localization in neuropsychology. Academic, New York, pp 1–20
Kertesz A (1985) Aphasia. In: Frederiks JAM (ed) Clinical neuropsychology. Elsevier, Amsterdam, pp 287–331 (Handbook of Clinical Neurology, vol 1/45)
Lashley KS (1963) Brain mechanisms and intelligence. A quantitative study of injuries to the brain. Dover, New York (Original 1929)
Levine AM (1988) Buspirone and agitation in head injury. Brain Injury 2:165–167
Luria AR (1970) The process of reflection under the light of modern neuropsychology. Psychologia 13:61–74
Marshall JF (1984) Brain function: neural adaptations and recovery from injury. Annu Rev Psychol 35:277–308
Meier MJ, Strauman S, Thompson WG (1987) Individual differences in neuropsychological recovery: an overview. In: Meier MJ, Benton AL, Diller L (eds) Neuropsychological rehabilitation. Churchill Livingstone, Edinburgh, pp 71–110
Merzenich MM, Kaas JH, Wall JT, Nelson RJ, Sur M, Felleman D (1983) Topographic reorganization of somatosensory cortical areas 3b and 1 in adult monkeys following restricted deafferentation. Neuroscience 8:33–55
Milner B, Teuber H-L (1968) Alteration of perception and memory in man: reflections on method. In: Weiskrantz L (ed) Analysis of behavioral change. Harper and Row, New York, pp 268–375
Ploog D (1980) Emotionen als Produkte des limbischen Systems. Med Psychol 6:7–19
Poeck K, Huber W, Kerschensteiner M, Stachowiak F-J, Weniger D (1977) Therapie der Aphasien. Nervenarzt 78:119–126
Pöppel E (1970) Excitability cycles in central intermittency. Psychol Forsch 34:1–9
Pöppel E (1977) Midbrain mechanisms in human vision. In: Pöppel E, Held R, Dowling JE (eds) Neuronal mechanisms in visual perception. Neurosci Res Program Bull 15:335–343
Pöppel E (1985a) Bridging a neuronal gap: perceptual completion across a cortical scotoma is dependent on stimulus motion. Naturwissenschaften 72:599
Pöppel E (1985b) Grenzen des Bewußtseins. Über Wirklichkeit und Welterfahrung. Deutsche Verlags-Anstalt, Stuttgart

Pöppel E (1988) Taxonomie des Subjektiven auf der Grundlage eines pragmatischen Monismus. In: von Böcker F, Weig W (eds) Aktuelle Kernfragen in der Psychiatrie. Springer, Berlin Heidelberg New York, pp 24–36
Pöppel E (1989) Taxonomy of the subjective: an evolutionary perspective. In: Brown JW (ed) Neuropsychology of visual perception. Erlbaum, Hillsdale, New Jersey, pp 219–232
Pöppel E, Richards WA (1974) Light sensitivity in cortical scotomata contralateral to small islands of blindness. Exp Brain Res 21:125–130
Pöppel E, Held R, Frost D (1973) Residual visual function after brain wouds involving the central visual pathways in man. Nature 243:295–296
Pöppel E, Brinkmann R, von Cramon D, Singer W (1978) Association and dissociation of visual functions in a case of bilateral occipital lobe infarction. Arch Psychiatr Nervenkr 225:1–22
Pöppel E, Stoerig P, Logothetis N, Fries W, Boergen K-P, Örtel W, Zihl J (1987) Plasticity and rigidity in the representation of the human visual field. Exp Brain Res 68:445–448
Pöppel E, Schill K, von Steinbüchel N (1990) Sensory integration within temporally neutral system states: A hypothesis. Naturwissenschaften 77:89–91
Pöppel E, Chen L, Glünder H, Mitzdorf U, Ruhnau E, Schill K, von Steinbüchel N (1991) Temporal and spatial constraints for mental modelling. In: Bhatkar VP, Rege KM (eds) Frontiers in knowledge-based computing. Narosa, New Delhi, pp 57–68
Poppelreuter W (1917) Die Störungen der niederen und höheren Sehleistungen durch Verletzung des Okzipitalhirns. Voss, Leipzig (Die psychischen Schädigungen durch Kopfschuß im Kriege 1914/16, vol 1)
Prigatano GP et al. (1986) Neuropsychological rehabilitation after brain injury. Johns Hopkins University Press, Baltimore
Prigatano GP (1987) Personality and psychosocial consequences after brain injury. In: Meier M, Benton AL, Diller L (eds) Neuropsychological rehabilitation. Churchill Livingstone, Edinburgh
Raisman G (1969) Neuronal plasticity in the septal nuclei of the adult rat. Brain Res 14:25–48
Risberg J (1986) Regional cerebral blood flow. In: Hannay HJ (ed) Experimental techniques in human neuropsychology. Oxford University Press, Oxford, pp 514–543
Sabel BA, Slavin MD, Stein DG (1984) GM1 ganglioside treatment facilitates behavioral recovery from bilateral brain damage. Science 225:340–342
Saper CP, Plum F (1985) Disorders of consciousness. In: Frederiks JAM (ed) Clinical neuropsychology. Elsevier, Amsterdam, pp 107–128 (Handbook of Clinical Neurology, vol 1/45)
Schneider G (1973) Early lesions of superior colliculus: factors affecting the formation of abnormal retinal projections. Brain Behav Evol 8:73–109
Scoville WB, Milner B (1957) Loss of recent memory after bilateral hippocampal lesions. J Neurol Neurosurg Psychiatry 20:11–21
Singer W, Zihl J, Pöppel E (1977) Subcortical control of visual threshold in humans: evidence for modality-specific and retinotopically organized mechanisms of selective attention. Exp Brain Res 29:173–190
Sprague JM (1966) Interaction of cortex and superior colliculus in mediation of visually guided behavior in the cat. Science 153:1544–1547
Stein DG (1988) Contextual factors in recovery from brain damage. In: Christensen A-L, Uzzell BP (eds) Neuropsychological rehabilitation. Klüwer, Boston, pp 1–18
von Cramon D (1979) Quantitative Bestimmung des Verhaltensdefizits bei Störungen des skalaren Bewußtseins. Thieme, Stuttgart
von Monakow C (1911) Lokalisation der Hirnfunktionen. J Psychol Neurol 17:185–200
von Steinbüchel N (1987) Therapie der zeitlichen Verarbeitung akustischer Reize bei aphasischen Patienten. Thesis, University of Munich
von Steinbüchel N, Pöppel E (1991) Temporal order threshold and language perception. In: Bhatkar VP, Rege KM (eds) Frontiers in knowledge-based computing. Narosa, New Delhi, pp 81–90
Teuber H-L (1975) Recovery of function after brain injury in man. Ciba Found Symp 34:159–186
Wall PD, Egger MD (1971) Formations of new connections in adult rat brains after partial deafferentation. Nature 232:542–545

Will BE, Rosenzweig MR, Bennett EL, Herbert M, Morimoto H (1977) Relatively brief environmental enrichment aids recovery of learning capacity and alters brain measures after postweaning brain-lesions in rats. J Comp Physiol Psychol 91:33–50

Woods BT, Teuber H-L (1973) Early onset of complementary specialization of cerebral hemispheres in man. Trans Am Neurol Assoc 98:113–117

Zeki SM (1978) Functional specialisation in the visual cortex of the rhesus monkey. Nature 274:423–428

Zihl J, von Cramon D (1979) Restitution of visual function in patients with cerebral blindness. J Neurol Neurosurg Psychiatry 42:312–322

# Cortical Representational Plasticity: Some Implications for the Bases of Recovery from Brain Damage

*W. M. Jenkins and M. M. Merzenich*

## Introduction

Over the past several decades, most forebrain neuroscientists have adopted an anatomically dominated view of the origins of brain functions. According to this view, neurons are assigned their functional roles through a critical period in early life; those roles are defined by the maturation of neurons and their connections, and once established, describe the operations of those neurons for a lifetime. There is a great body of evidence that reveals this general viewpoint to be incorrect.

One of the most common methodologies in neurophysiology has been the detailed study of the response properties of individual neurons. Such studies have usually been conducted within only a brief window of time in the life of an animal or human. Much has been learned from this approach. However, a different approach is needed to understand the complex behaviorally relevant neurological processes occurring within the neocortical mantle. It is precisely these variable interactions within and between neural networks and the consequent use-driven changes in the neural networks themselves that underlie human cognitive functions such as language, speech, recognitions, judgement, remembering, and the acquisition and execution of motor skills.

The results presented in this paper represent the initial results of an attempt to develop model systems with which we can look for experience-dependent functional changes over time, across a network of neurons located within a small sector of the neocortex.

## Methodological Approach

Our approach has been to define the topography of selective response properties of neurons within a sector of neocortex that represent either the skin surface of hands or the movements evoked by intracortical microstimulation in adult monkeys. Responses within this small neocortical patch, on the order of 2–4 mm across, are defined with a dense sampling on the order of every 100–150 μm. "Maps" of neuronal responses and/or evoked movements are

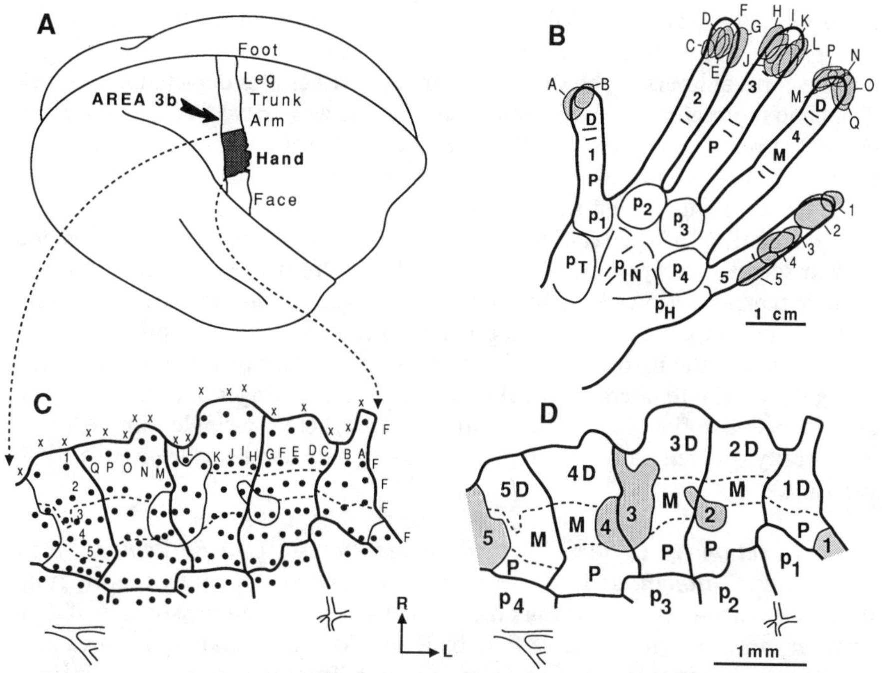


**Fig. 1 A–D.** Location and topographic representation of the hand within area 3b in a normal adult owl monkey. **A** Lateral view of the right neocortex. The approximate location of area 3b is outlined. The large cutaneous representation of the hand is indicated by *stippling* and is located medial to the representation of the face and lateral to that of the remainder of the body surface representation. **B** Outline of the glabrous hand surface in a normal adult owl monkey, with two typical sequences of receptive fields (from sites *1–5* and *A–Q* in **C**) drawn. The large numbers *1–5* denote the digits (e.g., *1*, thumb; *D*, *M*, and *P* are distal, middle, and proximal phalanges, respectively); *p 1–4* are the palmer pads at the base of the digits; *pH* is the hypothenar eminence; *pT* is the thenar eminence; and *pIN* refers to the three insular pads. **C** Locations of 174 penetration sites from which the topographic representation of the hand surfaces shown in **D** were reconstructed. Numbers *1–5* and letters *A–Q* adjacent to penetration sites indicate locations at which the cutaneous receptive fields shown in **B** were obtained. *Lines* are boundaries between the territories of representation of different hand surfaces shown in **D**. Note that the map has been rotated 90° counterclockwise with respect to **A**. **D** Diagrammatic illustration of the representation of hand surfaces. *Stippled zones* indicate dorsal (hairy) skin on the digits. *Solid lines* outline territories of representation of the digits and palmer pads. *Broken lines* mark the borders between phalangeal representational zones. The distal digit tips are represented along the rostral margin of area 3b. More proximal portions of the digits and palm are represented at successively more caudal locations within area 3b. (From Jenkins et al. 1990)

obtained prior to, immediately after or long after some experimental manipulation, e.g., the behavioral training of the animal subject. The basic approach for this kind of mapping experiment is illustrated in Fig. 1. In Fig. 1 A, the location of area 3 b or primary somatosensory cortex in the forebrain is indicated with the location of the hand representation within the lateral parietal strip indicated by stippling. Figure 1 B illustrates typical cutaneous receptive fields (e.g., A–Q and 1–5) which were defined by stimulation of the skin with fine probes and whose stimulation evoked discharges in neurons within the middle cortical layers at the similarly marked cortical sites depicted in Fig. 1 C. The hand representation map depicted in Fig. 1 D was drawn by outlining cortical areas over which receptive fields were centered over given skin surfaces. The delimiting lines were drawn between penetration sites with receptive fields centered on different labeled skin areas.

Examination of the relationships between the cortical recording sites and their associated receptive fields indicates that there is a highly ordered topographic representation of the hand in Area 3b (for details see Merzenich et al. 1987). Thus for example, there is a distal to proximal finger representational gradient along the rostral to caudal cortical axis within this region. Similarly, along the medial to lateral cortical axis there is a little finger to thumb progression in receptive field locations. In other words, there is a single, simple, topographically ordered pattern of representation of the hand surface in this cortical zone.

*These Functionally Defined Cortical Representations Can Be Remodeled by Experience, Throughout Life.* We know that sources of inputs, the distributions of cortico-cortical and thalamocortical afferents, and the spreads of dendritic arbors are highly variable field by field. Nonetheless, any given area provides a variable anatomical repertoire of inputs, from which an almost infinite number of forms of functional representations can be created. Some examples of the variability in hand representations in adult owl monkeys within area 3b were described by Merzenich et al. (1987). It was hypothesized by these investigators that such variations in hand representations were at least partly, attributable to the different histories of functional hand use experienced by these monkeys. It was further hypothesized that this "differential use" provided a basis for the selection of the subset of inputs that activate neurons at any given cortical site. In other words, the cumulative effects of behaviorally relevant hand use altered the effectiveness of existing synapses and thus continually dynamically remodeled representational topographies. Within the neocortex, area 3b has the smallest spatial distribution of afferent endings of any somatosensory field. Thus, we would expect it to be the least alterable of any of the numerous somatosensory cortical fields.

Earlier studies from several laboratories on the effects of various forms of peripheral denervation of selected skin surfaces revealed that cortical maps reorganized (Franck 1980; Kalaska and Pomeranz 1979; Merzenich et al. 1983 a, b; 1984; Wall and Cusic 1984). Furthermore, those results could not be completely explained by simple "unmasking" phenomena since the ensuing functional cortical representational reorganization was progressive over several months. Those studies and others suggested the functional organization of cortical representations was "use dependent" moreover, the temporal structure of neural inputs (i.e., depending on correlation-based mechanisms) appeared to be a critical component to this remodeling (Clark et al. 1988; Jenkins et al. 1990).

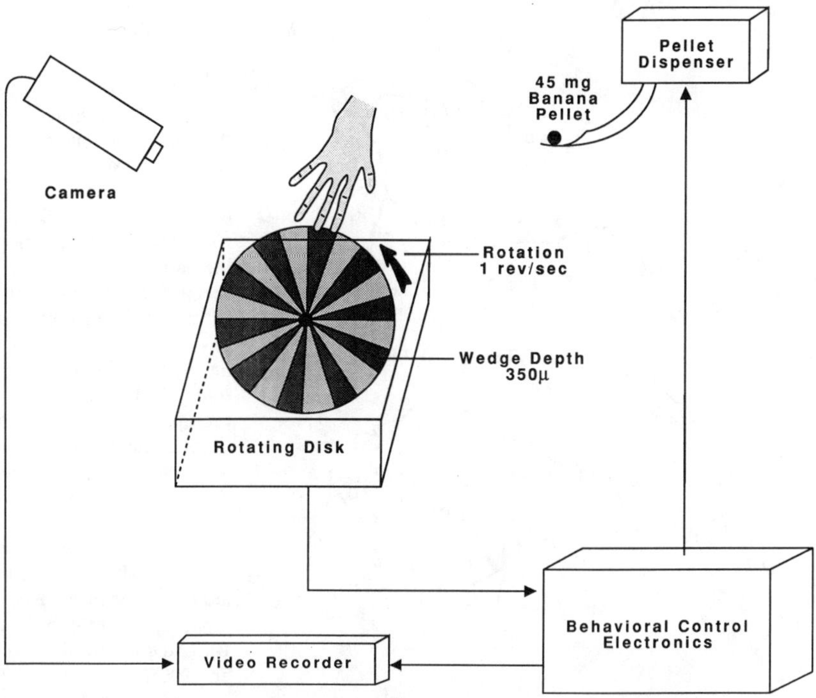


**Fig. 2.** Behavioral apparatus which required the monkey to maintain contact with a rotating stimulus disk for about 10–15 s per banana pellet reward. Only the distal aspect of the distal segment of one or more digits contacted the disk. Ten wedge-shaped groves 350 μ deep were machined into the metal disk. The disk in most experiments was continuously rotating at 1 rev/s, providing the contacted digital skin with edges moving across the digit at a rate of 20 Hz. (From Jenkins et al. 1990)

To directly attack the question of "differential use", we asked: what happens to these cortical representational maps if we train an adult primate to differentially use a restricted patch of skin (see Jenkins et al. 1990)? The apparatus and method used for this purpose are illustrated in Fig. 2. The tactile stimulus delivery device consisted of a round metal disk that had an alternating pattern of raised and lowered surfaces. The pattern consisted of 20 pre-shaped wedges that alternated in depth by 350 μm. The disk was rotated by a motor at the rate of 1 rev/s. The apparatus was mounted in a frame on the animal's home cage and arranged so that the distal aspect of the longest digits could contact the disk. The monkeys' task was to maintain contact withthe rotating disk for about 15 s in order to receive a banana-flavored food pellet. These procedures resulted in about 600 banana pellets being delivered per day. The task itself required the animal to regulate contact force with the disk in order to maintain disk contact and produced a high degree of temporally coherent stimulation of limited sectors of skin on the contacting digits.

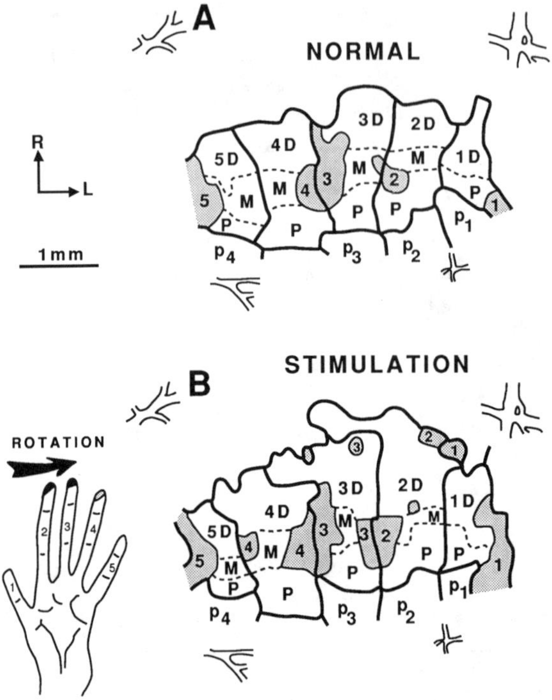


**Fig. 3. A** Reconstruction of the hand representation in area 3b for OM 1 prior to differential stimulation. Map labels as in Figure 1. **B** Post stimulation reconstruction of the hand representation. Skin surfaces differentially stimulated during the disk contact behavior are indicated in *black* on the hand inset at the *bottom left*. The skin surfaces on the tips of digit 2 and 3 and occasionally the tip of digit 4 were stimulated in the behavior in this monkey. The cortical representation of the stimulated skin surfaces expanded greatly in all such experiments (compare the distal aspects of digits 2, 3, and 4 in **A** and **B**). (Adapted from Jenkins et al. 1990)

The question then is does such differential use produce changes in neocortex? The representational maps from one case are shown in Fig. 3. Figure 3A illustrates the area 3B hand representation obtained prior to "differential use" and that in Fig. 3B the representation obtained immediately after 109 days of "differential use". The hand inset depicts the skin surfaces stimulated during the behavioral task (shown in black). Note that there is a great enlargement in the cortical representation of the stimulated phalanges. What about a specific behaviorally engaged skin surface? One such comparison is shown in Fig. 4. Of course there are other distortions in the post behavior map, Figure 4 simply highlights the nearly 500% increase in the cortical area of representation of the behaviorally engaged skin surface.

Receptive field sizes were observed to be significantly smaller within the enlarged cortical representation of stimulated skin surfaces. Thus, for example, Fig. 5 shows the outlines of glabrous cutaneous receptive fields obtained prior to and immediately after behaviorally controlled stimulation. Note that in the histogram (Fig. 5, bottom) that receptive sizes were significantly smaller on the distal phalanges of digits 2 and 3, but not for other digits. These results suggest that there is a roughly inverse relationship between area of cortical representation and receptive field size (see Sur et al. 1980). It has earlier been argued that this inverse relationship is apparently maintained actively, as cortical representations are remodeled by use (Merzenich et al. 1984).

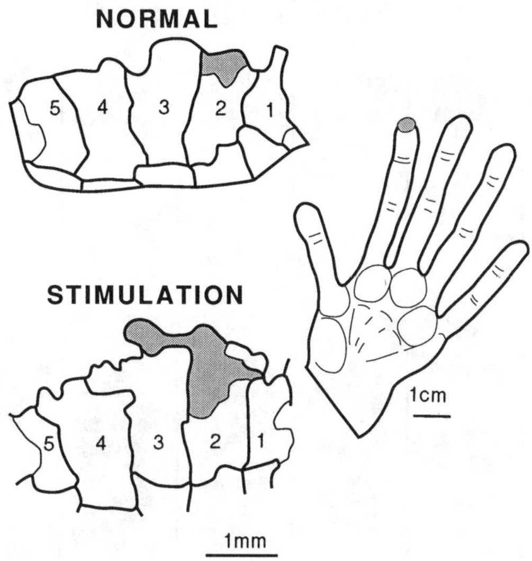


**Fig. 4.** Outlines of the area 3b cortical territories representing the surfaces of the digits for OM 1 prior to differential stimulation (normal, *top*) and after differential stimulation (stimulation, *bottom*). Most of the differentially stimulated skin surface on digit 2 is indicated by *stippling* in the hand drawing at the right. The zones of representation of the struck skin surface on the distal phalanx of digit 2 is *stippled* in both drawings, i.e., in this zone, all defined receptive fields overlapped onto this heavily stimulated surface. Note that after a period of differential digit tip stimulation in this monkey – as in other monkeys studied with this paradigm – there was a substantial enlargement of its territory of representation. In this monkey, most of the gain in territory was from across the area 3b-3a border as defined functionally prior to the initiation of this digital stimulation behavior. (From Jenkins et al. 1990)

Another way to view these receptive field size changes is by showing their sizes and cortical location simultaneously. Figure 6 shows a three-dimensional surface plot of cortical location (x and y dimension) and inverse receptive field size (z dimension).

The smallest receptive fields have high z axis values while the largest receptive fields have low z axis values. Note that for the normal map the largest receptive fields are located towards the palm and that the smallest receptive fields are found toward the digit tips. Note that after differential stimulation there is a large cortical region corresponding to the representation of stimulated skin surface that has much smaller receptive fields.

What are the potential consequences for perceptual capacities of such changes? One obvious suggestion is increased spatial resolving capacity. Several psychophysical studies in monkeys and man have suggested a site-specific progressive improvement in spatial discrimination with extended practice (Dresslar 1894; Jones et al. 1973; Vierck and Jones 1970; Volkmann 1858). In studies conducted in our laboratory, adult monkeys trained on either auditory or somatosensory discriminations exhibit marked improvement in discrimination abilities with experience that are restricted to the trained sensory surface

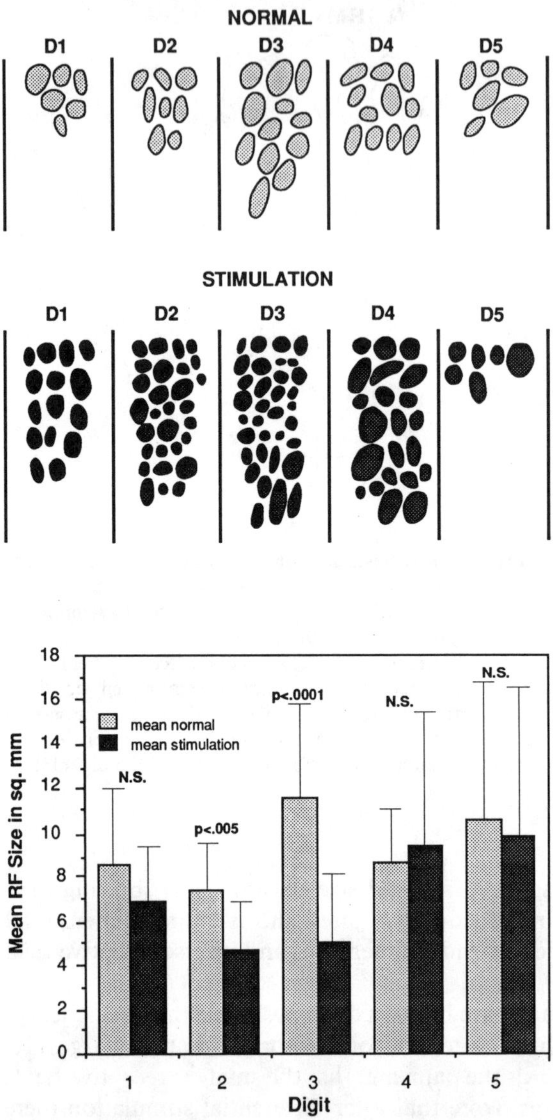


**Fig. 5.** Receptive fields from the distal phalanges of a normal monkey (OM 1) are outlined at the *top* (normal). Receptive fields from the post stimulation map are shown in the *middle* (stimulation). The receptive fields from both experiments are drawn to the same scale. These data are summarized at the *bottom* where the *bars* indicate mean receptive field size in $mm^2$ in the normal map (*black*), and after differential stimulation (*grey*). *Error bars* indicate standard deviations. Receptive fields representing skin surfaces heavily engaged (distal phalanges on digits 2 and 3) in these differential stimulation behaviors in area 3b are significantly smaller (digit 2, $F(1,35) = 9.416$, $p < 0.005$; digit 3, $F(1,44) = 32.54$, $p < 0.001$) than those recorded in the same representational zones prior to the behavior. (From Jenkins et al. 1990)

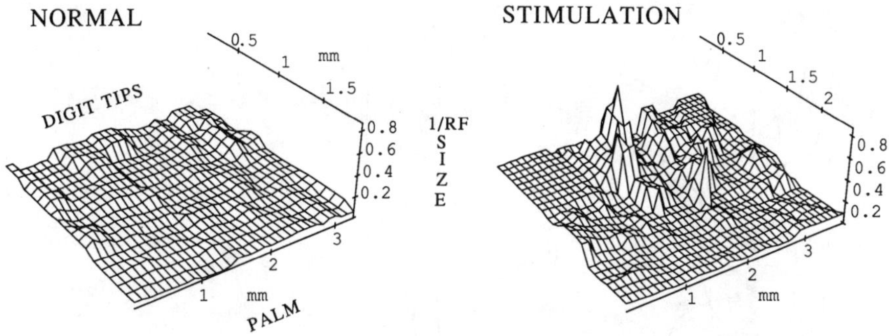


**Fig. 6.** The distributed effects of behaviorally controlled skin stimulation for OM 1 are shown by a three-dimensional surface plot of cortical location (x and y dimension) and inverse receptive field size (z dimension). The smallest receptive fields have high z axis values while the largest receptive fields have low z axis values. Note that for the normal map the largest receptive fields are located towards the palm and that the smallest receptive fields are found toward the digit tips. Note that after differential stimulation there is a large cortical region corresponding to the representation of stimulated skin surface that has much smaller receptive fields. (Data from Jenkins et al. 1990)

(Recanzone et al. 1989). Furthermore evidence from combined quantitative mapping electrophysiological studies in these same animals reveal not only changes in "representational maps", but also substantial changes in temporal details and in magnitudes of distributed suprathreshold neuronal responses (Recanzone et al., unpublished observations). We conclude that the specific responses of cortical neurons – and cortical "maps" – are shaped by our experiences (Merzenich et al. 1988). We conclude that these use-dependent changes reflect operation of *the* basic adaptive neocortical process. We conclude that this use-dependent remodeling of cortical maps accounts for the rich variety in experience-derived abilities that mark human kind.

*Temporal Coincidences of Behaviorally Significant Stimuli Play a Crucial Role in Shaping Cortical Representations.* We have a half dozen experimental examples that reveal the capacity for significant representational translocations, and that reveal a critical role for temporal input coincidence for generating such representational changes (Allard et al. 1985; Clark et al. 1986; Jenkins et al. 1990; Merzenich et al. 1983 a, b; Recanzone et al. 1989). For example, we have altered the spatiotemporal structure of afferent inputs into the cortex by moving a segment of the sensory surface into a new physical location – thus altering the timing relationships inputs from this surface have with the surrounding sensory surface at its old location and its new location. We accomplished this by moving an always-innervated vascularized patch of skin from one digit to another, by a "neurovascular island transfer" (Clark et al. 1986). An example of such an experiment is shown in Fig. 7. When such neurovascular Island transfers are preformed in experimental adult monkeys, we have observed that the representation also shifts to new cortical locations with receptive fields commonly overlapping both the island pedicle skin and the skin of the recipient site.

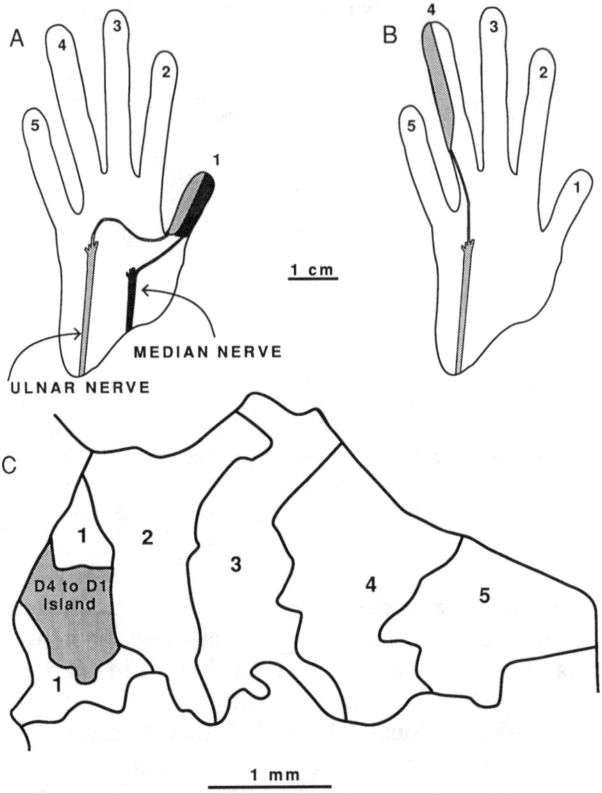


**Fig. 7.** The consequence of moving an innervated vascularized skin flap (i.e., a neurovascular island flap) from ulnar digit 4 to the ulnar half of digit 1. Six months after such a skin transfer, a cortical representation of this transferred skin surface emerged within the zone of representation of digit 1. This represents a transcortical representational movement of over 1.5 mm. (From Merzenich et al., unpublished observations)

By analogy, movements in representation such as that depicted in Fig. 7 (i.e., over 1 mm in this case) imply that skin surface representations destroyed by a cortical lesion should in principal have the ability to regain cortical representation(s) at a new site(s). Presumably such post lesion representational reorganization would be constrained by the size of lesion, the underlying anatomy of the specific field, and would be experience dependent.

## Changes in Motor Cortex

Are representational changes seen in other cortical fields? For example what are the effects of training an animal to perform a motor task? In another series of experiments we have observed changes in the representation of movements in area 4 in adult monkeys as a consequence of a simple digit skill acquisition paradigm (Nudo et al., unpublished observations). In those experiments movement representation maps of the hand, wrist, arm and shoulder were obtained by use of the intracortical microstimulation technique and by observing stimulus-evoked movements. Such motor "maps" were obtained prior to and after training on a motor task. In one such task, animals were trained to retrieve small food rewards from a Plexiglass board containing food wells of diminishing size, the smallest of which (h1) necessitated insertion of only one finger for successful retrieval. The question was: are there consequences of practicing these movements for movement maps in the motor cortex? The results of one such experiment are shown in Fig. 8. This digit skill acquisition paradigm again resulted in a differential enlargement of the cortical zone of representation of digit movements in adult monkeys. As shown in Fig. 8C, retrieval from the largest three wells (h 2–4) was nearly flawless without training, requiring only one attempt (i.e., involving digit flexion) per reward even on the first day. By contrast, efficient retrieval from the smallest well (h1) required several days of training. Digit exercise resulted in significant changes in the topography of movement representations in motor cortex (compare Fig. 8A, B). Cortical regions whose stimulation evoked digit movements are shown in black. As illustrated in D, the entire digit area (d1-5) was enlarged by almost 20%. When digit movements were subdivided further, it can be seen that the representation of thumb movements (not used extensively in the retrieval task) decreased in area by almost 20%, while representation of movements involving digits 2–5 (primary movements in the retrieval task) were enlarged by about 40%. We conclude that this evident representational plasticity in motor cortex again manifests the adaptive processes underlying the improvement of perceptual abilities or the acquisition of motoric skill with practice.

## Functional Reorganization Induced by Cortical Lesions

Consider the specific case of the recovery from brain injury. How can mechanisms of representational plasticity contribute to recovery? We believe that "representational recovery" parallels functional recovery (Jenkins and Merzenich 1987). Some examples of cortical lesions and consequent representational changes in the hand region of 3b in adult owl monkeys are shown in Fig. 9. For case 1, most of the representation of digit 3 and that of a small portion of digits 2 and 4 representations were within the zone of the lesion (indicated in black) on the day it was made. After 94 days, the cortex medial to the lesion was mapped once again. We observed a reemergence of nearly all of the representation of digit 3, although receptive fields located on digit 3 were now unusually large. Furthermore, in this case we observed a reversal in topographic sequence of represented digits. That is, normally as one moves from lateral to medial in cortex the normal representational sequence is from radial to ulnar (e.g., thumb to little finger) whereas we observed the reversed

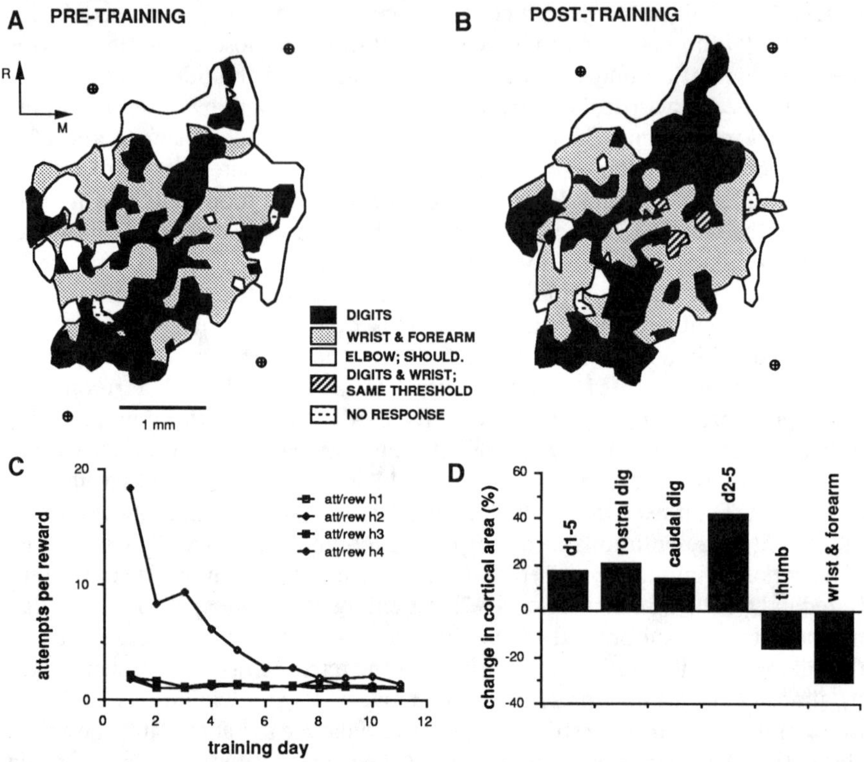


**Fig. 8 A–D.** Digit skill acquisition differentially enlarges the cortical representation of digit movements in adult monkeys. This animal was trained to retrieve small food rewards from a Plexiglass board containing food wells of diminishing size, the smallest of which (h4) necessitated insertion of only one finger for successful retrieval. **A** Motor map prior to, and **B** after training. As shown in **C**, retrieval from the largest three wells (h1–3) was nearly flawless without training, requiring only one attempt (digit flexion) per reward even on the first day. In contrast, efficient retrieval from the smallest well required several days of training. After 11 training days, a second map was derived using the same mapping procedure as before. Digit exercise resulted in significant changes in the topography of movement representations in motor cortex (**B**). As illustrated in **D**, the entire digit area (d1–5) was enlarged by almost 20%. When digit movements were subdivided further, it can be seen that the representation of thumb movements (not used extensively in retrieval task) *decreased* in area by almost 20%, while representation of movements involving digits 2–5 (primary movements in retrieval task) were enlarged by about 40%. (From Nudo et al., unpublished observations)

sequence from digit 5 to digit 4 to digit 3. Case 2 (Fig. 9) also illustrates an abnormal and somewhat jumbled topographical representation. Furthermore, all three cases illustrated in Fig. 9 had large sectors of cortex in which receptive fields were abnormally large.

The representational plasticity we have observed in these and other post-lesion cases and the neural mechanisms that underlie such plasticity almost certainly account for a significant part of the recovery of function after stroke. We hypothesize that the capacity of any given cortical field for representational re-

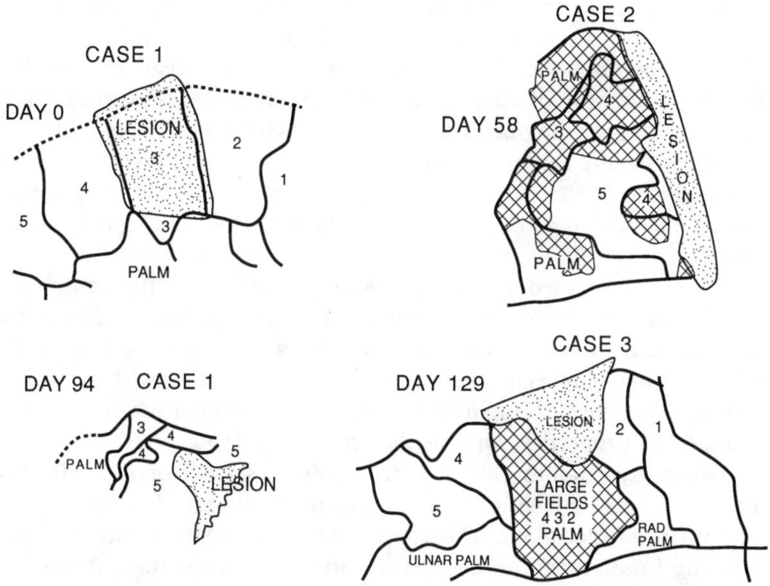


**Fig. 9.** Three cases illustrating some of the effects of small cortical lesions within the area 3b hand representation. For case 1 (*left, top*) the location of the cortical lesion is shown in *stippling* and included most of the zone of representation of digit 3 and a part of the digit 2 and 4 representations on the day the lesion was induced. Note that 94 days later (*left, bottom*) there is a reversal in the topographical sequence of digit representations and that a cruder digit 3 representation emerges in the cortex medial to digits 4 and 5. Another feature of maps obtained several weeks after cortical lesions in 3b is illustrated for cases 2 and 3 on the *right*. After these cortical lesions the skin surface representations initially destroyed by the lesion reemerge in adjacent intact cortex but the receptive fields are abnormally large (*cross-hatched* region). (Adapted from Jenkins and Merzenich 1987)

covery will reflect the anatomical distributions of inputs to that field. A field with anatomically restricted connections like area 3b has a correspondingly space-limited capacity for representational recovery. A given frontal or posterior parietal or temporal cortex field many of which have very widespread, virtually all-to-all anatomical distributions of their inputs should have a correspondingly greater capacity for representational recovery after its partial destruction. Cerebral strokes or injury should generate an almost infinite variety of behavioral consequences of disruptions of the more than 100 functional cortical areas of humans, each of which has field-specific inputs and outputs, each of which makes field-specific perceptual and motor contributions to behavior, and each of which is itself a source of inputs to other cortical fields. Representational recovery will be played out field by field, at each area limited by the spreads of anatomical inputs and the integrity of input sources and output destinations. To the extent that sectors of key cortical areas survive the injury, representational recovery and hence functional recovery can occur, and can potentially be greatly facilitated by appropriately controlled post-lesion behavioral training.

One facet of these intrinsic dynamic cortical mechanisms impacts heavily on the course of recovery after brain damage: *These self-organizing mechanisms are competitive*. Strong inputs dominate over weak inputs. This domination is presumably often exaggerated by a rehabilitation strategy that employs heavy training of fragmented, distorted surviving behaviors, that would hypothetically swamp lesion-weakened cortical representations and functions. As a consequence of these dynamic competitive processes *and* fragmented post-lesion behaviors, new cortical representations and functional constructs will emerge.

On the basis of our findings, we hypothesize that the neural mechanisms that account for learning and memory in a normal individual make a primary contribution to functional recovery after a brain injury. Learning, a lasting change in behavior as a consequence of our interaction with stimuli in the environment, has been thought to depend on lasting changes in the structural and functional properties within the central nervous system for more than 100 years (e.g., James 1890; for recent reviews see Woody 1986; Brown et al. 1990). With the advent of modern electrophysiological techniques and the development of special model preparations, much progress has been made in elucidating fundamental mechanisms responsible for various forms of learning. One enduring notion, described most completely in the hippocampus is that learning results in a long term change in effectivenesses of synapses, i.e., long-term potentiation (LTP) (Lømo 1966). Numerous studies have suggested a variety of pre- and post-synaptic mechanisms that might account for these input- and learning-induced neuronal changes in the hippocampus and in other anatomical regions (for recent reviews see Anderson 1987; Kandel et al, 1987; Brown et al. 1990). LTP has also been described particularly elegantly at the cellular level at the cortico-rubral synapse and has been demonstrated there during one form of classical conditioning in cats (e.g., Tsukahara 1987). In this particular example, Tsukahara (1987) suggested that a movement of the contact sites of corticorubral synapses to more effective cellular loci accounts for the classically conditioned behavior. The pioneering work of Woody et al. (1978) demonstrated that motor cortex neurons can also exhibit LTP if acetylcholine is iontophoretically administered when the neuron is depolarized by its inputs. Furthermore, this early study suggested that this effect is mediated by cyclic GMP acting as a second messenger, and results in persistent increases in input resistances mediated via potassium channels. In a number of other LTP models, other second messengers have been proposed that act on the potassium channels (c.f. Kandel et al. 1987). There exist numerous other specific examples of LTP occurring at other locations within the central nervous system or in the ganglia of invertebrates that involve different learned behaviors and different specific proposed cellular and molecular mechanisms (for reviews see Woody 1986; Andersen 1987; Kandel et al. 1987; Ito 1987). Nearly all of these examples suppose that these mechanisms operate in a normal adult animal during the course of learning or memory. Furthermore, it can be reasonably assumed that these cellular model preparations represent exemplary changes in the distributed responses of neurons in the large forebrain neural networks that are cooperatively engaged in any specific learned behavior. These same cellular mechanisms presumably also account for the functional representational reorganization that we have observed after brain damage. In both instances, there must be changes in the input-output relationships of complexly interconnected groups of neurons. At the cellular level, the effectiveness of individual synapses *must* change, whether they be by pre- or postsynaptic mechanisms or both, whether they be by long term potentiation or long term depression or both, or whether they involve one or many classes of transmitters, receptors, second messenger systems, etc. In all instances, enduring changes are driven by activating the system in a behaviorally significant way, and measured changes in representational topography reflect distributed changes in synaptic efficacy originating at the cellular level.

Cortical representations and the functions they subserve are undoubtedly also altered by mechanisms that are not explicitly involved in learning. Cortical representations arise in part because of the complex interplay of excitatory and inhibitory influences in any given cortical region. While these constructs are refined by learning, they may also make immediate and wholly passive adjustments after brain injury. Such passive cortical network responses are presently a subject of intense study in our laboratory. Functional reorganization in cortical areas not directly damaged by brain injury can also be expected. Brain damage will result in alteration of a lesion specific set of functional areas that constitute input sources to many other non-damaged cortical areas. New, fragmented distributions of input sources to other cortical fields should create novel representational constructs, some of which must be unique to brain injured-patients. In instances in which there are "weaker" or parallel representations in other cortical areas, these zones may develop novel representational constructs. For example, the second somatosensory cortical area (SII) in primates is known to receive its principal inputs from primary somatosensory cortex (SI). If a large but partial lesion of SI is made, then there is a major functional reorganization of SII (Pons et al. 1988). This reorganization presumably reflects the now-dramatically-altered inputs from SI.

Another important implication of our findings is that even if a cortical lesion was anatomically identical in its locus and extent in any two individuals, the resultant representational and functional defects would be idiosyncratic, as would the course of subsequent functional recovery. Cortical representations are an emergent property of a dynamic self-organizing neural network, and are not attributable to a fixed "hard wired" system. The representational constructs that emerge in such a system reflect the cumulated stored histories of the patterns of neural inputs and the behavioral contexts in which the networks have evolved over the lifetime of a given individual. The constructs of no two individuals will be identical.

Behavioral substitutions can also be expected to occur after brain injury. A new behavior can be substituted for a behavior that is lost or defective as a result of damage to requisite brain structures. And in these instances, distorted brain representations and substituted behaviors reciprocally feed each other. The brain damage distorts behaviors, which in turn further drive brain regions to consolidate the distorted representations subserving novel emergent compensatory behavior. Finally, in another class of substitution a new cortical area can be the primary source of a behavior, while before injury it only contributed secondarily.

We are no longer in the province in which recovery from brain injury can be studied using only pharmacological techniques, or by behavioral methods and measures of deficits, or by looking for anatomical defects. The brain in its physiology is *dynamic*. We should study its self-organization more directly if we are to arrive at a clear understanding of the best solutions for the treatment of brain injury.

## References

Allard T, Clark SA, Jenkins WM, Merzenich MM (1985) Syndactyly results in the emergence of double-digit receptive fields in somatosensory cortex in adult owl monkeys. Soc Neurosci Abstr 11:965

Andersen PO (1987) Properties of hippocampal synapses of importance for integration and memory. In: Edelman GM, Gall WE, Cowan WM (eds) Synaptic function. Wiley, New York, pp 403–429

Brown TH, Kairiss EW, Keenan CL (1990) Hebbian synapses: biophysical mechanisms and algorithms. Annu Rev Neurosci 13:475–511

Clark SA, Allard T, Jenkins WM, Merzenich MM (1986) Cortical map reorganization following neurovascular island skin transfers on the hands of adult owl monkeys. Soc Neurosci Abstr 12:391

Clark SA, Allard T, Jenkins WM, Merzenich MM (1988) Syndactyly results in the emergence of double digit receptive fields in somatosensory cortex in adult owl monkeys. Nature 332:444–445

Dresslar FB (1894) Studies in the psychology of touch. Am J Psychol 6:313–368

Franck JI (1980) Functional reorganization of cat somatic sensory-motor cortex (SmI) after selective dorsal root rhisotomies. Brain Res 186:458–462

Ito M (1987) Longterm depression as memory process in the cerebellum. In: Edelman GM, Gall WE, Cowan WM (eds) Synaptic function. Wiley, New York, pp 431–445

James W (1890) The principles of psychology. Holt, New York

Jenkins WM, Merzenich MM (1987) Reorganization of neocortical representations after brain injury: a neurophysiological model of the bases of recovery from stroke. Prog Brain Res 71:249–266

Jenkins WM, Merzenich MM, Ochs MT, Allard T, Guíc-Robies E (1990) Functional reorganization of primary somatosensory cortex in adult owl monkeys after behaviorally controlled tactile stimulation. J Neurophysiol 63:82–104

Jones MB, Vierck CJ, Graham RB (1973) Line-gap discrimination of skin. Percept Mot Skills 36:563–570

Kalaska J, Pomeranz B (1979) Chronic peripheral nerve injuries alter the somatotopic organization of the cuneate nucleus in kittens. Brain Res 236:35–47

Kandel ER, Klein M, Hochner B, Shuster M, Siegelbaum SA, Hawkins RD, Glanzman DL, Castellucci VE, Abrams TW (1987) Synaptic modulation and learning: new insights into synaptic transmission from the study of behavior. In: Edelman GM, Gall WE, Cowan WM (eds) Synaptic function. Wiley, New York, pp 471–518

Lømo T (1966) Frequency potentiation of excitatory synaptic activity in the dentate area of the hippocampal formation. Acta Physiol Scand (Suppl) 68:128

Merzenich MM, Kaas JH, Wall JT, Nelson RJ, Sur M, Felleman D (1983a) Topographic reorganization of somatosensory cortical areas 3b and 1 in adult monkeys following restricted deafferentation. Neuroscience 8:33–55

Merzenich MM, Kaas JH, Wall JT, Sur M, Nelson RJ, Felleman D (1983b) Progression of change following median nerve section in the cortical representation of the hand in areas 3b and 1 in adult owl and squirrel monkeys. Neuroscience 10:639–665

Merzenich MM, Nelson RJ, Stryker MP, Cynader MS, Schoppmann A, Zook JM (1984) Somatosensory cortical map changes following digit amputation in adult monkeys. J Comp Neurol 224:591–605

Merzenich MM, Nelson RJ, Kaas JH, Stryker MP, Jenkins WM, Zook JM, Cynader MS, Schoppmann A (1987) Variability in hand surface representations in areas 3b and 1 in adult owl and squirrel monkeys. J Comp Neurol 258:281–296

Merzenich MM, Recanzone G, Jenkins WM, Allard TT, Nudo RJ (1988) Cortical representational plasticity. In: Rakic P, Singer W (eds) Neurobiology of neocortex. Wiley, New York, pp 41–67

Pons TP, Garraghty PE, Mishkin M (1988) Lesion-induced plasticity in the second somatosensory cortex of adult macaques. Proc Natl Acad Sci USA 85:4279–4281

Recanzone GH, Jenkins WM, Hradek GT, Schreiner CE, Grajski KA, Merzenich MM (1989) Frequency discrimination training alters topographical representations and distributed temporal response properties of neurons in SI cortex of adult owl monkeys. Soc Neurosci Abstr 15:1223

Sur M, Merzenich MM, Kaas JH (1980) Magnification, receptive field area and "hypercolumn" size in areas 3b and 1 of somatosensory cortex in owl monkeys. J Comp Neurol 44:295–311

Tsukahara N (1987) Cellular basis of classical conditioning mediated by the red nucleus in the cat. In: Edelman GM, Gall WE, Cowan WM (eds) Synaptic function. Wiley, New York, pp 447–469

Vierck CJ, Jones MB (1970) Influences of low and high frequency oscillation upon spatio-tactile resolution. Physiol Behavior 5:1431–1435

Volkmann AW (1858) Über den Einfluß der Übung. Leipz Ber Math Phys Cl 10:38–69

Wall JT, Cusic CG (1984) Cutaneous responsiveness in primary somatosensory (S-I) hindpaw cortex before and after partial hindpaw deafferentation in adult rats. J Neurosci 4:1499–1515

Woody CD (1986) Understanding the cellular basis of memory and learning. Annu Rev Psychol 37:433–493

Woody CD, Swartz BE, Gruen E (1978) Effects of acetylcholine and cyclic GMP on input resistance of cortical neurons in awake cats. Brain Res 158:373–395

# Biological and Psychosocial Considerations in Recovery from Brain Damage

*P. Bach-y-Rita and E. Wicab Bach-y-Rita*

## Neurobiological Mechanisms of Recovery

During the past 20 years there has been an increasing interest in brain plasticity and the capacity for recovery of function following brain damage. The capacity of the brain to reorganize following damage had not been generally recognized before that time for many reasons (discussed in Bach-y-Rita 1988). This new surge of interest in recovery of function has led to a series of therapeutic approaches to the brain-damaged patient.

The degree of functional improvement is dependent on many factors including age, area damaged, amount of tissue damaged, rapidity of the damage, as well as the rehabilitation program and environmental and psychosocial factors. These have been extensively examined elsewhere (e.g., Bach-y-Rita 1980, 1981; Bach-y-Rita and Balliet 1987; Boyeson and Bach-y-Rita 1989; much of the following has been adapted from Bach-y-Rita 1991).

While individual neurons do not appear to regenerate, there are a number of potential mechanisms of reorganization. The plasticity of neuronal processes appears to extend into advanced old age: the length of the terminal dendritic segment of cortical pyramidal neurons is 25% longer in non-senile 80-year-old humans than in normal 50-year-old persons; this might represent growth to compensate for normal cell loss (Buell and Coleman 1979).

Boyeson and Bach-y-Rita (1989) have summarized a 3-day conference, The Determinants of Brain Plasticity (Praglia, Italy, June, 1988), in which a number of relevant mechanisms were evaluated, in particular those related to neurotransmitter and neuroactive substances. Some points raised at the Praglia conference include the following:

Varon reported that, following frontal cortex damage, the contralateral cerebellum shows reduced activity, recently confirmed in PET scan studies, from our lab of persons with long-standing post-traumatic hemiparesis (Perlman et al. 1988). Boyeson noted that, if the rat contralateral cerebellum is made supersensitive by a unilateral locus coeruleus lesion 2 weeks before a sensorimotor cortex injury, total permanent recovery from hemiplegia is noted as little as 1 h post infusion of noradrenaline (24 h after the cortical lesion), and suggested that the anatomical basis for the effect is the simultaneous projection of individual locus coeruleus cells to both contralateral cerebellum and ipsilateral sensorimotor cortex.

Glial cells are now considered to be determining the microchemical environment that the neuron sees, including trophic factors such as those relating to cellular outgrowth and mechanisms of functional recovery.

In regard to the therapeutic roles of pharmacological agents, Fuxe considers that many of the effects of exogenous ganglioside are via the lipid part of the membrane. Animal studies revealed that, if gangliosides are administered during the first 48 h, there seems to be an increase in TH-immunoreactive cell bodies and increased cell survival, with increased functional recovery.

Agnati discussed gangliosides in relation to interactions between neurons and glia. Gangliosides, by modulating polyamine biosynthesis, can in some way increase the efficacy of the transformation of putrescine into GABA. In a rat model, gangliosides protected 40% – 50% of the striatal neurons and produced a large activation of astroglia, noted7 days later.

Stein noted that ganglioside treatment prevented loss of body weight following large cortical transections in rats, and produced early positive behavioral responses. However, 39 days after injury, the treated and untreated animals were not distinguishable. Combining ganglioside and amphetamine treatment was not beneficial. Stein noted that both beneficial and disruptive effects of ganglioside treatment can be noted. Convulsive activity can be increased. A frontal cortex transplant model revealed that successfully ganglioside-treated rats are actually worse 1 year later. He cautioned that, when clinical trials are planned, a number of factors (such as location, extent, and type of the lesion, how long treatment is continued, and how long afterwards treatment behavior is assessed) must be taken into consideration (Boyeson and Bach-y-Rita 1989). Other neuroactive substances such as protein kinase C, nerve growth factors, glutamate and others may play a role in the reorganization. In the future pharmacological therapy may target several mechanisms, with specific drugs affecting specific intra- and extracellular, and glial, mechanisms.

## Physical Rehabilitation

Procedures and techniques for the rehabilitation of persons with brain damage have been extensively described elsewhere (e.g., DeLisa 1988; Goodgold 1988) and will not be detailed here. The techniques have developed out of practical experience rather than evolving from experimental evidence.

As early as possible, often within the first few days, physical rehabilitation is begun. We use this term to include the various therapeutic approaches undertaken by members of a interdisciplinary rehabilitation team, such as physical therapy, occupational therapy, speech therapy, and recreational therapy. Rehabilitation nurses, psychologists, vocational rehabilitators, and others are included on the team in addition to the physician trained in rehabilitation who is the team leader. This program continues through the hospitalization and is often continued when the patient is discharged.

Rehabilitation does appear to improve the functional outcome (Lehmann et al. 1975). However, there is little or no demonstrated scientific basis for most of the procedures, and few of the procedures have been validated by controlled studies. The importance of the intervention of the various therapies (e.g., speech, occupational, physical, recreational, etc.) has not been demonstrated sufficiently. The requirements of neurorehabilitation are great, and the heavy demand for services has led to a considerable growth of neurorehabilitation facilities and professional groups. Yet there is a dearth of evaluation data.

Environmental factors must be considered when evaluating neurorehabilitation. Patients kept in a rehabilitation ward are in unfamiliar, often hostile environments, deprived of family and home. Often rehabilitation facilities are located in the basement or in other harsh settings. These and other environmental factors may influence rehabilitation outcome. Recent evidence has shown that even the view through the window may influence recovery from surgery: Ulrich (1984) showed that surgical patients assigned to rooms with windows looking out on a natural scene had shorter postoperative hospital stays, received fewer negative evaluative comments in nurses' notes, and took fewer potent analgesics than matched patients in similar rooms with windows facing a brick building wall.

The therapeutic environment also includes the home and social environments. A supportive family member may be able to undertake rehabilitation interventions that, although less technically developed than professional therapy, may be able to achieve significant functional gains in the familiar and supportive environment of the home; specific therapeutic activities may be more closely related to the patient's particular interests (Bach-y-Rita 1980). Research into the effects of the various therapy environments may lead to the most appropriate use, at different stages of evolution of the brain-damaged patient, of acute hospital bedside rehabilitation, rehabilitation units in acute hospitals, late (chronic) rehabilitation units, specific rehabilitation hospitals, community rehabilitation facilities, nursing homes, and home programs.

## Late Rehabilitation

We have designed rehabilitation programs which can be provided after the "spontaneous" recovery ceases to be a factor. One of our successful models of late rehabilitation is facial paralysis rehabilitation. With such patients we have evaluated rehabilitation programs specifically designed to obtain reorganization of function by reprogramming the motorneurons of the XII nerve on the operated side to become included in the facial motor programs (Balliet 1985; Balliet et al. 1982).

## Adaptation to Ability

Psychosocial factors are of considerable relevance to the recovery from brain damage. We have recently discussed this elsewhere, and the following section is taken from that discussion (Bach-y-Rita and Wicab Bach-y-Rita 1990).

Patients with long-standing disability who show significant recovery must adapt to the increasing function. Studies on how physically disabled persons perceive their disability (Campbell et al. 1986; Weinberg and Williams 1978) and how they assess the quality of their lives and the possibility of gaining abilities (Weinberg 1984) revealed that stages of adjustment to disability, learned helplessness, and perceived interference of disability with the attainment of goals may influence the perception and the desirability of partial or complete recovery of abilities. The family system and the culture may influence both the outcome of rehabilitation and the desirability of recovery (Bach-y-Rita and Wicab Bach-y-Rita 1990).

The following is a theoretical framework for our studies in this area: following an illness or accident that produces an impairment, there is a process of adaptation to the disability. However, a rehabilitation program that produces an increase in ability also requires adaptation to a relatively non-disabled status. The adaptation to loss will include a process of mourning (shock, denial, anger, sadness, depression; Hughes 1984), and will trigger individual coping mechanisms such as denial and compensation that will contribute to the nature of the adaptation to an impairment and consequent disability. Psychological processes such as cognitive appraisal and coping (Lazarus and Folkman 1984) and social dimensions such as roles, status, support networks, and institutional and cultural definitions of disability should be considered mediating variables that contribute to the outcome of the rehabilitation process (i.e., adaptation to disability and adaptation to ability).

## Conclusions

Following brain damage, significant recovery of function is possible. Patients recover better with neurorehabilitation than without it. Functional recovery potential persists for many years after the brain damage occurs, and specific late rehabilitation procedures have been developed to take advantage of that potential. Factors that appear to be of importance in recovery include brain plasticity, the therapeutic program, the environment, and psychosocial factors. Much remains to be determined in regard to which specific procedures are most effective. Scientifically based studies are of great need in the field.

*Acknowledgement.* The work was supported in part by NIDRR Grant G 0087 C 2008.

## References

Bach-y-Rita P (1980) Recovery of function: theoretical considerations for brain injury rehabilitation. Huber, Bern

Bach-y-Rita P (1981) Brain plasticity as a basis for the development of rehabilitation procedures for hemiplegia. Scand J Rehabil Med 13:73–83

Bach-y-Rita P (1988) Brain plasticity. In: Goodgold J (ed) Rehabilitation medicine. Mosby, St. Louis, pp 113–118

Bach-y-Rita P (1991) Applications of principles of brain plasticity and training to restore function. In: Young RR, Delwaide PJ (eds) Principles of restorative neurology. Butterworth, London (in press)

Bach-y-Rita P, Balliet R (1987) Recovery from stroke. In: Duncan PW, Badke MB (eds) Motor deficits following stroke. Year Book Medical Publishers, New York, pp 79–107

Bach-y-Rita P, Wicab Bach-y-Rita E (1990) Biological and psychosocial factors in recovery from brain damage in humans. Can J Psychol 44:148–165

Balliet R (1985) Motor control strategies in the retraining of facial paralysis. In: Portman M (ed) Proceedings of the 5th international symposium on the facial nerve, 1984, Bordeaux. Masson, Paris, pp 465–469

Balliet R, Shinn JB, Bach-y-Rita P (1982) Facial paralysis rehabilitation: retraining selective muscle control. Int J Rehabil Med 4:67–74

Boyeson MG, Bach-y-Rita P (1989) Determinants of brain plasticity. J Neuro Rehabil 3:35–57

Buell S, Coleman P (1979) Dendritic growth in aged human brain and failure of growth in senile dementia. Science 206:854–856

Campbell ME, Cull JG, Hardy RE (1986) Disabled persons' attitudes toward disability. Psychol Q J Hum Behav 23(2–3):16–20

DeLisa JA (ed) (1988) Rehabilitation medicine: principles and practice. Lippincott, Philadelphia

Goodgold J (1988) Rehabilitation medicine. Mosby, St Louis

Hughes F (1984) Reaction to loss: coping with disability and death. In: Marinelli PR, dell'Orto EA (eds) Psychological and social impact of physical disability. Springer, New York, pp 131–136

Lazarus SR, Folkman S (1984) Stress, appraisal, and coping. Springer, Berlin Heidelberg New York

Lehmann JF, DeLateur BJ, Fowler RS, Warren CG, Arnhold R, Schertzer G, et al. (1975) Stroke: does rehabilitation affect outcome? Arch Phys Med Rehabil 56:375–382

Perlman S, Wilson MA, Blood K, Balliet R, Turaki PA, Sunderland JJ, Rowe B, Sackett JF (1988) Cerebellar metabolism of FDG in patients with brain damage. 35th Meeting of the Society of Nuclear Medicine, San Francisco. J Nuclear Med 29:822

Ulrich R (1984) View through a window may influence recovery from surgery. Science 224:420–421

Weinberg N (1984) Physically disabled people assess the quality of their lives. Rehabil Lit 45(1–2):12–15

Weinberg N, Williams J (1978) How the physically disabled perceive their disabilities. J Rehabil 44:31–33

# Discussion: Environmental and Experiential Factors Play a Key Role in Determining the Outcome of Injury to the Central Nervous System

*D. G. Stein*

Studies of recovery from injury to the central nervous system are entering a revolutionary stage as changes in both conceptual thinking about the brain and rapid-fire discoveries about mechanisms appear almost on a daily basis. The traditional notion of the brain as a "hard-wired", genetically determined collection of structures, each with a predetermined function, is gradually giving way to a much more dynamic and holistic view based on principles of development plasticity, and change.

The doctrine of *localization of function* has held the field of neuropsychology in its grip for almost two centuries and has led to the pessimistic view that once an area of the brain has been damaged or destroyed, the functions it subserves must be irretrievably lost. Ramon y Cajal (1928), the Nobel prize-winning neuroanatomist, best expressed this view when he stated that:

"Once development was ended, the fonts of growth and regeneration of the axon and dendrites dried up *irrevocably*. In adult centers, the nerve paths are something fixed and immutable; everything may die, nothing may be regenerated (p. 750)."

Significant medical and social consequences stemmed directly from this static doctrine of neuronal organization and function. Most importantly, if the view was correct, would it make sense to seek expensive, time-consuming treatment for patients who had little hope for a positive outcome? Would medical, rehabilitative and social resources be better spent on other diseases where there was better possibility of success?

This meeting itself demonstrates that beliefs and attitudes can and do change. Kuhn (1970) in discussing how scientific paradigms evolve writes:

..."the early developmental stages of most sciences have been characterized by continual competition between a number of distinct views of nature, each partially derived from, and all roughly compatible with the dictates of scientific observation and method. What differentiated these various schools was not one or another failure of method – they were all "scientific" – but what we shall come to call their incommensurable ways of seeing the world and practicing science in it.

Normal science, the activity in which most scientists inevitably spend almost all of their time, is predicated on the assumption that the scientific community knows what the world is like. Much of the success of the enterprise derives from the community's willingness to defend that assumption, if necessary at considerable cost. Normal science often suppresses fundamental novelties because they are necessarily subversive of its basic commitments. Nevertheless, so long as those commitments retain an element of the arbitrary, the very nature of normal research ensures that novelty shall not be suppressed for very long" (p. 4).

These last 10 years have witnessed the "revolutionary" paradigm shift that Kuhn has referred to, and although there is now overwhelming evidence that recovery alter traumatic injury to the brain does occur, there are still many questions and puzzles about its biochemical, physiological, anatomical and behavioral concomitants. This conference is but one of the many steps that will be needed to unravel the mysteries of recovery which will then lead to effective treatments and new rehabilitation strategies.

A major problem that must be answered as we try to generalize from basic research using animals as subjects, to the clinical situation with patients, is: what do we mean by the term "recovery"? Why is recovery seen in some laboratories and clinics and not others? One simple reason for the discrepancy is that no one has come up with an agreed-upon definition of the term "recovery". Different groups have different meanings for both rehabilitation and recovery. For example, in discussing recovery from brain injury, Laurence and Stein (1978) stressed that the phrase "recovery of function" can refer to the straightforward accomplishment of certain goals by the subject (achieving an "end") or it can refer to the strategies (or "means") by which organisms accomplish their goals. For the working therapist and his patient, the issue may simply be to improve the latter's quality of life and there is little concern about the particular strategies or underlying physiological substrates. Thus the question of "how" may be less important than "whether" the goal is obtained. Yet, if each group or clinic sets its own arbitrary definition of "recovery" it is not surprising that there are so many differences of opinion concerning whether or not a given function is said to be "recovered"; not to mention what might satisfy the patients or their families.

A parallel question to that of defining what is meant by recovery, is what is meant by the term "function". How is the function of a given brain area to be defined? In the past, many functions of brain regions were defined by the loss or impairments of behaviors that accompanied damage to the structure in question. For example Pöppel (1989) recently defined (CNS) functions "as those that, in principle, can be lost after circumscribed injuries of the brain" (p. 6). But there are numerous cases in which "circumscribed injuries" do *not* lead to significant, functional impairments. For example, there is a large literature demonstrating that slow growing, bilateral injuries to the brain (e.g., serial lesions), often spare the complex behaviors thought to be mediated by the injured structures (Finger et al. 1973; Finger and Stein 1982, for examples). In these cases involving rats, cats and monkeys, bilateral damage does not lead to behavioral symptomatology. How, then, is the "function" to be defined according to the 'classical' definitions provided above?

Behavioral descriptions of deficits following circumscribed CNS injuries are the forte of neuropsychologists whose specialized tests are designed specifically to localize "deficits" to specific brain regions. But what constitutes an adequate definition of a "deficit" or its localization to a particular brain region in the context I have just described? What is the appropriate behavioral test to identify when and how a function is lost? For example, although Pöppel (1989) has argued that "the integrity of local neuronal structures is essential for the availability of specific psychological functions (p. 222);" the serial lesion data argue against that view.

In addition, in the clinic, Pöppel et al. (1973) and others (e.g. Zihl 1981; Pommerenke and Markowitsch 1989) have demonstrated that patients with cerebral 'blindness' following posterior cortical injuries, have residual vision and *can* make visual discriminations if they are properly trained; a phenomenon they refer to as "blindsight". In this case are visual functions lost or are they suppressed or 'blocked' by the neural insult? Animal research on this topic as well as the blindsight data, can be taken to indicate that 'inhibition' of function rather than loss, may be one result of 'localized' brain injury. Under the circumstances, the problem becomes how to "unlock" or "unmask" the repressed function.

Some time ago, Meyer (1972) and his colleagues showed that cats with massive, bilateral, posterior cortical lesions could be rendered almost totally blind. However, following an injection of amphetamine, a potent neuroleptic, the "blind" cats were able to make visually guided placing responses as long as they were under the effects of the drug. Meyer argued that the lesions blocked access to the visual "engrams" which could be "derepressed" by the activating properties of the amphetamine. More recently, Feeney and Sutton (1988) showed that cats and rats could recover almost normal limb movements and gait following bilateral sensorimotor cortex lesions if they were given a single injection of amphetamine at the time of the injury. Without recourse to any drugs Held et al. (1985) were able to show that enriched sensory activity and opportunity to explore the environment, could lead to better (although not complete) recovery of gait in adult rats which had received extensive injury to the sensorimotor cortex. In combination, these studies reveal that the 'functions' of a given area may be altered (or determined?) by the organism's experience and not just by its genetically 'fixed' neuronal connections (or their disruption).

William Jenkins' elegant and sophisticated research presented at this meeting most directly speaks to this important issue. He, Michael Merzenich and their colleagues have repeatedly demonstrated that the classical view suggesting that maturation of neuronal connections determines their 'functions' for a lifetime, is simply not true. Using precise, electrophysiological recording of single neurons in the sensorimotor cortex to map their receptive fields, Jenkins and his colleagues have shown that such fields can be modeled and remodeled by experience and training. More importantly for this discussion, following loss of sensory inputs, these same neurons may change their receptive fields dramatically (i.e., skin surface representation shifts). In some cases after cortical damage, the representation of skin sensory areas may shift to undamaged, previously unused portions of the remaining cortex. Likewise, as animals are trained on a sensory discrimination task, there are continuous shifts in the locus of cortical representation as well as in specific, receptive field characteristics. These are just a few of the dramatic instances of context-induced, neuronal plasticity, that could never be explained or understood from the localizationist paradigm.

Under these circumstances, is it not likely that rehabilitation training, or even the patient's pre-injury experience, could alter neuronal activity in a similar fashion? If Jenkins and Merzenich are correct in thinking that individual experience plays such an important role in determining CNS activity and function, we should be concerned with the issue of whether it makes sense to 'standardize' rehabilitation therapy such that all patients with a 'given' type of injury receive the same treatments. Such standardization could probably, in many cases, be beneficial, but at the same time, without taking into consideration the patient's past experience, motivational state, etc., rote training might also lead to an enhanced deficit (e.g., spasticity) – if the wrong neurons and/or behavioral strategies were 'stamped in'. Later in this book, Anne-Lise Christensen will discuss how more individualized therapeutic strategies may be employed – a point of view which has not yet received appropriate attention of either researchers or clinicians working in this area.

Although there are many questions that could be addressed in more detail, two with particular clinical relevance will close my discussion. The first is concerned with how soon after injury the treatment should begin. Thanks to a large body of recent laboratory research, it is now quite clear that early and aggressive intervention and therapy may lead to the best prognosis for recovery. It has to be emphasized that brain injury and the concomitant cell loss is not a single, unitary event. Rather, a cascade of processes, some of which may last for years, is the complex result of neural damage. To give but a few examples, in the first stage(s) of injury, both neurotoxins and excitotoxins may be released into the brain parenchyma (Nieto-Sampedro 1988). As a result, neurons initially spared by the trauma itself could begin to die in massive numbers resulting in cell loss more devastating to the patient than the initial injury itself.

Fortunately, there is a growing literature demonstrating that pharmacologic intervention to block some of these 'negative' processes is now possible. For example, calcium channel antagonists given in the early stages of injury can block the damaging effect of calcium ions on protein degradation and subsequent loss of cell membrane (LeVere et al. 1989; Pickard et al. 1989). Likewise, administration of glutamate antagonists in the early stages of trauma, can also prevent the excitotoxicity that causes neuronal death when this substance is stimulated and released in large quantities following the injury (Boast et al. 1988; Faden et al. 1989). Thus, blocking some of the secondary consequences of brain injury may be as important to the recovery process(es) as providing neurotransmitter replacement or other forms of pharmacotherapy later in the course of treatment.

Finally, research on how much time should be devoted to rehabilitation or other forms of post-injury 'therapy' is another area that needs careful investigation. Geschwind (1985) felt that most clinicians not only did not pay sufficient attention to "seeking the right maneuvers" to elicit recovery, they also did not give enough attention to the time necessary for the processes leading to recovery to become manifest. Referring to the aphasias, he said that:

"Most neurologists are gloomy about the prognosis of severe adult aphasias after a few weeks and pessimism is reinforced by a lack of prolonged follow-up in most cases. I have, however, seen patients severely aphasic for over one year, who then made excellent recovery. One patient returned to work as a salesman, the other as a psychiatrist. Furthermore, there are patients who continue to improve over many years, for example, the patient whose aphasia is still quite evident six years after onset, cleared up substantially by 18 years" (p. 3).

I take Geschwind's observations to suggest that perhaps we are not doing enough to provide long-term therapy and rehabilitation to patients whose progress through the spectrum of recovery may be arduous and long. There is no principle of neuronal organization that demands that functional recovery occur immediately or not at all. The decision to withold or terminate either pharmacological treatments or rehabilitation therapy is probably based more on economic (i.e., it would cost too much to continue) and social factors (let's get on to something with a more rapid, personal payoff; i.e., seeing a quick recovery) than it is on purely physiologic grounds; i.e., what we know about how the nervous system actually works.

The time course of recovery can also be taken to mean that the therapy itself may need to change as the CNS endogenous response to the trauma progresses. As the underlying physical substrates change over time, so should the therapy. Thus, for example, in the earliest stages, it might be appropriate to give drugs which block edema and reduce excitotoxicity, then shortly follow this regimen with neurotrophic factors that could enhance neural sparing or reduce neuronal loss by repairing damaged membranes. In this context, nerve growth factor (Will et al. 1988) and gangliosides (Dunbar and Stein 1988) have been proposed as potentially important therapeutic agents, to name only a few. Days to weeks later, it might then be necessary to begin neurotransmitter replacement therapy or even under some circumstances, cell replacement through fetal brain tissue grafts.

Still much more research needs to be done to determine what specific types of cognitive and behavioral rehabilitation should be provided. As Bach-y-Rita (1991) pointed out in his presentation, and elsewhere, "there is little or no demonstrated scientific basis for most of the (rehabilitation) procedures, and few of these procedures have been validated by controlled studies. The importance of the intervention of the various therapies has not been demonstrated".

The section on basic hypotheses concerning recovery of function has opened the door to many important and exciting questions, with the subject of each easily deserving of an entire symposium in its own right. I believe that the contextual approach to "recovery of function" is a revolutionary paradigm in the process of its own development. It puts aside the traditional, mechanistic and reductionistic view in favor of a more holistic approach to patients and their potential therapy. Weiss (1967), a leading developmental systems biologist tried to make this point years ago when he said that:

"In trying to restore the loss of information suffered by thus lifting isolated fragments out of context, we have assigned the job of reintegration to a corps of anthropomorphic gremlins. As a result, we are now plagued – or blessed, depending on one's party view – with countless demigods, like those in antiquity, doing the jobs we do not understand: the organizers, operators, inductors, repressors, promotors, regulators, etc., – all prosthetic devices to make up for the amputations which we have allowed to be perpetrated on the organic wholeness, or to put it more innocuously, the "systems" character, of nature and our thinking about nature" (p. 821).

Just as no one has been able to predict the monumental and historic changes now occurring in Europe, no one may be able to predict where this current neuroscientific revolution will lead, but it is certain that brain-injured patients who only too recently had nothing to hope for, may soon come to expect a dramatic turn for the better.

## References

Bach-y-Rita P (1991) Applications of principles of brain plasticity and training to restore function. In: Young RR, Delwaide PJ (eds) Principles of restorative neurology. Butterworth, London (in press)

Boast CA, Gerhardt SC, Pastor G, Lehmann J, Etienne PE, Liebman JM (1988) The N-methyl-D-aspartate antagonists CGS 19755 and CPP reduce ischemic brain damage in gerbils. Brain Res 442:345–348

Dunbar GL, Stein DG (1988) Gangliosides and functional recovery from brain injury. In: Stein DG, Sabel BA (eds) Pharmacological approaches to the treatment of brain and spinal cord injury. Plenum, New York, pp 195–218

Faden AI, Demediuk P, Panter SS, Vink R (1989) The role of excitatory amino acids and NMDA receptors in traumatic brain injury. Science 244:798–800

Feeney DM, Sutton RL (1988) Catecholamines and recovery of function after brain damage. In: Stein DG, Sabel BA (eds) Pharmacological approaches to the treatment of brain and spinal cord injury. Plenum, New York, pp 121–142

Finger S, Stein DG (1982) Brain damage and recovery: research and clinical perspectives. Academic, New York

Finger S, Walbran B, Stein DG (1973) Brain damage and behavioral recovery: serial lesion phenomena. Brain Res 63:1–18

Geschwind N (1985) Mechanisms of change after brain lesions. Ann NY Acad Sci 457:1–11

Held JM, Gordon J, Gentile AM (1985) Environmental influences on locomotor recovery following cortical lesions in rats. Behav Neurosci 99:678–690

Kuhn T (1970) The structure of scientific revolutions. University of Chicago Press, Chicago, p 4

Laurence S, Stein DG (1978) Recovery after brain damage and the concept of localization of function. In: Finger S (ed) Recovery from brain damage: research and theory. Plenum, New York, pp 369–407

LeVere TE, Brugler T, Sandin M, Gray-Silva S (1989) Recovery of function after brain damage: facilitation by the calcium entry blocker nimodipine. Behav Neurosci 103:561–565

Meyer DR (1972) Access to engrams. Am Psychol 27:124–133

Nieto-Sampedro M (1988) Growth factor induction and order of events in CNS repair. In: Stein DG, Sabel BA (eds) Pharmacological approaches to the treatment of brain and spinal cord injury. Plenum, New York, pp 301–338

Pickard JD, Murray GD, Illingworth R, Shaw MDM, Teasdale GM, Foy PM, Humphrey PRD, Lang DA, Nelson R, Richards P, Sinar J, Bailey S, Skene A (1989) Effect of oral nimodopine on cerebral infarction and outcome after subarachnoid haemorrhage: British aneurysm nimodopine trial. Br Med J 298:636–642

Pommerenke K, Markowitsch HJ (1989) Rehabilitation training of homonymous visual field defects in patients with postgeniculate damage of the visual system. Restor Neurol Neurosci 1:47–64

Pöppel E (1989) Taxonomy of the subjective: an evolutionary perspective. In: Brown JW (ed) Neuropsychology of visual perception. Erlbaum, Hillsdale, pp 219–232

Pöppel E, Held R, Frost D (1973) Residual visual function after brain wounds involving the central visual pathways in man. Nature 243:295–296

Ramon y Cajal S (1928) Degeneration and regeneration of the nervous system. Oxford University Press, London

Weiss P (1967) When one plus one does not equal two. In: Quarton GC, Melnechuk T, Schmitt FO (eds) The neurosciences: a study program. Rockefeller University Press, New York, pp 801–821

Will B, Hefti F, Pallage V, Toniolo G (1988) Nerve growth factor: effects on CNS neurons and on behavioral recovery from brain damage. In: Stein DG, Sabel BA (eds) Pharmacological approaches to the treatment of brain and spinal cord injury. Plenum, New York, pp 339–360

Young W (1985) The role of calcium in spinal cord injury. CNS Trauma 2:109–114

Zihl J (1981) Recovery of visual field associated with specific training in patients with cerebral damage. In: van Hof MW, Mohn G (eds) Functional recovery from brain damage. Elsevier, Amsterdam, pp 189–202

# Controversial Concepts of Rehabilitation

# A Neurobehavioural Approach to Brain Injury Rehabilitation

*R. L. Wood*

## The Organisation of Rehabilitation for Patients with Brain Damage

A neurobehavioural approach attempts to address the problems of social outcome as opposed to clinical recovery per se. Many patients who make good progress according to clinical criteria still do not become integrated into the community, irrespective of the nature and level of their disability. This often occurs because traditional rehabilitation focuses too much on physical recovery and not enough on the patient's social behaviour, or their ability to recognise and adapt to changing situations.

Unlike other forms of serious trauma (e.g., spinal injury), brain damage alters personality and behaviour while simultaneously, imposing damage to the cognitive system which, under normal circumstances, mediates many forms of learning and allows individuals to maintain an awareness of their behaviour and exercise emotional control. Unless rehabilitation procedures address these important issues, many patients will fail to achieve their potential in terms of utilising skills and abilities needed for employment and social independence.

Clinical experience of rehabilitating individuals with traumatic brain injury, supported by the psycho-social follow-up studies of Brookes et al. (1986, 1987), Thomsen (1984) and Oddy (1984), clearly indicates a need to re-appraise the conceptual and operational basis of specialised rehabilitation services for brain-damaged patients in order to address the cognitive, emotional and behavioural sequelae of brain injury. In many cases, these legacies prove to be a greater obstacle to community re-entry and re-employment, than physical disability (Brookes et al. 1986). Therefore, any specialised comprehensive rehabilitation service for brain-damaged patients, must include methods of cognitive rehabilitation and behaviour management as primary forms of treatment within the spectrum of rehabilitation services.

The neurobehavioural approach attempts to achieve this by identifying the neurological or neuropsychological constraints which can interfere with learning and behavioural control (see Wood 1988, 1989). A behavioural paradigm is used to control and eliminate inappropriate or unacceptable social behaviour while principles of conditioning provide a framework for learning which reduces the impact of cognitive deficits and frontal lobe abnormalities on the acquisition of skills, abilities, or compensatory strategies which are important for independent living.

## The Importance of Learning in Rehabilitation

Learning is important to success in rehabilitation but brain injury interferes with learning by reducing information processing ability and disrupting many of the cognitive functions which integrate information and allow learning to occur, e.g., disorders of attention, memory, perception, insight and judgement (Wood 1988; Wood and Fussey 1991). Consequently, brain damage imposes serious constraints on the brain's ability to process information and (by implication) the ability to learn. This means that a specialised brain injury rehabilitation programme needs to:

1. Determine the extent and nature of a patient's learning disability
2. Devise strategies or techniques to help patients learn abilities or skills important to independent living
3. Consider alternative ways of learning and remembering such skills and abilities so that severe cognitive impairment or the problems imposed by frontal brain injury can be avoided or minimised
4. Generalise from the clinic into the community those skills and abilities that help translate good clinical recovery into good social outcome.

The neurobehavioural approach to brain injury rehabilitation promotes learning by:

1. Identifying and isolating those aspects of cognitive impairment that will interfere with learning and reduce the patient's potential for recovery
2. Adopting a procedural learning model (as opposed to a declarative model) to help patients acquire skills that will improve their level of social and functional independence
3. Reducing complex tasks to a sequence of discrete units of activity which the patient rehearses sequentially with the aid of verbal mediation to regulate performance
4. Consolidating each stage of learning before adding additional stages, allowing the patient to combine a number of discrete units of behaviour of activity into a *complex action sequence* that fulfils some functional requirement
5. Generalising skills learned in the clinic to the community by allowing patients to practice life skills in an environment comparable to one in which the skills will need to be displayed.

## Controlling Unacceptable Behaviour

The studies of families who have a head-injured relative all show that behaviour problems are the most enduring of all brain injury sequelae. They impose a great burden upon families who have to care for such individuals and there is a high incidence of psychological disorder, marital conflict and divorce in such families (especially when the wife is the victim of serious head injury, see Willer in preparation). Behaviour problems interfere with both the quantity and quality of rehabilitation a patient is likely to receive (see Eames and Wood 1985), and the experience of many American rehabilitation centres has been that staff feel very intimidated by brain-injured patients who display aggressive, threatening or sexually disinhibited behaviour.

The neurobehavioural approach has successfully reduced the frequency of such unacceptable behaviours by providing a rationale to help clinicians discriminate between threatening behaviour which is learned or employed purposefully (for vicarious reward) and those which are organically determined and require specific forms of chemotherapy in combination with behaviour management techniques (see Wood 1987).

The neurobehavioural approach has adapted traditional forms of behaviour modification in order that they can be applied to a brain-injured population, both to control undesirable behaviour and shape socially appropriate and adaptive behaviour. Techniques for controlling behaviour include time-out room procedures, response-cost paradigms, and other methods of reinforcement which influence a patient's motivation to conform to social norms. These methods have proved successful where other techniques, such as psychological counselling or sedative medication, have failed. Neurobehavioural methods have proved effective in both specialised (closed) treatment settings (Eames and Wood 1985), day centres for rehabilitation (Wood 1988) and community residential centres, which mainly address the needs of patients with frontal injuries (Goll and Hawley 1988).

Research procedures to evaluate such treatment methods include single-case design studies as well as group studies, using repeated measures analysis of variance to establish response trends.

## References

Brookes N, Campsie L, Symington C et al. (1986) The five year outcome of severe blunt head injury: a relative's view. J Neurol Neurosurg Psychiatry 49:764–770

Brookes N, Campsie L, Symington C et al. (1987) The effects of severe head injury on patient and relative within 7 years of injury. J Head Trauma Rehabil 2(3):34–45

Eames P, Wood RL (1985) Rehabilitation after severe brain injury: a follow-up study of a behavioural approach. J Neurol Neurosurg Psychiatry 48:613–619

Goll S, Hawley K (1989) Social rehabilitation: the role of the transitional living centre. In: Wood RL, Eames P (eds) Models of brain injury rehabilitation. Chapman and Hall, London, pp 142–163

Oddy M, Coughlin T, Tyerman A, Jenkins D (1985) Social adjustment after closed head injury: a further follow-up 7 years after injury. J Neurol Neurosurg Psychiatry 48:564–568
Thomsen IV (1984) Late outcome of very severe blunt head trauma: 10–15 year second follow-up. J Neurol Neurosurg Psychiatry 47:260–268
Wood RL (1987) Brain injury rehabilitation: a neurobehavioural approach. Croom Helm, London
Wood RL (1988) Clinical constraints affecting human conditioning. In: Davey G, Cullin C (eds) Human operant conditioning in behaviour modification. Wiley, London
Wood RL (1989) Salient factors approach to brain injury rehabilitation. In: Wood RL, Eames P (eds) Models of brain injury rehabilitation. Chapman and Hall, London
Wood RL, Fussey I (1991) A model of cognitive rehabilitation. In: Wood RL, Fussey I (eds) Cognitive rehabilitation in perspective. Chapman and Hall, London (in press)

# Neuropsychological Rehabilitation and the Problem of Altered Self-Awareness

*G. P. Prigatano*

## Introduction

Neuropsychological rehabilitation can be defined as those teaching or training activities aimed at improving cognitive and personality functioning following brain injury. Elsewhere, I have attempted to define the terms "cognition" and "personality" and the two complementary activities constituting neuropsychological rehabilitation: namely, *cognitive retraining* and *psychotherapy* (Prigatano et al. 1986). The focus of this presentation will be to discuss the problem of altered self-awareness after brain injury and briefly relate it to the various goals and activities involved in neuropsychological holistically oriented rehabilitation.

Five points will be developed:

1. The problem of altered self-awareness after brain injury has been poorly understood. Yet, this problem may substantially contribute to the poor long-term psychosocial difficulties frequently seen after brain injury.
2. Assuming that a given brain-njured patient has enough residual cerebral function to seriously consider a return to a productive lifestyle, the problem of altered self awareness must be actively addressed in order to maximize the possibility of *maintaining* that productive lifestyle after formal rehabilitation ends.
3. Both cognitive retraining and psychotherapy can help the patient improve self-awareness after brain injury. Carrying out these activities in the context of a therapeutic milieu environment may be crucial for patients to realistically understand their residual deficits and reestablish purpose and meaning in life in the face of sorrow.
4. Intense interaction with brain injured patients produces anxiety and depression in the family as well as the rehabilitation staff. Neuropsychological rehabilitation programs can lose their vitality and creativity if the needs of the family and staff are not actively addressed.
5. There is tentative evidence that neuropsychological rehabilitation may improve the long-term psychosocial outcome (including employment statistics) after brain injury. The central problem for the patient, however, is dealing with a sense of "lost normality". It is for this reason that psychotherapy is a crucial component to neuropsychological rehabilitation.

## The Problem of Altered Self-Awareness and Psychosocial Outcome

The manifestations of altered self-awareness are common after brain injury, but precisely defining and measuring this class of disturbance is difficult. Stuss and Benson (1986) defined "self-consciousness or self-reflectiveness as that attribute of the human which not only allows awareness of the self, but also realizes the position of the self within the social milieu" (p. 246). I will define self-awareness as the capacity to consciously represent or perceive the "self" in relatively "objective" terms while maintaining a sense of subjectivity. This is a paradox of human consciousness. On the one hand, it strives for "objectivity" – that is, perceiving a situation, object, or interaction in a manner quite similar to other's perceptions. While at the same time, maintaining a sense of private, subjective, or unique interpretation of an *experience*.

Given the subjective nature of experience, self-awareness emerges from the interaction of "thoughts" and "feelings". It is perhaps the highest integrated function of the brain and, I believe, is heavily dependent on the integrity of what Mesulam (1985) has termed heteromodal cortex. That is, cortical association areas that integrate inputs from primary sensory-motor systems with limbic or paralimbic systems are crucial for self-awareness.

Thus, human self-awareness is the simultaneous thought/feeling interaction that allows an experience to be objectively described and subjectively felt at the very same time. Because of this intimate connection of thoughts and feelings, the phenomenon has a lot to do with what we call intentions and intentionality, as Pribram (1980) has suggested. To intend some action or to prefer to perceive some event means that a subjective conscious force "wants something". That "wanting something" means a combination of knowing what is "out there" and what one perceives needing "in here".

Damage to the brain, particularly involving heteromodal regions, will produce varying types and degrees of altered self-awareness. Our discussion will focus primarily on traumatic brain injured (TBI) patients, but patients with various brain disorders may demonstrate this class of neuropychological impairment (Prigatano and Schacter 1991), as witnessed by usual object agnosis (Bauer and Rubens 1985), anosognosia for jargon aphasia (Lebrun 1987) and anosognosia for hemiplegia (Weinstein and Kahn 1955).

Observe the severe TBI patient during the recovery course. Several weeks after coma, the patient may walk around the rehabilitation unit in a zombie-like state. He may respond to questions, carry on limited dialogue, and be partially – or fully oriented to his environment. However, the patient lacks spontaneity and a range of affective expression. The ability to actively engage another in conversation is limited as is the ability to emphasize with others' feelings. The patient is extremely "concrete" in his thinking process (Goldstein 1942) and can be described as self-centered and difficult to manage. Like a computer, the patient, at best does exactly what he or she is told and finds it difficult to modify a behavior or a thought process in light of unexpected information. The patient's "interactions" with others are seen as rudimentary and primitive with the patient being unable to show much self-reflection.

It should not surprise us that during this time many patients wish to leave the hospital and return home or to work against medical advice. The patient does not recognize his or her altered higher cerebral functions and complains that their needs are not being adequately met.

While the acute manifestations of disturbed self-awareness are striking and often appear to recover with time, it is suggested that residuals of this problem exert important influences on the patient's behavior several weeks, months, and even years post-brain injury. Oddy et al. (1985) studied both patients' and families' descriptions of residual neuropsychological deficits seven years post-injury. Uniformly, the patients underestimate many behavioral problems compared to their relatives' report. Moreover, the relatives emphasized that the patient often seems unrealistic and unwilling to admit (i.e., deny) their residual deficits. This "denial" may very well have a neuropsychological basis to it and not be a pure form of psychiatric or "defensive" denial (McGlynn and Schacter 1989).

The research of Thompson (1984) reports that 10–15 years postinjury many TBI patients show greater sensitivity to distress, less tolerance for noise, and a loss of interest in the environment compared to 2 1/2 years postinjury. These problems may well be based on the brain injured patient's inability to grasp how their higher cerebral functions have changed; consequently they become disillusioned with life and show greater signs of social withdrawal and depression with the passage of time. Helping them understand the residuals of their higher cerebral deficits and how to establish a productive lifestyle in the face of brain injury undercuts this poor psychosocial outcome.

Initial pilot data (Prigatano 1991 c) obtained nearly 10 years ago, further documented the importance of altered self-awareness after brain injury. As Table 1 illustrates, TBI patients who were considered rehabilitation "successes" reported that they were not totally aware of their higher cerebral deficits *after* extensive and intensive rehabilitation. In contrast, every treatment "failure" insisted that they were fully aware of the effects of their brain injury. Fordyce and Roueche (1986) later observed that patient's ratings of their own abilities did not correlate with vocational outcome, whereas the relatives' and staff ratings did.

This type of data and other observations (Prigatano 1991 c) clearly demonstrate that the problem of self-awareness needs to be addressed within the context of neuropsychological rehabilitation to enhance psychosocial outcome.

## Improving Self-Awareness After Brain Injury and Maintaining Work

Aggressive treatment of altered self-awareness should be done in accordance with the overall clinical management of a given patient. If the patient remains

**Table 1.** Comparison of staff and patient ratings on awareness of implication after brain injury. (From Prigatano 1991c, p. 114)

| | Patient ratings | Scaff ratings |
|---|---|---|
| "Success" | | |
| DB (6 months) | 9 | 9 |
| BW (6 months) | 9 | 9 |
| ML (12 months) | 9 | 9 |
| AM (6 months) | 8 | 6 |
| "Failure" | | |
| SD (6 months) | 10 | 2 |
| (12 months) | 10 | 6 |
| TW (6 months) | 10 | 4 |
| (12 months) | 10 | 8 |
| CP (6 months) | 10 | 6 |
| (12 months) | 9 | 4 |

severely impaired several months postinjury, it is difficult to develop a rationale for aggressively working on the problem of altered self-awareness. One could legitimately ask the question, self-awareness for what? How will it serve the patient?

If, however, during any phase of recovery, it appears that the patient has a potential for independence, voluntary and/or gainful employment, it may be extremely useful for the patient to progressively learn how his higher cerebral functions have been altered.

Learning to approach the patient over altered-awareness is a delicate process and requires clinical sensitivity. Over the last ten years, I have come to appreciate that not every patient should be approached in the same manner. Initially, we placed all traumatic brain injured patients into a group setting as well as providing them individual therapies. This approach, however, led to some patients dropping out of the rehabilitation program prematurely. They seemed to be overwhelmed with group confrontation.

Consequently, we have reapproached patients with the attitude that we will begin with whatever rehabilitation needs the patient self-perceives. Within this context, one can then establish a therapeutic alliance with the patient which eventually allows them to trust our judgment. Elsewhere (Prigatano 1988), I have described how the problem of self-awareness can emerge in physical therapy as well as speech and language therapy. This can be a good beginning "place" to establish this therapeutic alliance.

Improved awareness, in our experience, can lead to the establishment of more realistic work activities and ultimately the acceptance of the existential situation. These are not simple words or platitudes. They reflect perhaps the most neglected aspect of neurological rehabilitation in technically oriented forms of medicine and psychology. The patient needs and deserves a time to place his or her tragedy into perspective and to construct their life not in spite of brain damage, but in the face of it. This allows them to make more realistic commitments which can then be maintained for longer periods of time.

At this point, psychotherapy, in its individual and group formats, can be indispensable as a major source of care.

Psychotherapy can be defined in many different ways (Prigatano et al. 1986). A basic definition, however, that I often teach patients is as follows. Psychotherapy is like turning the lights on in a dark room full of bear traps. It does not take away or remove the bear traps of life; it simply allows you to see where not to step if you hope to avoid further pain in your life. Having the patients understand how they have been affected and what steps to take in order not to further hurt their adjustment is extremely important. Even in patients with severe memory difficulties, problems in abstract reasoning and impulse control, they can be taught to understand those realities of life. Psychotherapy is not limited to those with an IQ of 120 or higher or who are so-called psychologically minded. In fact, it is the responsibility of the therapist to determine how to best approach a patient within the context of psychotherapy. This means entering the patient's phenomenological world and using whatever ethical strategies are necessary for the patient to begin to understand themselves.

We have found many sources of intervention to be helpful in this regard. Not only has artwork been useful, but actually having patients bring in the music or the songs that they relate to in their day-to-day life, has been a very provocative method by which we can enter their phenomenological world. Patients may not be able to directly tell us about their depression, their anger, their loneliness, etc. However, their songs reflect these themes and many other important issues in their life.

Within the context of our neuropsychological rehabilitation program, patients receive at least 1–2 h of individual psychotherapy each week. They are also involved in daily group psychotherapy. If the patient becomes overwhelmed by this latter activity (or does not seem to benefit from it), they are not forced to continue. However, they can return to this hour as they and various therapists perceive the need to do so. Patients thus can come back into group psychotherapy at a time that they feel better prepared to deal with this issues in a group setting.

In the context of group psychotherapy, many patients discuss their work trials, an important component to the rehabilitation day (Prigatano et al. 1986). They talk about their frustrations in taking reduced job responsibilities. They talk about worry over being evaluated by the treatment team. They talk about concerns over making less of an income than they had prior to the injury. Some will talk about a feeling of lost hope or concern that they will no longer be successful in life. Gradually, however, some patients begin to talk about whatever success they are experiencing during the work trial. They emphasize that this is the first time that they have felt valuable since their brain injury. They can talk about their sense of growing dignity and the respect that they are starting to recapture from others. Patients who are not yet working and who are struggling with these same issues can benefit from hearing how others are dealing with these sensitive topics.

Perhaps one of the best ways to determine the efficacy or usefulness of group psychotherapy, or any form of psychotherapy, for brain injured patients is to compare statistics regarding those patients who maintain employment after rehabilitation programs that incorporate this type of treatment versus those who do not. In our setting, the individuals that have been able to maintain either voluntary or paid employment have dealt with these affective issues within the context of individual and/or group psychotherapy. There is something quite powerful about the group experience which allows the individual to face problems in a more realistic manner. We have not gathered systematic statistics at this point to document this claim, but existing data in the literature are supportive of it.

Certainly the long-term follow-up study by Thompson (1984) indicates that less than 10% of severe traumatic brain injured patients may be working 10–15 years postinjury. Our own research (Prigatano et al. 1984) as well as that of Ben-Yishay et al. (1987), suggests that approximately 30%–50% of our patients may be maintaining gainful employment several years postinjury. In Phoenix, we have statistics that suggest that the percentage may increase from 50% to 70% if voluntary employment is included. That is, even in severe traumatic brain injured patients another 20%–30% of the patients can be helped to maintain a productive lifestyle if given an opportunity to deal with the affective issues involved in maintaining voluntary work.

Indirect evidence in favor of this point of view has recently been described by Ben-Yishay and Prigatano (1990). Attempting to predict vocational outcome, Ben-Yishay and his colleagues noted that three factors accounted for 42% of the variance in their regression equation. These factors were involvement with others, regulation of affect, and acceptance. They state:

> "These three predictor variables reflect the patient's ability to relate to others, to effectively regulate the expression of emotion in everyday functional life situations and to assimilate various remediated therapy interventions designed to improve self-awareness and self-acceptance". (Ben-Yishay and Prigatano 1990)

It is our belief that it is precisely this latter dimension which is so important for individuals maintaining employment. Patients cannot maintain a productive lifestyle unless they have come to face the realities of their life and this means improving self-awareness and self-acceptance.

## The Importance of the Therapeutic Milieu in Neuropsychological Rehabilitation and Dealing with the Problem of Self-Awareness

The historical insights of Goldstein (1942, 1958) and Luria (1948) clearly established a rationale for the importance of understanding a brain injured patient's altered personality and emotional (catastrophic) reactions as well as systematically analyzing the nature of a neuropsychological symptom and syndrome for re-educational purposes. Luria's (1948) outstanding work (and those of his students, e.g., Christensen 1989) emphasizes the need to give the patients systematic practice at improving those components of a functional cerebral system that has been rendered unoperational. Modern cognitive retraining can only develop when taking to heart the ingenious insights of Luria and adopting them to a growing body of literature found in cognitive psychology and the neurosciences, particularly as it relates to the pharmacology of manipulating nervous system activity.

These insights not withstanding, however, the work of Ben-Yishay et al. (1987) for the first time demonstrated the tremendous importance of the therapeutic environment or milieu for teaching patients how to socially adapt to their residual deficits. It is not easy for many therapists to work intensively with severe TBI patients and to expose their own strengths and weaknesses on a day-to-day basis. Yet, as we follow patients several years after neuropsychological rehabilitation, we are often impressed with how they can progressively gain insights into their disabilities several months or years after brain injury. The process by which this is accomplished is difficult to identify, but when patients are worked with from a purely individual approach, we often do not see the same gains that are achieved using a milieu or holistic approach.

What does the milieu or the therapeutic environment provide to help with the problem of altered self-awareness?

1. The milieu actively focuses on the awareness problem from different vantage points. Awareness regarding problems in gait, alterations in hand writing, changes in voice, as well as in other areas can be approached before giving feedback on more "sensitive" areas.
2. The milieu experience makes public (in a protected way) what is "wrong" and allows patients to face their deficits in a realistic way. Facing a problem in a group setting allows for multiple feedback. A patient may need to "hear the message". Also, there is something about facing a problem in this environment that gives the individual greater freedom from that problem.
3. The milieu provides patients an opportunity to see that they are not alone in their struggles. They see other patients making progress, as well as struggling with important issues.
4. The milieu provides positive role models. Patients "graduating" from the neuropsychological rehabilitation program who reconstruct a meaningful life despite the inevitable disappointments in employment and personal life are powerful incentives. They reinforce the idea that patients can reconstruct their life.
5. The milieu provides for ongoing recognition and social reinforcement to accept one's state in life and to not give up hope. This flows from the preceding contributions of milieu.
6. Milieu gives full recognition that a loss of brain functions does not have to mean a loss of personal dignity and meaning in life. Brain injury does not affect all strengths or skills. Yet, in learning their residual strengths and weaknesses individuals have to face their problems despite the sorrow that is inevitable.

As great as the insights of Dolstein (1942, 1958) and Luria (1948) were, their discussions of rehabilitation do not seem to adequately address the psychotherapeutic needs of brain dysfunctional patients. It is for this reason that I feel we must go beyond the traditional insights of these individuals and develop rehabilitation programs that actively involve a psychotherapeutic component.

## Family and Rehabilitation Staff Needs in Neuropsychological Rehabilitation

An interesting study by Franzen and Myers (1973) provides a type of animal model for gaining insight into the social adjustment problems of TBI patients, their family, and the rehabilitation staff. After bilateral ablations of prefrontal or anterior temporal cortex in rhesus monkeys, Franzen and Myers (1973) observed the social behavior of these animals and of unoperated monkeys placed in proximity with them. They concluded the following:

1. "With reintroduction to their social groups these operates (i.e., operated monkeys) approached without hesitation any animal irrespective of that animal's dominance status" (p. 144), a clear problem in social judgment.
2. "These lesioned animals failed to re-establish relationships with their family members" (p. 144).
3. "The prefrontal and anterior temporal operates largely lost the use of their facial expressions, posturings, and gesturings in social interactions.... Other group members could no longer predict the behavior of the lesioned animals. These alterations together led to losses of social status in the group hierarchy and often actual exclusion of the operates from most group interactions" (p. 144).
4. "... pronounced emotional disturbances (occurring in the nonoperated, normal animals) followed the reintroductions of the lesioned animals due to their decreased and inappropriate social signaling" (p. 153).

Parenthetically, it should be noted that recent PET scan findings in TBI patients provide evidence of frequent disturbance of the anterior tips of the temporal lobes even when such damage is not seen on CT or MRI (Ruff et al. 1989; Langfitt et al. 1986). These studies are compatible with postmortem studies which demonstrate a high frequency of both prefrontal and anterior temporal lobe injury in TBI patients. Thus, the description of Franzen and Myers (1973) is extremely relevant to our patient population.

Distress in family members of TBI patients has been studied and summarized by various authors (Bond 1983; Klonoff and Prigatano 1987). Clearly, the major stress on family members appears to be personality change (McKinlay et al. 1981). Loss of temper, social withdrawal, and "unreasonableness" are commonly reported as producing "high burden" in families (Brooks and

McKinlay 1983). Also, immaturity, insensitivity to others, and inability to handle unexpected changes are commonly reported as greatly distressing to families.

These difficulties often clinically appear in patients who seem to lack insight into the extent of their behavioral problems and the impact it has on those around them. Recently, we have reported (Prigatano et al. 1990) that TBI patients frequently tend to underestimate problems they have in social interaction. Of special importance was the observation that patients greatly underestimate their ability to recognize when something they have said or done upsets someone else. This problem plus trouble controlling negative affect, I believe, is at the core of the stress experienced by others when interacting with brain injured people.

Our treatment staff, despite their best intentions, frequently find themselves frustrated and irritated with the apparent lack of sensitivity TBI patients show in social interaction. This can produce a fair amount of professional "burnout" in staff as well as burnout in families (if not managed). Elsewhere (Prigatano 1989), I have tried to describe how we attempt to work with the staff to avoid these problems and keep them creative in their therapeutic activities. Rehabilitation staff and families need to better understand the problem of impaired awareness in patients to adequately work with them.

## The Efficacy of Neuropsychological Rehabilitation

No matter what scientific criteria are established to measure the efficacy of neuropsychological rehabilitation, *for the patient* the primary problem is that of lost normality (Prigatano 1991 b). Patients want to regain whatever loss of function they have suffered. Except in "mild" injuries, this is seldom if ever possible.

We can measure how many people return back to work after severe TBI (Prigatano et al. 1987), their degree of social isolation (Kozloff 1987), and the impact of neuropsychological rehabilitation on employment statistics (Prigatano et al. 1986; Ben-Yishay et al. 1987). We can measure the use of leisure time after brain injury (Christensen 1989). But the central measure of efficacy from a purely neuropsychological perspective is, does the mind (i.e., the integrated function of brain) actually behave in a manner similar to preinjury status as a result of rehabilitation efforts? The second question is, can such rehabilitation substantially help brain injured patients re-establish a sense of altered or "new" normality?

Only modest restoration of higher cerebral functioning appears to be achieved via our present scientific and clinical methods [despite the revolutionary ideas of Luria (1948)]. Patients do improve in their higher cerebral functioning with time, as well as with intervention strategies, but we still do not know how to manipulate the relevant variables in any systematic way to achieve a greater degree of functional cerebral restitution. Neuropsychological rehabilitation, however, may impact on altered self-awareness and, therefore, successfully impact on three criteria of normality: the ability to work, to love, and to play (Prigatano 1991b). That is, with neuropsychological rehabilitation, a greater proportion of individuals can return to a productive lifestyle. Some can establish more mutually satisfying interpersonal relationships. And, in some patients, there can be an acceptance or better an "integration" of a sense of self which has been altered, but still has many of the old phantasies, hopes, and desires. Brain injured individuals can indulge in personal and social forms of play to help reconstruct an altered sense of individuality after their tragedy.

How we learn to deal with this problem in both a scientific manner as well as in a manner of human concern for another will serve to enrich our own lives and the lives of the patients who we are entrusted to care for.

## References


Bauer RM, Rubens AB (1985) Agnosia. In: Heilman KM, Valenstein E (eds) Clinical neuropsychology, 2nd edn. Oxford University Press, New York, pp 187–241

Ben-Yishay Y, Prigatano GP (1990) Cognitive remediation. In: Griffith E, Rosenthal M (eds) Rehabilitation of the adult and child with traumatic brain injury, 2nd edn. Davis, Philadelphia

Ben-Yishay Y, Silber SM, Piasetsky E, Rattok J (1987) Relationship between employability and vocational outcome after intensive holistic cognitive rehabilitation. J Head Trauma Rehabil 2(1):35–48

Bisiach E, Vallar G, Perani D, Papagno C, Berti A (1986) Unawareness of disease following lesions of the right hemisphere: anosognosia for hemiplegia and anosognosia for hemianopia. Neuropsychologia 24(4):471–482

Bond MR (1983) Effects on the family system. In: Rosenthal M, Griffith E, Bond M, Miller JD (eds) Rehabilitation of the head injured adult. Davis, Philadelphia, pp 209–217

Brooks DN, McKinlay W (1983) Personality and behavioral change after severe blunt head injury – a relative's view. J Neurol Neurosurg Psychiatry 46:336–344

Christensen A-L (1989) The psycho-social outcome – study of 46 patients. Meeting of The Danish Association for Rehabilitation Medicine, Copenhagen

Fordyce DJ, Roueche JR (1986) Different perspectives of disability among patients, staff and relatives during rehabilitation of brain injury. Rehabil Psychol 31:217–224

Franzen EA, Myers RE (1973) Neural control of social behavior: prefrontal and anterior temporal cortex. Neuropsychologia 11:141–157

Goldstein K (1942) Aftereffects of brain injury in war. Grune and Stratton, New York

Goldstein K (1958) The effect of brain damage on the personality. Psychiatry 15:245–260

Klonoff PS, Prigatano GP (1987) Reactions of family members and clinical intervention after traumatic brain injury. In: Ylvisaker M, Gobble EMR (eds) Community re-entry for head injured adults. College-Hill, Boston, pp 381–402

Kozloff R (1987) Networks of social support and the outcome from severe head injury. J Head Trauma Rehabil 2(3):14–23

Langfitt TW, Obrist WD, Alavi A, Grossman RI, Zimmerman R, Jaggi J, Uzzell B, Reivich M, Patton DR (1986) Computerized tomography, magnetic resonance imaging, and positron emission tomography in the study of brain trauma. J Neurosurg 64:760–766

Lebrun Y (1987) Anosognosia in aphasics. Cortex 23:251–263

Luria AR (1948) Restoration of functions after brain trauma (in Russian). Academy of Medical Science Press, Moscow (Pergamon, London 1963)

McGlynn SM, Schacter DL (1989) Unawareness of deficits in neuropsychological syndromes. J Clin Exp Neuropsychol 11:143–205

McKinlay WW, Brooks DN, Bond MR, Martinage DP, Marshall MM (1981) The short-term outcome of severe blunt head injury as reported by relatives of the injured persons. J Neurol Neurosurg Psychiatry 44:527–533

Mesulam M-M (1985) Principles of behavioral neurology. Davis, Philadelphia

Oddy M, Coughlan T, Typerman A, Jenkins D (1985) Social adjustment after closed head injury: a further follow-up seven years after injury. J Neurol Neurosurg Psychiatry 48:564–568

Pribram KH (1980) Mind, brain, and consciousness: the organization of competence and control. In: Davidson J, Davidson R (eds) The psychobiology of consciousness. Plenum, New York, pp 47–61

Prigatano GP (1988) Emotion and motivation in recovery and adaptation to brain damage. In: Finger S, LeVere T, Almli C, Stein D (eds) Brain injury and recovery: theoretical and controversial issues. Plenum, New York, pp 335–350

Prigatano GP (1989) Bring it up in milieu: toward effective traumatic brain injury rehabilitation interaction. Rehabil Psychol 34(2):135–144

Prigatano GP (1991 a) Deficits in social and vocational functioning after TBI. In: Brooks N (ed) Closed head injury: psychological, social, and family consequences, 2nd edn. Oxford University Press, New York (in press)

Prigatano GP (1991 b) Work, love, and play after brain injury: observations from the neurosciences, art and literature. Menninger Bull (in press)

Prigatano GP (1991 c) Disturbances of self-awareness of deficit after traumatic brain injury. In: Prigatano GP, Schacter DL (eds) Awareness of deficit after brain injury: clinical and theoretical issues. Oxford University Press, New York, pp 111–126

Prigatano GP, Schacter D (eds) (1991) Awareness of deficit after brain injury: theoretical and clinical implications. Oxford University Press, New York (in press)

Prigatano GP, Fordyce DJ, Zeiner HK, Roueche JR, Pepping M, Wood B (1984) Neuropsychological rehabiliation after closed head injury in young adults. J Neurol Neurosurg Psychiatry 47:505–513

Prigatano GP et al (1986) Neuropsychological rehabilitation after brain injury. The Johns Hopkins University Press, Baltimore

Prigatano GP, Klonoff PS, Bailey I (1987) Psychosocial adjustment associated with traumatic brain injury: statistics BNI neurorehabilitation must beat. BNI Q 3:10–17

Prigatano GP, Altman IM, O'Brien KO (1990) Behavioral limitations that brain injured patients tend to underestimate. Clin Neuropsychol 4:143–176

Ruff RM, Buchsbaum MS, Troster AI, Marshall LF, Lottenberg S, Somers LM, Tobias MD (1989) Computerized tomography, neuropsychology, and positron emission tomography in the evaluation of head injury. Neuropsychiatry Neuropsychol Behav Neurol 2(2):103–123

Stuss DT, Benson DF (1986) The frontal lobes. Raven, New York

Thompson IV (1984) Late outcome of very severe blunt head trauma: a 10–15 year second follow-up. J Neurol Neurosurg Psychiatry 47:260–268

Weinstein EA, Kahn RL (1955) Denial of illness. Thomas, Springfield, IL, USA

# Setting up a Neurorehabilitation Unit

*N. Brooks*

## Introduction

Within Europe and the United States many new neurorehabilitation services have been set up in recent years. Some have evolved from units dealing with other populations such as those with a spinal injury, or those with a range of disabling conditions, but whether setting up de novo, or evolving from an already existing service, a number of central issues will face those responsible for the unit (Diller 1987). These are clinical, organisational, and numerical. The clinical issues deal with the nature of the clinical population and the services delivered to it (Christensen 1987; Aronow 1987). The organisational problems concern the structure of service delivery and related matters, and the numerical issues concern the most appropriate ways to quantitate the process and effectiveness of service delivery.

## Clinical Aspects

The two central concerns here are the nature of the clinical population, and the nature of the clinicians hired to service that population (Rimel et al. 1990). Assuming that the unit is to service those with severe brain injury, this population can be divided into three according to time after injury. The first time period is that immediately after the injury, when the patient may not yet be medically stable, and may be heavily dependent upon acute medical and nursing input (Miller et al. 1990). The second stage begins when the patient is medically stable and no longer dependent upon medical and nursing support, and the third stage involves re-entry back into the community (Jacobs et al. 1990). Clearly these stages overlap, but the needs of the patient are very different in each of the three stages. At the first stage, the need is predominantly for skilled medical and nursing staff. Nevertheless, rehabilitation can begin here, even if it is only a process of assessing the patient. Conscious level, recovery in orientation, and recovery in primitive communication can all be assessed here, and so there is already a role for the classic therapists and neuropsychology. More specialist services such as teaching/education, and vocational/recreational services are not yet appropriate, but social work will certainly be appropriate for members of the patient's family.

During the next stage, the patient is medically stable, and this may be considered as the classic rehabilitation phase. Here the classic rehabilitation professionals (physiotherapy, occupational therapy, speech therapy) are centrally involved in intensive, daily, and prolonged service delivery. In addition, neuropsychologists will be involved working with cognitive, emotional, and behavioral issues, and social workers will be working with the family and may well be dealing with many issues of counselling with the patient. During this stage, active plans should be made for re-entry back to the community, even though this may not be appropriate for many weeks or months. This means that specialists involved in recreational and vocational matters should begin to be involved during this period, although their involvement will not peak until the time when discharge becomes an increasing reality (Wehman et al. 1989). Medicine may be involved on a consulting basis here, or in a leadership role. There is certainly no logical necessity why the team at this stage should be directed by a physician or surgeon, unlike the first stage where the team *must* be directed by such a person.

During the third phase, the patient is achieving re-entry back into the community. This can be run from the same unit which houses the patients at the second stage, or may be in a quite separate unit (Cope et al. 1985; Cerveli 1990). This "transitional rehabilitation" is designed to ensure that the skills developed during the first phase do not deteriorate on community re-entry, and specialists involved in recreation and vocational re-entry (particularly "job coaches") may be crucial here (Wehman et al. 1989, 1990).

While it would be a wonderful outcome if all patients returned to fully independent living, this is not a reality for many patients, and this means that there is yet a further phase of patient management (it could no longer be considered to be rehabilitation), and this is long term living. For many patients, return to independent (or any) employment is not a feasible option, and for many of these return home may be problematic. In this case there is an enormous need for focussed housing options involving sheltered or supported living. This may be for the lifetime of the patient, and can be carried out in small units where patients can have differing degrees of supervision, and have access to community and other resources to give them the most productive and dignified lifestyle possible (Dixon et al. 1988).

The exact mix of staff chosen will, of course, depend upon the severity of the patient and the stage after injury at which rehabilitation is taking place. This is discussed further in the next section.

## Organisational Aspects

The organisation aspects centre around staff; what kind of staff should be hired?; what proportions of different staff should be hired?; how should the activities of the different staff members be allocated and controlled?; how can skilled staff be found?; if skilled staff cannot be found, how may unskilled staff be trained and supported?

For the director of a new unit, these aspects may be the most crucial of the many with which he/she has to deal. A failure to find appropriately qualified and motivated staff can have a devastating effect on the quality and morale of a unit, and unit directors have to be prepared to carry out considerable staff training and support. All too often staff members of a particular profession may be available, but lack any experience of acute brain injury, and bring with them inappropriate experience which they try to generalise to head injury. When they find that this fails, they feel unhappy, and may blame themselves or the unit. The key in this situation is for the director to ensure that a coherent and "rolling" course of stall training is set up involving different facets including case presentations, formal lectures, seminars, informal case discussions, attendance at meetings/conferences, etc. Unit directors may argue that the cost of this is prohibitive, but the cost of failing to do it may be even more prohibitive in terms of increased staff turnover and reduced quality of outcomes in the patients being managed.

In many units, there are high quality clinical staff working, but not as a team. The individual clinicians each spend their own time with the injured person, and no one person has an overview of the patient's progress. In this situation, a "Case Manager" is crucial (Dixon et al. 1988; Rapp 1986; McMillan et al. 1988). Such a person has the responsibility for ensuring that individual initial evaluations of the patient are carried out, and that from these evaluations a coherent and appropriate treatment programme is set up. The Case Manager then ensures that progress is maintained during treatment, and if progress is not being maintained, it is the Case Manager's responsibility to ensure that steps are taken to remedy the situation. In many units in the United States, Case Managers are hired with no responsibilities other than case management (Henderson and Wallack 1987). In others, members of the different professions take on case management in addition to their day-to-day clinical responsibilities. In practice this can work quite well providing that any individual staff member does not have more than one or two "case management" patient, and provided also that such staff members are well supported by senior staff. In practice, this arrangement tends to break down, and every unit should consider having designated Case Managers with direct individual clinical responsibilities.

## Numerical Aspects

In setting up a unit, the first stress is always, and understandably, on getting patients in, getting treatment started, and setting up a good organisation system. It is very easy to forget that there is a professional and moral obligation to demonstrate that the treatment is or is not effective. Clinicians often feel that simply to make statements about effectiveness is enough, but it is increasingly realised in Europe and the United States, that a unit has a responsibility to set up a database or databases to demonstrate the effectiveness and cost effectiveness of service delivery (Brooks 1991). In this situation, one person should be responsible for numerical issues, and will then be faced with a number of problems including the format of the database, how extensive it is, how "user friendly" it is, and who has access to it, how, and for what purpose.

A range of different options appear in clinical service, with some units setting up central databases that are controlled and managed by a data manager, and with others having databases that while controlled centrally are accessible (often in part rather than in total) by any of the individual clinicians working in the unit. The second option is much more difficult to set up in terms of computing and software requirements, but is infinitely more rewarding to individual staff members, and is greatly to be recommended if at all possible. The problem with a central database is that individual staff feel distant from it, and have no commitment in maintaining quality or accuracy of data.

The unit manager will find that setting up a database raises its own kind of problems. Individual clinicians will often have little idea about translating their clinical observations into quantitative information, or may propose quantification schemes that are grandiose, inappropriate, and inaccurate. This is an issue that needs very sensitive handling, as failure to involve individual clinicians can have a very serious negative effect on the quality of information in a database.

## Conclusions

Setting up a new unit is a daunting task. The range of issues facing the director are large, and decisions made early in the life of a unit can have repercussions for many years to come. While some decisions are easily changed (numbers and distribution of different kinds of staff), others are not (architectural structure of the unit, design of a database). Appropriate decisions taken early on can ensure that services delivered to an appropriate population with high quality, and the ability to demonstrate numerically the quality of outcome. Failure to make these decisions, or making inappropriate decisions early on can lead to poor quality clinical input, and a complete inability to demonstrate the effectiveness of clinical process or outcome.

## References

Aronow HV (1987) Rehabilitation effectiveness with severe brain injury: translating research into policy. J Head Trauma Rehabil 2(3):24–36

Brooks DN (1991) The effectiveness of post acute rehabilitation. Brain Injury 5(2):103–109

Cervelli L (1990) Re-entry into the community and systems of posthospital care. In: Rosenthal M, Griffiths ER, Bond MR, Miller TD (eds) Rehabilitation of the adult and child with traumatic brain injury. Davis, Philadelphia, pp 463–475

Christensen A-L (1987) Program for rehabilitation of brain damage in Copenhagen. In: Christensen A-L, Uzzell B (eds) Neuropsychological rehabilitation. Kluwer, London, pp 115–124

Cope JE, Cope DN, Cervelli L (1987) Rehabilitation of the severely brain-injured patient: a community-based, low-cost model program. Arch Phys Med Rehabil 66:38–40

Diller L (1985) Rehabilitation in traumatic brain injury – observations on the current U.S. scene. In: Christensen A-L, Uzzell B (eds) Neuropsychological rehabilitation. Kluwer, London, pp 53–68

Dixon TP, Goll S, Stanton KM (1988) Case management issues and practices in head injury rehabilitation. Rehabil Counsel Bull 31:325–343

Henderson M, Wallack SS (1987) Evaluating case management for catastrophic illness. Business Health 7–11

Jacobs HE, Blatnick M, Sandhurst JV (1990) What is lifelong living, and how does it relate to quality of life? J Head Trauma Rehabil 5(1):1–8

McMillan TM, Greenwood RD, Brooks DN et al (1988) An introduction to the concept of head injury case management with respect to the need for service provision. Clin Rehabil 2:319–322

Miller JD, Pentland B, Berrol S (1990) Early evaluation and management. In: Rosenthal M, Griffith ER, Bond MR, Miller TD (eds) Rehabilitation of the adult and child with traumatic brain injury. Davis, Philadelphia, pp 21–51

Rapp D (1986) Brain injury casebook. Thomas, Springfield, IL, USA

Rimel RW, Jane JJ, Bond MR (1990) Characteristics of the head-injured patient. In: Rosenthal M, Griffith ER, Bond MR, Miller TD (eds) Rehabilitation of the adult and child with traumatic brain injury. Davis, Philadelphia, pp 8–16

Wehman PH, Kreutzer JS, West MD et al (1989) Employment outcomes of persons following traumatic brain injury: preinjury, postinjury, and supported employment. Brain Injury 3:307–412

Wehman PH, Kreutzer JS, West MD et al (1990) Return to work for persons with traumatic brain injury: a supported employment approach. Arch Phys Med Rehabil 71:1047–1052

# Discussion: Controversial Concepts of Rehabilitation

*A.-L. Christensen*

The first presentations this morning of the basic hypotheses clearly gave evidence of a vast amount of new information that needs to be incorporated in the actual rehabilitative work. How far away is the practical application from the basic knowledge of the plasticity of the brain and how do the possibilities of strengthening the recovery versus avoiding maladaptive development influence the rehabilitative work? In which way can concepts like the contextual approach suggested by Donald Stein influence the concepts behind the planning of rehabilitation programs?

How does the shift in the cerebral circuitry that can be claimed to arise due to the function of environmental, hormonal and other organismic events influence the therapy or treatment given?

Again with reference to Donald Stein, it seems to me that the most important new knowledge is that factors that are a consequence of an injury to the CNS are seen as a dynamic series of events in which many different variables play a role in determining the outcome. The complexity of this notion can be seen from a table, that is shown in Donald Stein's Heinz Werner Lecture series: *Development and Plasticity in the CNS: Organismic and Environmental Influences* (1988) (see Table 1). The table is from a paper by Norman Geschwind (1985).

It is not an easy task to incorporate these factors in the planning of the content of a rehabilitation program. It also seems to call for a new approach in research within the area.

What is the present state of the art? The concepts that have been presented to us by the three speakers in this part of the program each dealt with a proposal for a rehabilitation set-up. The factors stressed were different, however. In Dr. Wood's and Dr. Prigatano's approaches, theoretical concepts were presented together with suggestions concerning the application of the ideas. The two approaches had distinct theoretical backgrounds, the first in learning theory and the second in personality and psychoanalytic theory. Dr. Brooks' presentation had a practical character where the daily life disturbances and their remediation were discussed. The initial statement in his paper stressed the demand both for a theoretical debate about the nature and administration of neuropsychological rehabilitation and clarification of the vast area of practical problems within the field.

The rehabilitative approaches presented were different and it is my impression that at the present stage of our knowledge more presentations would have

**Table 1.** Change after lesions of the nervous system

I. Mechanisms (listings are not necessarily exclusive)

*A. Biochemical*
- Nonspecific
  - Edema and disappearance of edema
  - Ischemia without destruction
  - Immune responses
  - Scarring
  - Pressure effects
- Specific
  - Increase or decrease in numbers of receptors
  - Induction or inactivation of enzymes
  - Viral alterations of specific cell function
  - Immune responses to specific neural components
  - Alterations in transmitter release
  - Transmitter reuptake by inactive neurons (Zigmond effect)
  - Alterations in membrane properties

*B. Structural*
- Disrupted organization
- Sprouting – collateral and terminal
- Anomalous connections
- Demyelination
- Transsynaptic and transneuronal degeneration
- Diminished cell death in other areas (in fetal and possibly early postnatal life)

*C. Physiological*
- Changes in facilitation, inhibition, and occlusion
- Loss of feedback effects
- Pacemaker shifts
- Slowed conduction
- Changes of synchrony
- Opening of ineffective synapses
- Changes of spatial or temporal summation
- Kindling and epilepsy

*D. "Psychological"*
- Perception of change by intact regions
- Alternate strategies

II. Factors influencing late change
- Age
- Species
- Previous learning
- Individual differences (type and size of structures, connection, biochemistry, individual talents, handedness)
- Previous exposure to drugs, hormones, and so forth (pre- and postnatal)
- Serial lesions
- Epilepsy
- Stimulation (such as skin lesions or deliberate stimulation)
- Emotional effects – motivation, hormones, circulating transmitters, and so forth
- Susceptibility to immune attack of areas formed abnormally in prenatal life

given an equal number of approaches, maybe alike in some respects but differing in emphasis. Neil Brooks' statement certainly is to the point.

Roger Wood differentiated between early stages of recovery after brain injury and the more long-lasting sequelae; an important point for discussion. Principles of learning were considered to be the main treatment method administered during the whole course of rehabilitation. Wood claimed that the "neuro part" of the neuro behavioral approach aimed at stabilizing behavior and diminishing emotional as well as cognitive "organic" disturbances following injury. The learning model was described as including the reduction of complex tasks to a sequence of discrete units of activity, where the patient has to rehearse sequentially with the aid of verbal mediation to regulate performance.

Furthermore, each stage of learning had to be consolidated before additional stages were added, allowing the patient to combine a number of discrete units of behavior of activity into a complex action sequence that fulfilled the purpose of functional requirements.

In addition the neurobehavioral approach was claimed to serve the purpose of control of behavior; threatening behavior which was learned or employed purposefully for vicarious reward and which intimidates staff can be eliminated by the techniques of behavior management or the methods of reinforcement of socially adaptive behavior. The strong effect inherent in the learning principles is the core of this method; however, the old battle from general psychology between learning theoreticians comes to mind: learning by insight or learning by conditioning.

In his autobiography *In Search of Mind*, Bruner (1983) describes the battle at Duke in the 1930s between Thorndike and Adams. Thorndike interpreted his cats' behavior in puzzle boxes as blind trial and error shaped by rewards and punishment from outside, whereas Adams proposed that adaptive behavior in puzzle boxes grew out of the hypotheses generated by the organism in response to the available cues in the environment. If the environment, according to Adams, contained relevant and combinable cues, animals would respond with insightful hypotheses. However, it would also be possible to design blind environments that would make their inhabitants look stupid.

What is the world of the brain-damaged person, how does he/she experience his or her surroundings, how do we reach him/her, by which cues, but most important how do we make him/her not look stupid, and how do we in Dr. Prigatano's words "reestablish purpose and meaning in life in the face of brain damage and the sorrow it wakes"?

As early as in the 1920s, Kurt Goldstein provided valuable insight into this understanding and today it is a rather well accepted notion, stressed especially by the work of Dr. Prigatano, that psychotherapy, both individual and group, is a most important part of rehabilitation.

A main purpose of therapeutic intervention is to help the patient in his/her basic need to make sense of the world. The therapist must understand the analogies which the patient will often use to express this need and he must understand that the patient's thinking does not lack sense. His/her experiences are not flat or dull, but they deeply evidence the fear and the loss. The brain is hurt, but the profile of abilities as measured by neuropsychological tests is typically a zig-zag curve. Some functions are nearly always preserved and it is the therapist's task to plan the rehabilitation in accordance with the resources. The method that according to my experience best helps to fulfill this need and provides a possibility for an analysis of the psychological functioning is Luria's Neuropsychological Investigation (Christensen 1974).

Luria's ideas about looking at intellectual processes in terms of functional systems instead of discrete abilities provide us with a possibility to analyse the component parts of a function. In *The Making of Mind* (1979) Luria writes that functional systems are considered a working constellation of activities with a corresponding working constellation of zones of the brain that support the activities developed and changed over time. An excellent example of such an activity is writing, which clearly could not have been coded in the human brain in a purely organic fashion because it involves the use of man made tools. Many different regions of the brain are involved in the complex functional system that underlies writing and each area is responsible for a particular part of the process under normal conditions. Disturbance in any one area will have distinctive effects on the subsequent performance.

In making a diagnosis we ask which link, or links, in the normal system of the working constellation of brain zones is disturbed. Once our analysis has integrated the dysfunction with an area lesion we can undertake treatment. Treatment and diagnosis are not as separated as they seem. In the course of trying to treat particular disturbances we often have to modify our diagnosis. In treating the disturbances we try to make use of the remaining links which we supplement with external aids to reconstruct the activity on the basis of a new functional system which may require a considerable period of retraining. But at the end of the period the aim is that it should be possible for the patient to engage in the activity without external assistance. During the process it is important to find a way to give the patient as much feedback as possible concerning both the defect and its effect on the patient's actions. The purpose of the feedback is to give the patient the information that is crucial to the reorganisation of the required functional system.

The introduction of an investigation method that can provide qualitative information regarding the effect on function caused by different lesions is meant to serve the purpose of individualizing treatment. If we want to pay attention to the contextual approach we must possess knowledge not only about the methods for rehabilitation, the right time for what kind of intervention, pharmacological or psychological, but we must also incorporate as many characteristics as can be identified about the person who is in need of treatment. The process needs to be dynamic.

Awareness of early intervention is very important. Pharmacological treatment needs to be planned in accordance with the notions of dynamic changes. Also stages in the rehabilitation procedure are recommendable. In the first stage it is important to give the most effective neurosurgical and medical treatment, but also to be aware of the acute needs of the patients and the families.

Secondly, psychological needs must be met. Once discharged from hospital possibilities for continuous development of the patient are asked for. This can be done within a work environment or it can be done in education. It can also be done by way of promoting social interaction and the leisure activities that the patient had before the trauma.

At the Center for Rehabilitation of Brain Damage at the University of Copenhagen we have implemented an approach whereby we have combined cognitive and learning theory training and a more psychosocially directed therapy. The application of these methods and follow-up outcomes has been described in detail elsewhere (Christensen et al. 1991). We find that the pattern of family life becomes normalized. The patients come to live independently of the care of others, and reliance on treatment and support from health service providers is markedly reduced. There is also a high incidence of patients returning to a working environment. The most interesting finding is the continuing general improvement manifested in three-year follow-up examinations.

The presentations under the heading of controversial concepts of rehabilitation evidenced strong and innovative efforts of rehabilitation specialists. The combination of the best parts from each or the cumulative experiences and insight make it realistic to expect progress in bettering the lives of the survivors of brain injury. As a closing remark, however, I want to add that the treatment must be provided by therapists not by family members, who need to stay what they are, spouses or children, mothers and fathers.

## References

Bruner J (1983) In search of mind. Harper and Row, New York

Christensen A-L (1974) Luria's neuropsychological investigation. Munksgaard, Copenhagen

Christensen A-L et al (1992) Psycho-social outcome following individualized neuropsychological rehabilitation of brain damage. Acta Neurol Scand (in press)

Geschwind N (1985) Mechanisms of change after brain lesions. Ann NY Acad Sci 457:1–11

Luria AR (1979) The making of mind. Harvard University Press, Cambridge

Stein DG (1988) Development and plasticity in the CNS: organismic and environmental influences. Clark University Press, Worcester

# Methodology

# Research Design in Neuropsychological Rehabilitation

*L.E. Trexler and J.D. Thomas*

## Introduction

Measuring the change attributable to a rehabilitative intervention is a complex enterprise from a number of independent but related perspectives. In order to review the complexity of this subject, we will present a number of key topics that must be considered in the design of rehabilitation research. A basic premise in our discussion is that empirical research is necessary but is reductionistic in nature and must be so. It must parse the world of observables and constructs so as to allow for the isolation of experimental manipulations and repeatable measurement. Rehabilitative intervention, by its nature, is holistic and does not respond kindly to reductionism. From this springs a tension that is difficult to resolve; however, it is also the case that the two may demonstrate a synergy so that the results of either endeavor may guide and positively affect the other (Oscar-Berman 1989; Wilson 1987). Moreover, scientifically sound data collection methods can be used in both clinical practice and research. We will present three key issues that exert a significant though typically hidden influence on research design in neuropsychological rehabilitation. Initially, we will consider a typology of neuropsychological interventions. This will be followed by a brief discussion of design and analysis issues and a suggestion for programmatic research.

## A Typology for Neuropsychological Interventions

Neuropsychological rehabilitation is a recent development and, as such, the issues of definition, philosophy, level of analysis, and techniques of intervention have not been resolved. The fundamental commonalities in neuropsychological rehabilitation involve the accepted use of cognitive tests for the measurement of cerebral impairment and the proposal that this knowledge (combined with models of information processing in uninjured individuals) can suggest treatment strategies. In spite of this foundation, differences in paradigms and philosophies can limit comparisons between seemingly similar research.

One possible correction for this is to make explicit the assumptions that underlie the measurement-intervention model. For example, Trexler (1987) and

Trexler and Zappala (1985) proposed an "onion" model where successive layers of the model represent successive levels of analysis. The innermost layers described intra-individual interventions, and the outermost represented those directed at the community. Another kind of example can be found in the work of Diller and Gordon (1981) where they differentiated remediation from rehabilitation. The term remediation described the restoration of impaired cognitive abilities and skills. Conversely, rehabilitation was defined as the approach of a multi-disciplinary team where a broad range of deficits and issues related to disability are addressed. Obviously, these levels of intervention are not orthogonal. This model was intended to support the view that cognitive deficits should be the focus of intervention. We believe that similar constructs can be incorporated into an alternative model that reflects the knowledge that has accumulated in the last 10 years.

## The Hierarchical-Factor Model of Intervention

The model we would propose is shown in Figure 1. Its form is taken from the model of intelligence proposed by Burt (in Vernon 1961) and the method of factorial construct validation described by Royce (1963).

At the highest and most abstract level of the model is the construct of *Multi-modal Rehabilitation.* Rehabilitation in this sense is a function of no particular professional orientation; however, it is neuropsychologically based in that it offers behavioral measurement via performance tests and a large knowledge-base of the effects of cerebral lesions. At this level, the model makes no assumptions about time since onset or etiology. Its general aim is the improvement in adaptation following injury. Research directed to this level of analysis would seek to answer the question of the efficacy of treatment generally (i.e., Do patients that received treatment have a better chance of working?, a better quality of life?, etc.). Investigations by Prigitano (1986), Ben-Yishay et al. (1987),

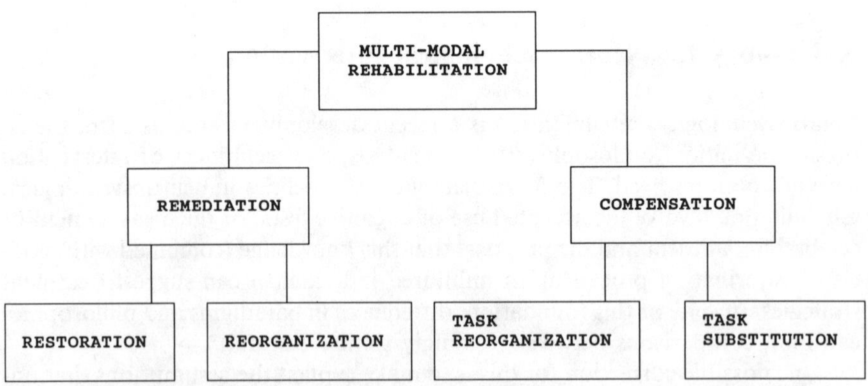


**Fig. 1.** The hierarchical-factor model of intervention

and Fryer and Haffey (1987) exemplify neuropsychological rehabilitation program research where interventions consisted of a variety of remediation, psycho-social, and functional components.

At the next lower level in the model we have identified the constructs of *remediation* and *compensation*. We view these as essentially orthogonal. Both refer to the reinstitution or return of a lost function; however, the former involves components of human abilities, and the latter involves complex skilled performances (e. g., Fleishman 1972). Both of these may be broadly defined as functions, but we would argue for the need for a formal distinction, as the convenience of the word "function" obscures the level of analysis issue. For example, different treatments could be designed to "fix" both the arithmetic operation of subtraction and the balancing of a checkbook ledger. They would have different methods and different end goals and yet they could both be said to be treatments for impaired functions. It is likely that in clinical practice, research will be aimed at a finer analysis for the validation of more specific intervention. The longer term purpose of this level of the hierarchy is to provide a method of characterizing these more specific methods of treatment.

At the lowest level of our model are four intervention types. They are all based on the premise that repetition or practice can improve task performance and that there is some level of generalizability between training tasks and "real-world" performances at all levels of complexity. The two factors subsumed under remediation differ in terms of the degree to which they attempt to reinstitute an existing relationship between structure and function. *Restoration* refers to the possibility that a particular function may be performed with the same elements following damage and subsequent intervention. The mechanisms responsible for this are as yet uncertain; however, disinhibition, strengthening "weak synapses", and nerve cell growth have been proposed (e. g., Laurence and Stein 1978). *Reorganization* refers to the possibility that undamaged cerebral structures may come to subserve impaired cognitive abilities much in the way that an animal with a surgically removed limb may learn to ambulate (e. g., Luria 1963). Thus impaired cognitive functions might be performed in a new way that reflects a reorganized neural apparatus.

The two factors subsumed under compensation both refer to the possibility that the learning of strategies may improve the performance of skilled tasks. They differ in terms of the degree to which existing skills are retained in the retrained behavior. The construct of *task reorganization* refers to the possibility that existing tasks may be modified with a minimum of changes to inputs, stages, and outputs. An example of this kind of intervention can be seen in our own clinical practice where an impulsive stroke patient was taught to use a second-check strategy with a calculator that gave a printed paper-tape output when balancing the checkbook ledger. The basic task was performed in the same way; however, there was a modification of the pre-existing self-checking strategy that reduced the frequency of errors. The final intervention type, *task substitution*, involves the institution of new strategies or skills that allow successful performance. With both of these, no claim is made regarding the underlying neural systems that mediate behavioral change. An example of this intervention type can be found in the work of Sohlberg and Mateer (1989) where memory impaired patients were trained to use a personal journal to improve their recall of daily events.

## Strategies of Design and Analysis

Before discussing the issues of design and analysis, it is necessary to consider potential sources of error that can obscure conclusions. These involve subject and task variables. As noted by Hiscock and MacKay (1985) neuropsychological research has many similarities to research in the area of individual differences. Thus to the typically confounded subject variables of gender, age, and education may be added the factors of lateral dominance, possible abnormalities of the aging process, and intra-individual differences in cerebral functional localization. To these factors can be added the complexities related to the neuropathology such as etiology, time since onset, relative focalness or diffuseness of lesion, size of lesion, completeness of lesion, etc. (Brooks et al. 1984; Smith 1981). From our own clinical practice in rehabilitation we would include the issues of premorbid psychopathology, awareness of injury, and adjustment to change in life circumstance. Regardless of the design one wishes to apply in the testing of an intervention, these factors may serve to limit the generalizability of findings.

A second problematic source of error involves task variables. By this we refer to outcome measures. These are typically scores derived from neuropsychological tests that have generally been developed in order to discriminate injured from uninjured individuals and localize sites of cerebral damage. Consequently, their ability to qualify deficits and describe the improvement that might follow an intervention is questionable. These variables are usually factorially complex and in all likelihood possess measurement error at high enough levels to severely reduce the power of statistical tests. This same charge may be leveled at "soft data" where subjective observations or ratings of behavior inflate within-group variance and thus reduce effect size (Kraemer and Thiemann 1989).

The solutions for these problems cannot be found in a broad, all encompassing injunction. It would seem obvious that there is a need for the accumulation of knowledge in the area of subject variables so that valid generalizations may be drawn regarding their effects. As will be suggested below, the ability to form homogenous groups in terms of some selected set of attributes is a requirement of group differences research. The issues related to task variables fall largely in the area of construct validation. As with psychology generally, progress in neuropsychology is dependent upon the ability to relate tests and test scores to specific abilities at various levels of abstraction and factorial purity. Confirmatory factor analysis offers a methodology in this area (Hunter 1977). Accordingly, we need to know more about these psychometric issues. Additionally, because statistical tests make assumptions about the underlying distributional properties of dependent variables, it is critical that these be explored in greater depth. To date, in intervention outcome research, it is common for outcome variables to be chosen on the basis of face validity or availability.

## The Application of Specific Experimental Designs

Research in neuropsychological rehabilitation will always be quasi-experimental, as damage to the brain in humans follows from "accidents of nature" and are not experimentally controlled. Therefore, true random selection of subjects to experimental groups remains a difficulty.

### Single Case Experimental Designs

Zurif et al. (1989) have commented on the recent resurgence of the single case methodology in neuropsychological research. Shallice (1979) has pointed out that recent popularity of the single case design may be attributable to increase recognition of some of the limitations of group design. Specifically, these limitations include (a) an inability to account for sample heterogeneity, in terms of "range of ages, premorbid intellectual skills and lesion sizes in patients forming a group and the interaction between etiology and lesion site" (p. 184) and (b) the inability to draw meaningful inferences about the nature of normal functional architecture from group designs. Wilson (1987) suggested that single case experimental techniques should, however, be differentiated from anecdotal and descriptive case reports, where the former allow for the systematic and rigorous study of the effects of intervention and control for spontaneous recovery.

While single case designs have traditionally been used to examine unique neuropsychological syndromes or investigate structure or functional architecture of normal human cognition, other studies in neuropsychological rehabilitation have demonstrated the utility of such designs (e.g., Gianutsos and Gianutsos 1979; Sohlberg and Mateer 1987). Advantages of the single case design include: (a) control of subject group heterogeneity, (b) experimental methodology more closely parallels clinical intervention, and (c) description of the trajectory of recovery. The main limitations, however, of single case designs are that (a) generalization across subjects is limited, (b) the nature of the recovery may not fall within the measurement period (late effects), and (c) the question of the statistical significance of any demonstrated improvement is difficult to determine.

### Group Experimental Designs

Adequate research in neuropsychological rehabilitation utilizing group designs is complicated by the requirements and assumptions of various statistical procedures. Subject-to-variable ratio requirements mandate very large sample sizes if many dependent variables are to be studied, particularly if several domains of inquiry are included for analysis. Further, large sample sizes are needed for adequate experimental power and to address measurement error. Further, ANOVA and MANOVA assume subject homogeneity, but as homogeneity increases, ability to generalize decreases.

Group designs do offer some distinct advantages, however. These designs permit assessment of the measurement error associated with the dependent variables. Further, more definite conclusions can be reached regarding the generalizability of findings from one subject to another. Finally, group designs permit direct analysis of the statistical significance of any change in neuropsychological or behavioral functioning.

The disadvantages of group methodologies in neuropsychological rehabilitation are the inverse of the advantages. Subject heterogeneity and between subject variance can minimize the significance of a treatment effect. Further, one cannot assume that statistical significance and clinical significance are comparable (Wilson 1987). Specific interventions may be of some benefit to certain patients and not to others. Group analysis, however, combines the data through either the derivation of means or through computation of variance, and the potential gain of a subset of the experimental group is lost. Further, some gains may be of considerable clinical significance in terms of the patient's functional adaptation, but because of subject and measurement error, not reach statistical significance.

A technical difficulty in the statistical determination of group differences involves the use of repeated measures. Whenever more than one assessment is made of a subject group, the experimentwise error rate increases. Additionally, the issue of correlated error variances limits the applicability of univariate repeated measures ANOVA designs (Shaffer 1979).

### Meta-Analysis

Effectiveness of neuropsychological rehabilitation cannot, of course, be answered in a single study. Differences in subject variables, differences in measurement, and differences in treatment methodology necessitate that multiple studies be performed through organized multi-center and multi-group programs of research. Meta-analysis (Hunter et al. 1982) provides for direct examination of effect size through analysis of error variance in relation to the significance of the results in many studies. These types of studies in neuropsychological rehabilitation are at the moment quite far away pending compilation of adequate group studies.

## Suggestions for Programmatic Research

Single case and group methodologies both offer advantages and disadvantages. The central issue, however, concerns selecting the right methodology for the right question. Even more important is the question of deriving theoretical formulations from which experimental design can be derived. The selection of the right subject and task variables, however, in context of the operating theoretical formulation, determines the scientific adequacy of any research. Subject and task variables are driven by the domain of inquiry in neuropsychological rehabilitation and level of analysis.

It is recommended that programs of research in neuropsychological rehabilitation evolve through a three stage process, initially focusing on single case or small-n designs, proceeding to group designs, and ultimately to meta-analysis of multiple group studies.

Single case and small-n studies are needed to derive the common constituent elements which comprise various neuropsychological syndromes as well as to determine what important sources of individual variability determine recovery and response to rehabilitation. It fact, at this stage of research, careful experimental analysis of atypical cases or "outliers" is crucial to discover subject or task variables which later can be experimentally studied in subsequent group designs. Further, case studies are needed to initially determine benefit from rehabilitation intervention and to differentiate spontaneous recovery from treatment effect. Lastly, case studies are important because they require that we clinically proceed with treating our patients based upon theoretical formulations and a methodology to determine if our interventions have clinically benefited the patient in a manner which was consistent with the original intent and theoretical formulation. These practices make for good science and good clinical intervention and promote a beneficial synergy between the two.

Group studies offer the possibility of examining the psychometric validity of the dependent measures, which cannot be performed in single case or small-n studies. Group studies can be constructed methodologically to study the impact of sample heterogeneity on size of treatment effect, once small-n and single case studies have determined the variables which significantly contribute to subject and task heterogeneity. This approach then permits an analysis of experimental power and error variance, thereby increasing the reliability and validity of diagnostic and rehabilitation efforts.

Following completion of well-designed group studies, meta-analysis of these studies will be able to assess the effect size attributable to natural recovery and rehabilitation. However, this stage of analysis will only be possible if organized programs of research are developed and implemented, sequentially rarifying hypotheses and subject and task sources of variability.

Neuropsychological rehabilitation from a clinical perspective is a relatively new endeavor. The research literature has grown exponentially in the last few years, but organized programs of research are still developing. It might be suggested that the process of scientific inquiry in neuropsychological rehabilitation will parallel the history of psychotherapy research. While clinical service delivery in psychotherapy has existed for over one hundred years, only recently have meta-analysis studies provided some reasonable statistical proof of the effectiveness of psychotherapy. Hopefully, we can learn from our history in the evolution of science and apply some of the successful strategies to the scientific study of the effectiveness of neuropsychological rehabilitation.

## References


Ben-Yishay Y, Silver SM, Piatesky E, Rattok J (1987) Relationship between employability and vocational outcome after intensive holistic cognitive rehabilitation. J Head Trauma Rehabil 2:35–48

Brooks DN, Deelman BG, van Zomeren AH, van Dongen H, van Harskamp F, Aughton ME (1984) Problems in measuring recovery after acute brain injury. J Clin Neuropsychol 6:71–85

Diller L, Gordon WA (1981) Interventions for cognitive deficits in brain injured adults. J Consult Clin Psychol 49:822–834

Fleishman EA (1972) On the relation between abilities, learning, and human performance. Am Psychol 27:1017–1032

Fryer LJ, Haffey WJ (1987) Cognitive rehabilitation and community readaptation: outcomes from two program models. J Head Trauma Rehabil 2:51–63

Gianutsos R, Gianutsos J (1979) Rehabilitating the verbal recall of brain injured persons by mnemonic training: an experimental demonstration using single-case methodology. J Clin Neuropsychol 1:117–135

Hiscock M, MacKay M (1985) Neuropsychological approaches to the study of individual differences. In: Reynolds CR, Willson VL (eds) Methodological and statistical advances in the study of individual differences. Plenum, New York, pp 117–176

Hunter JE (1977) Cluster analysis: reliability, construct validity, and the multiple indicators approach to measurement. Available from the Department of Psychology, Michigan State University, East Lansing, MI 48824, USA

Hunter JE, Schmidt FL, Jackson GB (1982) Meta-analysis: cumulating research findings across studies. Sage, Beverly Hills

Kraemer HC, Thiemann S (1989) A strategy to use soft data effectively in randomized controlled clinical trials. J Consult Clin Psychol 57:148–154

Laurence SL, Stein DG (1978) Recovery after brain damage and the concept of localization of function. In: Finger S (ed) Recovery from brain damage: research and theory. Plenum, New York, pp 369–407

Luria AR (1963) Restoration of function after brain injury. Pergamon, New York

Oscar-Berman M (1989) Links between clinical and experimental neuropsychology. J Clin Exp Neuropsychol 11:571–588

Prigitano GP (1986) Neuropsychological rehabilitation after brain injury. Johns Hopkins University Press, Baltimore

Royce JR (1963) Factors as theoretical constructs. Am Psychol 18:522–528

Shaffer JW (1979) On the analysis of repeated measures over time in medical, pharmacological, and behavioral research. J Behav Med 2:221–238

Shallice T (1979) Case study approach in neuropsychological research. J Clin Neuropsychol 3:183–211

Smith A (1981) Principles underlying human brain functions in neuropsychological sequelae of different neuropathological processes. In: Filskov SB, Boll TJ (eds) Handbook of clinical neuropsychology, vol 1. Wiley, New York, pp 175–236

Sohlberg MM, Mateer CA (1987) Effectiveness of an attention training program. J Clin Exp Neuropsychol 9:117–130

Sohlberg MM, Mateer CA (1989) Training use of compensatory memory books: a three stage behavioral approach. J Clin Exp Neuropsychol 11:871–891

Trexler LE (1987) Neuropsychological rehabilitation in the United States. In: Meier MJ, Benton AL, Diller L (eds) Neuropsychological rehabilitation. Livingstone, London

Trexler LE, Zappala G (1985) Emerging trends in neuropsychological rehabilitation. In: Formica MM (ed) Tratto di neurologia riabilitative. Marrapese, Rome

Vernon PE (1961) The structure of human abilities. Wiley, New York

Wilson B (1987) Single-case designs in neuropsychological rehabilitation. J Clin Exp Neuropsychol 9:527–544

Zurif EB, Gardner H, Brownell HH (1989) The case against the case against group studies. Brain Cogn 10:237–255

# Evaluation of Neuropsychological Therapies: The Importance of Measurement

*D. T. Wade*

## Introduction

Rehabilitation is a problem solving process focusing on disability, with four specific components: assessment of the problem(s); formulation and planning of a course of management; intervention which may be simple observation, active treatment or supportive care; and reassessment and evaluation of the effects of the intervention. This chapter concentrates upon evaluation. It introduces briefly a model of rehabilitation, and discusses evaluation, study designs, and principles and practice of measurement. Its main message is that investigators should spend more effort on choosing appropriate measures, particularly measures that demonstrate the clinical utility of the intervention being studied.

## Rehabilitation and the WHO Model

Evaluation of rehabilitative strategies is most easily understood in the context of the World Health Organisation (WHO) model of the consequences of disease (WHO 1980). This recommends that any illness should be considered at four levels which, although not easily distinguished in practice, are conceptually quite distinct.

Any illness stars with *pathology,* a malfunction or structural abnormality within an organ or organ system. Pathology is more or less equivalent to 'disease' or medical diagnosis, and is the major focus of medical attention and the hospital system.

Significant pathology will usually manifest itself eventually at the level of the whole body as a series of symptoms and/or signs. These disruptions of the physiology of the body are termed *impairments.*

The third level is that of *disability,* the loss or reduction of ability ot undertake normal functions. Disability is manifest at the level of the person within his or her own physical environment. It is (or should be) the focus of rehabilitative effort.

Finally there is *handicap,* the most difficult concept to define and measure. Handicap refers to the reduction in freedom experienced in a person's ability to undertake social functions and roles expected of them. It is the social and society consequences of disease. The most important features of handicap are that 'normality' is judged entirely with reference to the individual and that handicap in this context refers to the change experienced as a consequence of the disease. For example loss of a finger would not inconvenience many people, but would devastate a pianist.

Within this model it is worth stressing that as one moves from pathology to handicap environmental factors become increasingly important. Rehabilitation consists of acting on pathology, impairment or disability in order to reduce handicap. Rehabilitation not only refers to doing something with the patient, but also attempting to alter their environment. The 'environment' refers not only to physical factors but also political, administrative, legal and financial factors and consequently those involved in rehabilitation are inevitably involved in matters outside strictly medical boundaries.

## Evaluation and Study Design

### General Considerations

When evaluating any intervention, a clinician or investigator will be asking a series of questions:

- Was there any change in the patient's state after interventions?
- Was the change seen simply part of natural variability?
- Was the change seen simply the natural history of the condition?
- Was the change seen specific to the particular intervention?

In order to answer these questions it is necessary to control for spontaneous recovery and for a placebo response. There are two further complicating factors: the natural variability in a patient's state, and the unpredictable extent and rate of change in any individual patient.

Various study designs have been developed to overcome these problems. The most scientifically pure is the randomised, double-blind placebo controlled study, but this requires large numbers of patients and is thereby excluded for most neuro-psychological interventions because it is difficult to recruit and treat sufficient patients to gain an answer. Therefore less demanding designs are usually used.

The simplest design, the basis of most "clinical experience" is the A–B single case study design, but this fails to control for most factors. Various improvements upon this simple design have been devised, using single cases or small groups (see Barlow and Hersen 1984). Other designs used include various types of small group studies with cross-over between treatments, and designs which utilise complex statistical analysis.

## Types of Study

Studies can be used to answer two completely different questions which are often confused. Firstly, does the intervention have some effect on a physiological or psychological process. In medical practice, a good example is evaluation of anti-hypertensive treatment where the aim is to establish that the drug lowers blood pressure.

The second and much more important question is whether the treatment actually benefits the patient as expected. In the example given above it is assumed from previous research that lowering blood pressure by any means is beneficial and so most studies do not investigate whether the new drug actually reduces the risk of stroke.

However in most instances it is not necessarily the case that changing some physiological measure will lead to the expected benefit. For example, reducing blood viscosity and coagulability should prevent progression of stroke, but there is strong evidence that treatment which undoubtedly has the required haematological effects does not in fact prevent progression. Therefore it is always vital to prove that the patient benefits clinically; disability should be reduced.

A third question, often overlooked once the effectiveness of intervention has been established in individual patients, is whether the *policy* of treatment by a specific means is beneficial. It is often possible that more patients will be harmed than benefitted, or that the resources could be more effectively used in other ways. It should not be assumed that neuropsychological treatments cannot cause harm: patients may become dependent on the intervention; it might hinder other treatments; failure might lead to severe depression; other staff might stop helping the patient; the patient might not adjust satisfactorily to their predicament etc.

## Specific Considerations

When evaluating a particular intervention, the investigator needs to go through the following processes. First, most important and often underrated, he/she must define the question as accurately as possible. Not "Does this help my patient?" but "Do three half hour sessions of a (specified) training lead to an improvement in walking speed?" Most research questions are too general, and time spent in simplifying the research question is always well-spent.

Second, which design is most appropriate for this study? Many investigators spend much time trying to devise new or improved designs. This is rarely necessary or profitable – innumerable manhours have been spent on design already, and it is best to rely on the work of other experts wherever possible.

Last, what is the least data needed and which measures will obtain that data? Unfortunately less effort is spent considering this question, and so many studies are weaker than they should be. Some investigators devise new measures of unproven reliability and validity when suitable measures already exist.

Others concentrate upon measuring impairment, ignoring disability (or handicap). Many use unreliable measures. The remainder of this chapter concentrates upon choosing measures.

## Identify Necessary Information and Data

The first most important step when choosing any measure is to decide precisely what information you wish to obtain and why. In general measures will be needed for three reasons. Firstly to define the type of patient entered into the study, particularly with regard to *prognosis*. The prognosis will certainly relate to the natural (untreated) outcome and it may include features which identify patients likely to respond to the treatment. Next one may wish to measure various parts of the *process* of treatment, such as the amount and timing of treatment given and effects on presumed intervening variables (usually impairments). Lastly one must measure the *outcome*, and this outcome should be at the level of disability or handicap if at all possible. Some studies only measure process and forget that process is separate from outcome.

Next, it is necessary to determine the specific data appropriate to your needs. This requires reasonable background knowledge of the illness being studied. For example, if it is necessary to establish that a patient's prognosis was good or bad, then one must choose the measure known to establish the best prognostic information, not a second-best measure. This often requires considerable research, especially if the topic is outside the investigator's own field of expertise. As an example, many investigators studying patients with stroke often seem to have little knowledge about stroke and its natural history and therefore choose inappropriate measures.

Therefore, before even considering specific measures, it is necessary to determine the *minimum* information needed on *prognosis, process,* and *outcome.* Then it is necessary to start identifying the data which are *relevant*, and it important to resist the temptation to collect other irrelevant data. Next the actual measures can be chosen.

## Choosing Measures – Specific Advice

The first step is to discover what measures already exist. It is much better to use an existing measure if at all possible, provided that it is valid and reliable. For a start, you will save effort in establishing validity and reliability. Moreover at least some other people (those familiar with the measure) will understand your results. When choosing an existing measure (or developing a new one) it is necessary to ask the following questions:

- Is it actually relevant to this study (see last section)?
- Is it a valid measure of what I wish to assess?

- What is its reliability?
- Is it sensitive enough to detect the change/difference expected?
- Is it simple enough to be used throughout the study?
- Can the results be communicated to others?
- Is there a better measure available?

*Validity* is a concept most neuro-psychologists are familiar with, given the attention it usually receives in their textbooks. Only one point will made here. In any valid measure all the component items should come from the same level of impairment disability or handicap. For example, the widely used Rankin scale is invalid, mixing as it does impairment disability and handicap in one scale.

There are three main sources of uncertainty when comparing two results using one measure: there may be random variation in the patient's state; different observers may have differing biases when measuring; and if there is a mechanical tool being used, it too may vary over time. Although *reliability* is now often assessed, there is little agreement on how to express reliability (as a kappa statistic, as a correlation coefficient etc.).

It is also important to realise that even when a statistically high level of reliability has been demonstrated, individual variability can be considerable. For example, we found timing walking over 10 metres to be 'reliable' on test-retest ($r = 0.98$) but nonetheless individual readings varied by as much as 25% (Collen et al. 1990).

Much less attention has been paid to the assessment of *sensitivity,* yet it is obviously necessary to choose a measure which can detect the change expected. For example if mortality is the only outcome measure, one cannot detect reductions in morbidity! Recently there have been attempts to assess sensitivity, being based upon the statistical variance found in groups of patients. Otherwise one has to make a clinical judgement, perhaps based upon pilot studies.

The likelihood of detecting change can be increased in two ways. First an intrinsically very sensitive single measure can be used. Unfortunately such tests are rare, are often very complex, and are often not very reliable. The alternative is to use several complementary outcome measures. For example in a study evaluating the reduction of neglect one could measure. Activities of Daily Living (ADL), speed and accuracy of reading, ability to negotiate doorways, and speed and ability of completing a simple jig-saw.

Wherever possible the measure used should be simple particularly if more than one person is going to use the measure. *Simplicity* will improve patient (and user) compliance and will increase reliability. Unfortunately sensitivity will often require more complex measures and there is always a trade-off between the three requirements of simplicity, reliability and sensitivity.

Next it is always worth choosing measures whose results will be *easily understood* by others. Readers of the study (or your clinical colleagues) cannot be expected to have the interest and innate understanding you have. Result which are presented numerically with zero representing the worst level and 10 or 100 the best level are most easily understood. It is unwise to design a mea sure where 57 is the worst level and 17 the best (Sheikh et al. 1979) – the readers will simply not get used to the meaning of the numbers. It is also worth ensuring that the readers can obtain some clinical meaning from the results, preferably by giving a readily available reference to the measure or by giving clinical illustrations.

Finally it is always worth considering whether there are other, *better measures.* Time spent asking colleagues and reading around is time well spent. If you do devise new measures or use two or more similar measures, publish the results of any comparison of the two measures so that others may know which is better.

## Some Specific Measures

Most severe impairments seen after brain damage eventually impinge upon physical Activities of Daily Living (ADL) such as dressing, mobility, and being continent. Therefore most evaluations should include a measure of overall ADL functioning, both to describe the patient(s) being studied and to evaluate the practical utility of the treatment in terms of reducing disability.

The Barthel ADL index (Collin et al. 1988) is now the best standard measure of ADL (Wade and Collin 1988): It is valid, reliability has been studied, it is simple, it is more widely known than most other indices and it is relevant to the patient and his carers. Its sensitivity is poor, and so it will usually need to be complemented by more specific measures of manual dexterity, mobility or whatever is the focus of interest.

Measures of impairment will tend to be specific to particular diseases. For example one symptom measure for use in Parkinson's disease (McDowell et al. 1970) concentrates upon the features of the disease – tremor, rigidity, akinesia etc. In the context of treatments aimed primarily at reducing impairment, notably L-Dopa treatment, it is a valuable measure of process (though the weighted scores are not particularly justified). However it would not be a satisfactory outcome measure because it does not include disability. McDowell et al. (1970) recognised this, and devised a second measure concentrating upon disability.

There are also measures of impairment that can probably be applied to most diseases. Motor loss, for example, can be measured simply using dynamometry (power measurement; Bohannon and Adrews 1987) or the Motricity Index and Trunk Control Test (Collin and Wade 1990).

The measurement of intelligence using the WAIS illustrates many good features of a measure such as an easily understood result and well established reliability. Measurement of other cognitive impairments is difficult. Firstly, there is no agreement as to the boundaries of any phenomenon. Unilateral neglect, for example, is not a single problem and there is now evidence of double dissociation of many components. Aphasia is a second example: what is the status of verbal apraxia? Therefore cognitive phenomena are often defined simply by the tests used.

Secondly, and of less importance, it can be difficult to draw distinctions between impairments and disabilities. For example is reduced attention the impairment underlying difficulty remembering, or is amnesia a second impairment. And, if so, what is the disability? Similar problems arise when considering behaviour. Theoretically one should distinguish between subjective internal states such as "depression", "anxiety", "irritability" and the more objective external manifestations of these states, actual behaviours such as avoiding social contacts, shouting at others or showing no initiative. Most of the available measures, such as the General Health Questionnaire (Goldberg and Hillier 1979), are trying to assess the impairments (internal states). One powerful reason for this is that observing actual behaviour takes much time and effort.

The most important single measure of physical disability, the Barthel ADL index has already been discussed. Other useful simple measures include gait speed (Wade et al. 1987), the functional ambulation categories (Holden et al. 1984) and the nine-hole peg test (Heller et al. 1987). However it is also important to measure more extended abilities, notably domestic Activities of Daily Living and activities outside the house. Two useful measures are the Nottingham extended ADL scale (Nouri and Lincoln 1987) and the Frenchay Activities Index (Wade et al. 1985).

Measuring handicap is difficult, in part because one important aspect of handicap is that it concerns the change in an individual's own life and so is not so amenable to measurement using standard assessments.

## Conclusion

When evaluating any neuropsychological intervention, the investigator has many unique contributions to make:

- Identifying the initial hypothesis to be tested
- Clarifying and simplifying the question(s) being asked
- Choosing a suitable study design
- Considering the information needed on:
  - Prognosis
  - Process
  - Outcome
- Identifying the minimum data needed to obtain the information
- Reviewing the measures already available, choosing (or developing) measures which are:
  - Relevant
  - Valid
  - Reliable
  - Sensitive
  - Simple
  - Easily understood by others

The investigator should avoid, if possible, devising new measures, using second-rate measures if better ones exist, using measures or outcomes which will not be accepted or understood by others, and collecting any more data than is absolutely necessary.

In order to achieve this ideal, the investigator should spend as much time as possible refining the study before starting and he/she should consult as widely as possible, accepting help and advice from all sources. Conducting the study, and analysing the results is then the easiest part of the study.

## References


Barlow DH, Hersen M (1984) Single case experimental designs, 2nd edn. Pergamon, New York

Bohannon RW, Andrews AW (1987) Interrater reliability of hand-held dynamometry. Phys Ther 67:931–933

Collen FM, Wade DT, Bardshaw CM (1990) Mobility after stroke: reliability of measures of impairment and disability. Int Disabil Stud 12:6–9

Collin C, Wade DT (1990) Assessing motor impairment after stroke: a reliability study. J Neurol Neurosurg Psychiatry 53:576–579

Collin C, Wade DT, Davis S, Horne V (1988) The Barthel ADL index: a reliability study. Int Disabil Stud 10:61–63

Goldberg DP, Hillier VF (1979) A scaled version of the General Health Questionnaire. Psychol Med 9:139–145

Heller A, Wade DT, Wood VA, Sunderland A, Langton-Hewer R, Ward E (1987) Arm function after stroke: measurement and recovery over the first three months. J Neurol Neurosurg Psychiatry 50:714–719

Holden MK, Gill KM, Magliozzi MR, Nathan J, Piehl-Baker L (1984) Clinical gait assessment in the neurologically impaired: reliability and meaningfulness. Phys Ther 64:35–40

McDowell F, Lee JE, Swift T, Sweet RD, Ogsbury JS, Kessler JT (1970) Treatment of Parkinson's syndrome with L Dihydroxyphenylalanine (Levodopa). Ann Intern Med 72:29–35

Nouri FM, Lincoln NB (1987) An extended activities of daily living scale for stroke patients. Clin Rehabil 1:301–305

Sheikh K, Smith DS, Meade TW, Goldenberg E, Brennan PJ, Kinsella G (1979) Repeatability and validity of a modified activities of daily living (ADL) index in studies of chronic disability. Int Rehabil Med 1:51–58

Wade DT, Collin C (1988) The Barthel ADL index: a standard measure of physical disability? Int Disabil Stud 10:64–67

Wade DT, Legh-Smith J, Langton-Hewer R (1985) Social activities after stroke: measurement and natural history using the Frenchay Activities Index. Int Rehabil Med 7:176–181

Wade DT, Wood VA, Heller A, Maggs J, Langton-Hewer R (1987) Walking after stroke: measurement and recovery over the first three months. Scand J Rehabil Med 19:25–30

World Health Organisation (1980) International classification of impairments, disabilities, and handicaps. World Health Organisation, Geneva

# Discussion: Evaluation in Constructing Neuropsychological Treatments

*N. Mai*

Each of the papers just presented discussed some selected aspects of methodology, and it is a little difficult to comment on such discussions. Probably no one would object to most of the statements and proposals made. Undoubtedly it is true "that investigators should spend more effort on choosing appropriate measures, particularly measures that demonstrate the clinical utility of the intervention being studied" (Wade). Therefore, one way out for a discussant is to concentrate on those aspects the speakers decided to put less weight on or to exclude.

In evaluating neuropsychological treatments, both papers seem to favour one particular design – the classical control group study with random assignment of patients to a treatment or a nontreatment control group. This design is well known to examine a treatment in toto and is praised as the only sound way to rule out alternative explanations of observed changes, such as spontaneous recovery or effects of repeated testing. In addition, comparable effect sizes can only be calculated from such studies, and these are required as input data for a meta-analysis across several studies. A meta-analysis was classified by Trexler and Thomas as a key method to judge treatment effectiveness.

Controlled trials, preferably under blind conditions, are claimed to solve controversies, such as wether focused stroke rehabilitation improves (Reding and McDowell 1989) or does not improve outcome (Dobkin 1989).

Setting aside how double-blind conditions could be realized in a neuropsychological rehabilitation programme, there is at least some agreement that the basic question: "Does neuropsychological rehabilitation work?" is not a very sophisticated question. The frequent reiteration of this question is presumably only a reflection of the scientific prestige of rehabilitation as a research area. Has anyone ever advised an investigation into the global benefits of neurology or neurosurgery by a random assignment of patients to non-treatment control groups?

Most authors admit that, in clinical tests of treatments, methodological compromises and sacrifices have to be made to meet practical and ethical demands. In fact, it is difficult to imagine that patients with obvious impairments would give their informed consent to be randomly assigned to a non-treatment group. The complete information of a patient about a planned clinical trial combined with a clear statement of the right to reject participation at any time without negative consequences for further treatment are the minimum requirements of agreed ethical conventions (e.g., the Helsinki-Tokyo declaration of 1975).

As a consequence, one should definitely give up the idea of proving the benefits of neuropsychological rehabilitation programmes by a random assignment of patients to treatment or non-treatment groups. We do not lose too much by giving up this randomized control group design. This "package strategy" (Kazdin 1986) cannot reveal which components of the treatment are necessary or, more generally, why a treatment works. Recognizing this, many advocates of a package strategy have called for a strict standardization of all treatment procedures. However, standardization itself is not a strategy for dismantling treatment components, which requires experimental variation of the different components involved. Standardization at an early stage of treatment development runs the risk of premature fixation on therapeutic ideas which may obstruct further progress in their development (Greenwald et al. 1986).

The package strategy is not a suitable approach for developing or constructing treatments. However, designing working treatments is what is most needed in neuropsychological rehabilitation. Despite the progress in recent years, the whole field can be characterized by a paucity of treatment procedures. In this respect, neuropsychological rehabilitation differs clearly from the development of psychotherapy. Right from the beginning of psychotherapy, alternative treatment methods emerged from different theoretical considerations, and this proliferation of procedures is still going on. A major part of treatment research in psychotherapy has been concerned with the comparison of different techniques in treating patients (Garfield and Bergin 1986). In neuropsychological rehabilitation, it would be difficult to find sufficient alternative treatments worth the effort of systematic comparison.

"Does the treatment work?" is not the first question to be asked in constructing new treatments. A working treatment is the final product to be designed. Development starts with some procedures believed to be effective and, most important, with some measures to evaluate change. Many questions follow: "What are the necessary components?"; "What components can be added to make treatment more effective?" or "What treatment parameters should be altered?" Other questions may focus on the treatment process: "Under which conditions should a treatment be started?"; "When should a treatment be stopped?" or "What are patients' perceptions of treatment progress?". In principle, answers to such questions can be found by using group procedures as well as single-case designs. An example of mixing both strategies can be found in the treatment studies of visual-field defects by Zihl (1981) and Zihl and von Cramon (1985). One of the advantages in these studies was the availability of a quantitative measure, namely dynamic perimetry, which allowed the immediate evaluation of treatment progress and the effects of modifications in procedures.

The availability of measures which reflect progress in treatment is a critical prerequisite for constructing new treatment procedures. An ideal measure would combine validity with easy accessibility to allow for frequent sampling. Given an immediate valid feedback, even "trial and error" methods can be very effective in shaping a working procedure. Needless to say, such measures are very rare in neuropsychological rehabilitation. However, due to the tremendous progress in transducer technology and the availability of personal computers, there is some hope that suitable measures can be developed, at least in some areas. As an example, consider the traditional neurological method of measuring grip strength (using some type of dynamometers) as an indicator for impaired motor function. Maximal grip force is only a crude measure of impairment in precision of grip control. The continuous registration of forces produced between fingers, using commercially available force transducers, revealed clear dissociations between maximal grip force and more specific aspects of force control, such as maintaining constant force or producing rapid force changes (Mai 1989; Mai et al. 1988, 1989). These additional measures are easy to access and provide a specific follow up of impaired hand function in close relation to experimental investigations of hand gripping (e.g., Johansson and Westling 1988). Monitoring and evaluating progress provides the guideline for the therapist in improving his treatment, and in many cases the same quantitative information about changes can be used as direct feedback for the patient.

Even when a significant reduction of a specific impairment after treatment can be demonstrated, one may question the general effects of these therapeutic gains. This point was stressed by Wade in his contribution, and he advised including some measure of overall functioning in Activities of Daily Living (ADL) in all evaluations to judge the practical utility of a treatment. However, the sensitivity of ADL indices is typically poor and changes in scores, particularly when observed in post-treatment follow-up assessments and cannot be traced back to a specific treatment, which is usually embedded in a series of standard treatments. An overall evaluation of a compound treatment programme in terms of ADL or other common tests may serve several important purposes (e.g., further funding of programmes). To a designer of specific treatments, such an overall evaluation usually indicates no more than that there is plenty of room for further improvements.

Research on constructing new treatments requires access to patients and is therefore usually implemented in rehabilitation centres with the primary function of providing treatment. Sometimes this may lead to discussions as to whether treatments should be adapted to scientific demands or the reverse. I would like to argue for a definite priority of therapeutic demands. Patients referred to a rehabilitation centre expect a treatment and improvement according to the state of the art, which implies a tailoring of treatments to their individual needs. This excludes any assignment to a control condition with a low probability of producing change. However, patients may be asked to give their informed consent to participate in additional clinical trials on circumscribed problems. Many patients are highly interested in "experimental" treatments of their deficits, even when the expected benefits are quite unclear.

It is almost a truism that we learn from our errors. However, in treatment research it is a common practice to report exclusively successes. Treatment failures are familiar to most therapists. Examples are a "premature" termination of treatment by the patient or an obvious discrepancy between actual and expected outcome, such as a paradoxical enhancement of anxiety in relaxation training (Heide and Borkovec 1984). Systematic analysis of failures could be of considerable value in improving procedures (Diller and Weinberg 1986). An open-minded discussion of possible sources of failures such as patient, treatment or context variables requires a cooperative climate, which is not characteristic of every institution. In addition, a change in the publishing policy of journals would encourage reports on such failures.

To summarize, neuropsychological rehabilitation needs the development of specific treatments. This requires an intensification of the search for measures which can help in the design of new treatment procedures. The common overall outcome measures do not offer much assistance because their sensitivity is too poor for the evaluation of specific procedures. The choice of experimental design, which has absorbed much of past discussions, is of secondary importance compared with the choice of measures.

## References


Diller L, Weinberg J (1986) Learning from failures in perceptual cognitive retraining in stroke. In: Uzzel BP, Gross Y (eds) Clinical neuropsychology of intervention. Nijhoff, Boston, pp 283–293

Dobkin BH (1989) Focused stroke rehabilitation programs do not improve outcome. Arch Neurol 46:701–703

Garfield SL, Bergin AE (eds) (1986) Handbook of psychotherapy and behavior change, 3rd edn. Wiley, New York

Greenwald AG, Pratkanis AR, Leippe MR, Baumgardner MH (1986) Under what conditions does theory obstruct research progress? Psychol Rev 93:216–229

Heide FJ, Borkovec TD (1984) Relaxation-induced anxiety. Mechanism and theoretical implications. Behav Res Ther 22:1–12

Johansson RS, Westling G (1988) Coordinated isometric muscle commands adequately and erroneously programmed for the weight during lifting tasks with precision grip. Exp Brain Res 71:59–71

Kazdin AE (1986) The evalulation of psychotherapy: research design and methodology. In: Garfield SL, Bergin AE (eds) Handbook of psychotherapy and behavior change, 3rd edn. Wiley, New York, pp 23–68

Mai N (1989) Residual control of isometric finger forces in hemiparetic patients. Evidence for dissociation of performance deficits. Neurosci Lett 101:347–351

Mai N, Bolsinger P, Avarello M, Diener HC, Dichgans J (1988) Control of isometric finger force in patients with cerebellar disease. Brain 11:973–998

Mai N, Diener HC, Dichgans J (1989) On the role of feedback in maintaining constant grip force in patients with cerebellar disease. Neurosci Lett 99:340–344

Reding MJ, McDowell FH (1989) Focused stroke rehabilitation programs improve outcome. Arch Neurol 46:700–701

Zihl J (1981) Recovery of visual functions in patients with cerebral blindness. Effect of specific practice with saccadic localization. Exp Brain Res 44:159–169

Zihl J, von Cramon D (1985) Visual field recovery from scotoma in patients with postgeniculate damage. Brain 108:335-365

# Diagnostics

# Psychometric Evaluation of Neuropsychological Test Performances*

*K. Willmes*

## Introduction

One characteristic of a developed scientific discipline is the availability of proper measurement models and instruments. Under this perspective, considerable progress has been made in psychology in general in the last three decades. Likewise, neuropsychology has to take up the challenge and has to incorporate these measurement models into its body of assessment procedures. Recent overviews are, however, still devoid of them (Lezak 1988). Several reasons can be offered for this state of neuropsychological assessment in general:

- Many of the refined measurement models require large samples for reasonable parameter estimation and tests of model fit.
- Procedures used to investigate aspects of construct validity, such as multidimensional scaling procedures (Borg 1981), also call for large samples for stable similarity coefficient estimation.
- Clinical populations often exhibit much more systematic interindividual variation than non-brain-damaged subjects along some ability dimension.
- Some neuropsychological syndromes or patterns of impairment are very rare.

Whereas these arguments pertain to neuropsychology in general, the particular approach of cognitive neuropsychology (Caramazza and McCloskey 1988; Ellis and Young 1988) introduces an additional problem. For an in-depth analysis of an individual patient, assessment procedures are often specifically tailored to reveal the nature of the deficit(s) hypothesized to be causing a patient's disorders. Obviously, no information on the reliability and construct validity of these tasks or normative data can be at hand.

In the following, psychometric procedures for three substantial assessment problems in neuropsychology will be described and applied to data from aphasiology:

- Evaluation of individual patients' performances in a standardized test serving as baseline information about patients' patterns of impairment

* This paper is dedicated to Professor Klaus Poeck on the occasion of his 65th birthday.

- Detection of (double) dissociations in performance when the selective impairment is only partial
- Investigation of the measurement properties of polychotomous items with ordered categories often to be found for the grading of impaired performances

## Evaluation of Individual Test Profiles

Test scores from standardized neuropsychological assessment procedures are often available for one or both of the following reasons. They provide standard diagnostic information both for a single as well as for repeated examinations possibly before, during and after some intervention phase. They serve as baseline information about a patient's pattern of levels of impairment across or within more or less broadly defined functional domains.

A simple description of the pattern of impaired test performances, expressed as a profile of standard scores, can be misleading without taking into account measurement errors inevitably present in any assessment procedure. Basically, two types of (diagnostic) questions are of interest: (a) Are ther *reliable* differences between (subsets of) subtest scores both within and across examinations? (b) Are these reliable differences '*diagnostically valid*', showing an exceedingly large discrepancy between performances compared with a certain reference population of patients or non-brain-damaged subjects? A little-known set of procedures was given by Payne and Jones (1957) with reference to the WAIS. It was confined to observed standardized scores and ignored the fact that statistical hypotheses are related to unobservable parameters, i.e., in this case true scores in the sense of the classical test-theory model (Lord and Novick 1968). Huber (1973) offered such a comprehensive approach (see also Willmes 1985). The diagnostic hypotheses are related to the equality of levels of ability/impairment in a given individual patient. These hypotheses imply statistical (null-)hypotheses about the identity of true standardized scores for the respective subtests. To construct test statistics related to a single subject's performances, one needs an estimate of the individual error variance, i.e., the variability of test results over hypothetical replications of assessments with the same test(s). Because of obvious reasons like fatigue or practice, sufficient numbers of replications are not feasible. Therefore, in Huber's approach the crucial assumption is that for a homogeneous population these individual error variances are identical and can be approximated by the square of the standard error of measurement, which in turn crucially depends on the reliability parameter. A second important feature is the introduction of $\tau$-standardization. Identity of true raw-scores only implies identity of true standardized scores if the reliability parameters of the mental tests are identical. True-score ($\tau$) standardization overcomes that problem and can be accomplished by transforming the common standard scores y with mean L according to the following formula, which crucially involves the reliability parameter:

$$y^{\tau} = y/\sqrt{\varrho} + L(1 - 1/\sqrt{\varrho}) \tag{1}$$

For some mental test, $\varrho$ has to be estimated, and the standardized norm-sample mean is only an estimate of the population parameter L (e.g., L = 50 for T scores). Therefore, large standardization samples of no less than 400 subjects and reliability estimates from samples of no less than 100 are required. The standard use of psychometric single-case analysis procedures comprises analyses for one individual test profile as well as the comparison of two profiles of the same subject. Examples for more specific applications are the following:

*1. Selective impairment* (or selective sparing) of performances in one subtest of a test profile: For an in-depth study, e.g., of an aphasic patient with particular repetition (or reading) disorders, one could require as a strict prerequisite screening criterion that the patient's performance in the subtest Repetition of the Aachen Aphasia Test (AAT, Huber et al. 1984) is not only reliably but also diagnostically validly poorer than that in the other subtests. The next formula serves to compute the diagnostic validity of a difference in two test performances for one patient i, i.e., the probability of obtaining a still larger difference in $\tau$-standardized T scores $y^{\tau}_{ij}$, j = 1, ..., 5 tests, under the null hypothesis that the particular patient belongs to the actual aphasic population for which the mean true standardized scores are identical for both abilities measured:

$$z = (y^{\tau}_{ij} - y^{\tau}_{iRep})/K(1/\varrho_j + 1/\varrho_{Rep} - 2\varrho_{jRep}/\varrho_j\varrho_{Rep})^{1/2} \tag{2}$$

K equals 10 for T-scores, $\varrho_j$ and $\varrho_{Rep}$ are the reliabilities of the two subtests – j:Token Test, Written Language, Naming or Comprehension – and $\varrho_{jRep}$, the respective intercorrelation. The diagnostic validity probability $p_j$ is obtained from:

$$p_j = 1 - \Phi(z) \tag{3}$$

where $\Phi(\cdot)$ indicates the cumulative standard normal distribution. As a conservative criterion, each of the four pairwise comparison probabilities $p_j$ of the repetition T-score with the other four T-scores has to be below 0.05 to ensure an overall probability of no more than 20%, which is the maximum acceptable value suggested by Huber (1973).

*2. Selection of homogeneous subsets of aphasic patients* can be accomplished by using the test profile comparison procedures for a single patient. The formulae are applicable for the comparison of one profile from each of two patients i and k as well. A global comparison sensitive to both profile level and profile shape differences is carried out using:

$$\chi^2_m = (1/2K^2) \cdot \sum_{j=1}^{m} (\varrho_j/(1-\varrho_j)) \cdot (y^{\tau}_{ij} - y^{\tau}_{kj})^2 \qquad \text{– m subtests –} \tag{4}$$

If the respective p-value is no smaller than a liberal type-I error level of 0.10, the subjects can be taken to be homogeneous with respect to these basic language impairments. If the identity of the profile shapes irrespective of the profile level is of interest, possible level differences must first be adjusted. The profile level is a reliability-weighted average of the subtest performances:

$$h_i^\tau = \left\{ \sum_{j=1}^{m} (\varrho_j/(1-\varrho_j)) \cdot y_{ij}^\tau \right\} \Big/ \sum_{j=1}^{m} \varrho_j/(1-\varrho_j) \tag{5}$$

Global identity of profile shapes is then tested via a modification of (4), taking into account the difference $h_i^\tau - h_k^\tau$ in profile level among the two patients:

$$\chi_m^2 = (1/2K^2) \cdot \sum_{j=1}^{m} (\varrho_j/(1-\varrho_j)) \cdot (y_{ij}^\tau - y_{kj}^\tau - (h_i^\tau - h_k^\tau))^2 \tag{6}$$

*3. Selection of homogeneous patients from different languages* for comparative aphasiological research: Cross-linguistic studies of language breakdown have gained special attention in the last years, and multilingual test batteries have been designed for the assessment of basic language impairments. The psychometric properties of these batteries still remain unknown. For an adaptation of the AAT in Italian (De Bleser et al. 1986), objectivity, reliability, and validity properties (Luzzatti et al. 1987) are very similar to the original in German, and single-case analysis procedures can be carried out as well (Willmes et al. 1988). Although reliability estimates for both versions of the test are almost identical and T-scores only differ by at most 2 for identical raw-scores except for the most extreme scores, the profile comparison procedures mentioned in (2) cannot be applied. Well-established methods for equating test scores (Holland and Rubin 1982) cannot be applied for obvious reasons, either. No common "anchor test" and no common "anchor sample" of patients with identical proficiency in both languages can be found in principle. It is, however, possible to select patients from different languages who show a very similar level and pattern of performance according to psychometric single-case analysis procedures applied to either of the individual profiles. This must be considered a definite improvement compared to the rather broad criteria used in cross-linguistic studies so far. The same procedures can be applied for baseline assessment of a bi- or multilingual patient, which is more adequate then counting the number of (very short) subtests for which a certain percentage of items was solved correctly for the different languages studied (Nilipour and Ashayeri 1989) for example.

## Detection of Dissociations

The demonstration of (double) dissociations in the performance for two (sets of) tasks, which can sensibly be related within some theoretical framework of cognitive functioning or processing, is considered to provide most valid evidence for the evaluation of models of normal cognitive functioning (Shallice 1979; Blanken 1988). Since the theoretically expected or predicted selective impairment of some functional subsystem or processing route, however, is not absolute but only partial, statistical and psychometric models and procedures are needed as well for a sound statement concerning a dissociation obtained from an in-depth experimental study for a single patient. Several conceptual and technical aspects of this problem together with some suggestions for solutions will be treated in the following:

1. Often, little or nothing is known empirically about the particular reliability and validity properties of items comprising some task as well as of the various tasks themselves used in some single-case study. The methological approach often leads to the theory-driven but ad hoc generation of items. Implicitly, *content validity* is taken to be the major criterion for item generation and selection. A test is called *content valid* (Berk 1980; Klauer 1987) if it contains or represents a universe of items (behavioral domain), e.g., the universe of legal neologisms for a particular language. Such a universe can be defined by complete enumeration of its members or, more often, by stating the properties for the generation of any item from the universe. An item is characterized by both a stimulus and a response component, i.e., an operation that has to be performed on the stimulus (e.g. to make a lexical decision). This general framework, which is well established in educational psychology under the heading of criterion-referenced measurement or mastery testing (Hambleton and Novick 1973; Hambleton 1978), could prove to be successful for cognitive neuropsychology as well. In fact, it has tacitly been employed in rudimentary form in exemplary applications of the cognitive neuropsychological approach. The degree of *competence* (ability) of an individual can be defined as the probability of solving items correctly from a particular universe of items. Empirically, the level of competence can be estimated from a representative sample of items from that universe. The properties of this ability estimate depend on the particular test model employed, the most simple of which is the binomial model (see below). *Mastery* for some type of criterion-referenced task/test represented via a (sample from an) item universe can be defined as sufficient if the level of performance for some individual subject is larger than some lower bound of e.g., $p_c = 0.90$. Criterion-referenced testing thus relates the individual test performance to a certain level of competence, not to a distribution of scores across some reference population as does a test constructed according to the classical test theory model. One way of defining a (relative) dissociation proper is to require a high level of competence for one domain (e.g., $p_c = 0.95$ for writing to dictation of neologisms) and a very low one for another domain (e.g., a *minimum* competence level of $p_o = 0.20$ for regular words).

In general, there is no one-to-one relationship between a task domain and one component or route in some processing model. Several types of tasks or subdomains within one domain may be relevant or informative (e.g., not only a lexical decision after visual presentation of words and non-words, but also writing to dictation). Thus, different aspects of *internal* and *external construct validity* (Klauer 1987) of a set of items have to be demonstrated as well. Guttman's facet theory (Canter 1985), with its nonmetric multidimensional scaling methods (for an application in aphasiology, see Willmes et al. 1983), as well as procedures for investigating psychometric hierarchies (Price et al. 1980), are examples for assessing construct validity. But both usually require sizable samples of subjects.

2. When comparing the performance, i.e., the number of correct solutions for two theoretically related tasks for an individual patient using the large sample chi-square test or Fisher's exact test for a $2 \times 2$ table, several crucial assumptions are made implicitly. Actually, the test provides a comparison of two binomial probability parameters. For this test to be statistically valid, the random variables related to the outcomes for each item have to be independent. Extensive theoretical and simulation studies have shown that the chi-square test can be highly anticonservative even for rather weak positive serial dependencies among trials (Tavare and Altham 1983). There is a considerable risk of falsely identifying patients with dissociations. The only way of keeping dependencies negligible is a proper randomization of items. Another assumption implicit in the application of the binomial model is the identity of difficulty for all items in a test. This assumption can only be relaxed if the items constitute a random sample with or without replacement for some finite or infinite universe of items. Lord and Novick (1968) have shown that with item sampling the distribution of the total score across subjects is binomial. Since language items of some well-defined domain still exhibit different levels of difficulty, only the latter argument for a binomial distribution can be applied. Technically, item sampling poses no difficulty when using a PC. Theoretically, it is less obvious how well item universes can be defined for language items, e.g., real words in a lexical-decision task have to be controlled for number of graphemes/phonemes, complexity of consonant clusters, word frequency, concreteness, etc. Finally, the number of items required to obtain sufficient statistical power for a comparison of two binomial proportions should be considered when designing a single-case study. The same argument applies to the investigation of mastery/non-mastery. A total of 27 items, for example, would be required for a type-I error of 5% and a type-II error of 20% to ensure that for a criterion probability of $p_c = 0.95$ the decision of mastery or non-mastery would be within the above-error limits using a cut-off value of 24.

3. When comparing the total score for two content-valid tests to detect some dissociation, it is tacitly assumed that both performances are commensurable. But the inherent difficulty of task domains must be taken into account (Sergent 1988). Thus, baseline data are required which provide information on the "general" difficulty of different tasks. As an example, results for the lexical discrimination supplement to the AAT (Poeck and Göddenhenrich 1988; Huber et al. 1988) will be discussed briefly. The supplement is composed of 5 parts with 80 items each, requiring either semantic discrimination between pictures or words or phonemic discrimination between pictures, words, or legal neologisms. In a sample of 61 aphasic patients, the difficulty grading was as follows: neologisms $<$ phonemic similarity words $<$ semantic similarity words

= semantic similarity pictures < phonemic similarity pictures. For an individual patient, a (partial) dissociation can be defined to hold if, according to the binomial model, performances in two of the five tasks lead to non-overlapping confidence intervals. For routine use, this is more convenient than carrying out exact tests for 2×2-tables. Among the 61 patients, the majority of "dissociations" (20 from 35 overall) was present for poorer performance for neologisms. But this task must be considered more difficult both theoretically and empirically. Two attempts at a solution can be offered. Based on a mastery-approach, a dissociation could be taken to hold only if the "preserved" ability is compatible with a competence of at least $p_c = 0.90$ (66/80 correct) and if the "non-preserved" performance does not exceed random guessing competence ($p_o = 0.20$ for this MC-task; no more than 24/80 correct). With this criterion only one aphasic patient with selective impairment for neologisms remains. Taking reference to the observed level and variation of scores within the aphasic sample by considering percentile ranks (or some other standardized scores) instead of raw scores, a partial dissociation could be taken to hold for a percentile rank difference of more than 20 percentile ranks, for example. This criterion reduces the number of dissociations for neologisms drastically to 2 in 17 dissociations overall.

It has, however, been argued (Blanken 1988) that only baseline data from healthy controls can provide strictly valid information for cognitive neuropsychological studies. For aphasia research, such data on the total correct score would be of no help because normal performance would be very close to perfect. Thus, these tasks would have no discriminatory power even though there might be differences in the underlying latent ability continuum for normal subjects also.

## Evaluating Scale Properties of Polychotomous Items with Probabilistic Test Models

For the vast majority of psychological test procedures in neuropsychology, only the classical test-theory model has been employed, although it is weak in terms of its measurement properties. Item parameters, like item difficulty or item discrimination, are dependent on the distribution of ability levels in the respective sample used to estimate them. Thus, no *specifically objective* comparisons of both, item difficulties and person abilities (Rasch 1961; Wright and Masters 1982), are possible. The basic properties of probabilistic test theory can be illustrated with the simple logistic model for dichotomously scored items. The probability for a correct solution ($X_{\nu i} = 1$) for person $\nu$ for item i from a well-defined set if items is expressed as a function of an item-difficulty parameter $\delta_i$ and a person-ability parameter $\beta_\nu$, both measured on the same latent continuum:

$$\Pr(X_{\nu i} = 1 \mid \delta_i, \beta_\nu) = \exp(\beta_\nu - \delta_i)/(1 + \exp(\beta_\nu - \delta_i)) \quad (7)$$

For a set of k items and a sample of n subjects, all relevant information for a sufficient estimation of $\beta_v$ and $\delta_i$ is contained in the total number of items solved correctly, irrespective of the patterns of 0/1, and in the absolute frequency of subjects solving item i correctly. Several tests of model fit are available. An application of this model to Token-Test data has been given by Willmes (1981).

In aphasia testing, it is often useful to require a more differentiated item scoring, expressing different degrees of deviation from a correct solution. Several probabilistic test models for graded responses have been developed (Wright and Masters 1982), all yielding ability estimates on a one-dimensional latent continuum. The *partial credit model* is the least restrictive of them. The basic equation relates the probability of scoring x rather than x−1 on a scale ranging from 0 to m to a person-ability parameter $\beta_v$ and a set of item step parameters $\delta_{ij}, j = 1, \ldots, m$:

$$\Pr(X_{vi} = x \mid \beta_v, \delta_{ij}) = \exp \sum_{j=0}^{x} (\beta_v - \delta_{ij}) / \sum_{l=0}^{m} \exp \sum_{j=0}^{l} (\beta_v - \delta_{ij}) \tag{8}$$

An example for m = 4 category probability curves is shown in Fig. 2. From left to right, there is always a certain interval on the latent ability continuum for which one particular category probability curve is highest, indicating the most probable score for a particular ability level. The threshold values on the latent continuum corresponding to the intersection of two neighboring curves pro-

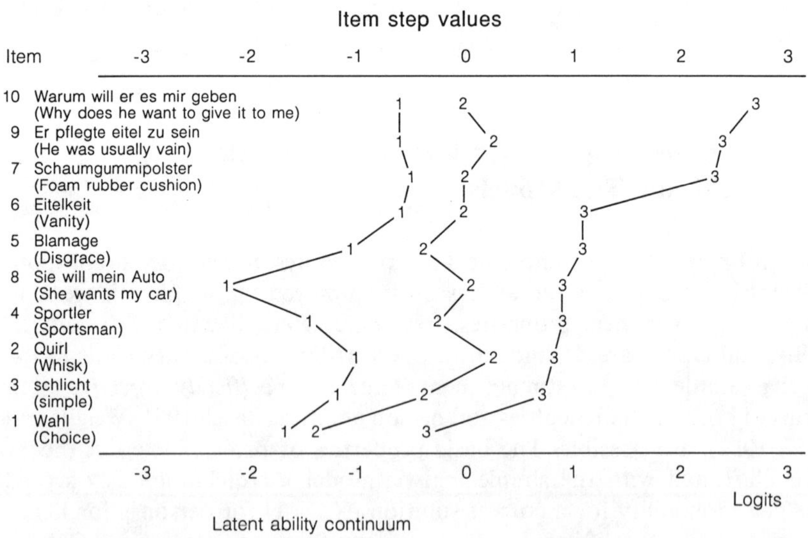


**Fig. 1.** CREDIT analysis (Masters et al. 1980) for the reading aloud part of the AAT subtest Written Language (Huber et al. 1984; Willmes et al. 1983): item step values for each of the ten items ordered according to increasing step values for a correct solution ($n$ = 378 aphasic patients; 87 persons excluded because of a total score of zero (75) or a perfect score of 30 (12); $n$ = 291 used in the analysis; 27 patients with insufficient person fit values)

vide information on how equidistant ability levels are on the *latent* continuum for adjacent *observed* grade scores. The common practice of using the total score for a set of items as the adequate ability indicator is strictly justified only if the differences between threshold values are identical both within and across items.

Application of the partial-credit model is demonstrated for the reading aloud part of the Written Language subtest of the AAT (see also Willmes et al. 1983). There are m = 4 grade scores for each of the k = 10 items. A large random sample of $n = 378$ aphasic patients was drawn from the AAT data base (Willmes and Ratajczak 1987), representing a wide range of severity levels and

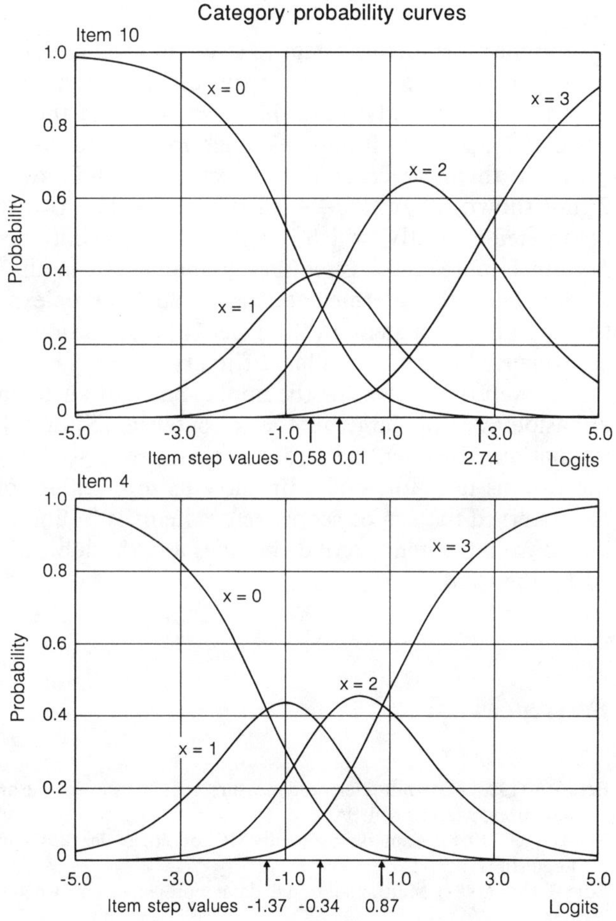


**Fig. 2.** Category probability curves from the partial credit model (Wright and Masters 1982) for item 10 ('Warum will er es mir geben' – 'why does he want to give it to me') and item 4 ('Sportler' – 'sportsman') with item step values taken from Fig. 1 for each of the four grade scores x = 0 to x = 3; item step values indicated by arrows

time after onset of the cerebro-vascular accident. The results of the analysis with the CREDIT program (Masters et al. 1980) are illustrated in Fig. 1.

For each item, those points on the latent ability continuum are indicated by successive integers 1,2,3, for which – from left to right – a score of 1 becomes more probable than 0, a score of 2 more probable than 1, and 3 more probable than 2. The items themselves are ordered according to the step value for score 3. Obviously, there are large differences in the relative placement of those step values, although the criteria for a particular score are identical for all 10 items. The step values 1 and 3 can be close together/far apart indicating a poorly discriminating/overdiscriminating item. The position of step value 2 can be close to 1 or 3 or just in the middle, providing information on the relative amount of ability that is required to be credited a particular score. Figure 2 shows the category probability curves for two items with rather different properties.

For the most difficult item 10 ("Warum will er es mir geben" – "Why does he want to give it to me"), it is plausible that it only requires a medium ability level to read correctly more than two thirds of the simple words (yielding a score of 2), but that it requires much more in terms of processing capacity to get all of them correct in the correct order. Quite to the contrary, if for item 2 (not shown) ("Quirl" – "whisk") more than two thirds of the graphemes are uttered correctly (which is difficult for the initial consonant cluster), then not much more ability is required to manage them all. Following the same line of argument, the intermediate step value 2 can be expected to be halfway between 1 and 3 for item 4 ("Sportler" – "sportsman") because there are two consonant clusters of similar difficulty.

A severe drawback for the applicability of such elaborated test models in aphasiology is the large number of subjects required for adequate parameter estimation. However, the verdict against group studies does not apply because the various tests for model fit allow us to examine for each subject whether the observed pattern of scores across items is in line with what would be predicted from the item (step) difficulties and the subject's ability level as indicated by the total score.

## References

Berk RA (1980) Criterion-referenced measurement: the state of the art. Johns Hopkins University, Baltimore, Maryland, USA

Blanken G (1988) Anmerkungen zur Methodologie der kognitiven Neurolinguistik. Neurolinguistik 2:127–147

Borg I (ed) (1981) Multidimensional data representations: when & why? Mathesis, Ann Arbor

Canter D (ed) (1985) Facet theory: approaches to social research. Springer, Berlin Heidelberg New York

Caramazza A, McCloskey M (1988) The case for single-patient studies. Cogn Neuropsychol 5:517–528

De Bleser R, Denes GF, Luzzatti C, Mazzucchi A, Poeck K, Spinnler H, Willmes K (1986) L'Aachener Aphasie Test (AAT). I. Problemi e soluzioni per una versione italiana del test e per uno studio crosslinguistico dei disturbi afasici. Arch Psicol Neurol Psichiatr 47:209–237

Ellis AW, Young AW (1988) Human cognitive neuropsychology. Erlbaum Hove

Hambleton RK (1978) On the use of cut-off scores with criterion referenced tests in instructional settings. J Educ Measure 15:277–290

Hambleton RK, Novick MR (1973) Toward an integration of theory and method for criterion-references tests. J Educ Measure 10:159–170

Holland PW, Rubin DB (eds) (1982) Test equating. Academic, New York

Huber HP (1973) Psychometrische Einzelfalldiagnostik. Beltz, Weinheim

Huber W, Poeck K, Willmes K (1984) The Aachen Aphasia Test (AAT). In: Rose FC (ed) Progress in aphasiology. Raven, New York, pp 291–303

Huber W, Willmes K, Göddenhenrich S (1988) Diagnose von Leistungsdissoziationen beim lexikalischen Diskriminieren. In: Günther KB (ed) Sprachstörungen. Schindele, Heidelberg, pp 306–329

Klauer KJ (1987) Kriteriumsorientierte Tests. Hogrefe, Göttingen, FRG

Lezak MD (1988) Neuropsychological test and assessment techniques. In: Boller FC, Grafman J (eds) Handbook of neuropsychology, vol 1. Elsevier, Amsterdam, pp 47–68

Lord FM, Novick MR (1968) Statistical theories of mental test scores. Addison-Wesley, Reading

Luzzatti C, Willmes K, Bisiacchi P, De Bleser R, Faglia L, Mazzucchi A, Posteraro L, Taricco M (1987) L' Aachener Aphasie Test (AAT). II. Proprietà psichometriche della versione italiana. Arch Pscicol Neurol Psichiatr 48:480–519

Masters GN, Wright BD, Ludlow LH (1980) CREDIT: item calibration and person management with ordered response categories. Computer program, University of Chicago

Nilipour R, Ashayeri H (1989) Alternating antagonism between two languages with successive recovery of a third in a bilingual aphasic patient. Brain Lang 36:23–48

Payne RW, Jones G (1957) Statistics for the investigation of individual cases. J Clin Psychol 13:115–121

Poeck K, Göddenhenrich S (1988) Standardized tests for the detection of dissociation in aphasic language performance. Aphasiology 2:375–380

Price LC, Dayton CM, Macready GB (1980) Discovery algorithm for hierarchical relations. Psychometrika 45:449–465

Rasch G (1961) On general laws and the meaning of measurement in psychology. Proceed 4th Berkeley Symp Math Statist Probab, pp 321–333

Sergent J (1988) Some theoretical and methodological issues in neuropsychological research. In: Boller FC, Grafman J (eds) Handbook of neuropsychology, vol 1. Elsevier, Amsterdam, pp 69–81

Shallice T (1979) Case study approach in neuropsychological research. J Clin Neuropsychol 1:183–211

Tavare S, Altham PME (1983) Serial dependence of observations leading to contingency tables, and corrections to chi-squared statistics. Biometrika 70:139–144

Willmes K (1981) A new look at the Token Test using probabilistic test models. Neuropsychologia 19:631–645

Willmes K (1985) An approach to analyzing a single subject's scores obtained in a standardized test with application to the Aachen Aphasia Test (AAT). J Clin Exp Neuropsychol 7:331–352

Willmes K, Ratajczak H (1987) The design and application of a data- and method base system for the Aachen Aphasia Test. Neuropsychologia 25:725–733

Willmes K, Poeck K, Weniger D, Huber W (1983) Facet theory applied to the construction and validation of the Aachen Aphasia Test. Brain Lang 18:259–276

Willmes K, Luzzatti C, Mazzucchi A, De Bleser R, Colombo C, Bisiacchi P (1988) L' Aachener Aphasie Test. III. Procedimento diagnostico per casi singoli. Arch Psicol Neurol Psichiatr 49:510–545

Wright BD, Masters GN (1982) Rating scale analysis. Mesa, Chicago

# Assessment of Mild, Moderate, and Severe Head Injury

*M. D. Lezak*

## Introduction

Despite the many different variables that can enter into the occurrence of brain damage in a moving vehicle accident (MVA), a similar pattern of deficits tends to emerge, differing among patients mostly with respect to the severity of the injury (Adams et al. 1985; Eisenberg and Levin 1989; Pang 1989; Teasdale and Mendelow 1984). This pattern of deficits should determine the core neuropsychological assessment program for persons with traumatic brain injury (TBI).

## Problems Which Affect Most TBI Patients

*Attentional Deficits.* Diminished mental efficiency affects most TBI patients regardless of severity of injury (Kay 1986; Rimel et al. 1981). Among the most prominent mental efficiency problems are attentional deficits resulting from slowed mental processing (Gronwall 1989; Rutherford 1989). These deficits may show up in a reduced attention span which limits the amount of information the patient can process at any given time. One important consequence of a reduced attention span is the inability to grasp and process meaningfully all that is heard in normal conversation so that these patients misunderstand much that is said to them. Impaired ability to focus (concentration) and to shift attention renders these patients both highly distractible and restricted in their ability to keep up with ongoing fast-paced events. Inability to think about or do more than one thing at a time has ramifications in almost every aspect of these patients' lives including difficulty doing mental computations, following a recipe, shopping in a highly stimulating place, carrying on a conversation with more than one person or with background noise, etc. With too much stimulation or when doing complex mental work, these patients become easily confused, their anxiety mounts as does distress and fatigue. Attentional deficits, even when seemingly mild, can have a significant impact not only on cognitive functioning, but on these patients' emotional well-being as well.

Each aspect of attention needs to be evaluated in itself as the presentation of these problems varies from one person to another. When a clear picture is obtained of the attentional deficits that trouble a patient and how they interfere with effective performance, then appropriate counseling and/or remediation techniques can be instituted. Assessment of attentional functions is relatively easy as there are many available methods and interpretations of the data is straightforward and immediately applicable (Lezak 1983).

*Verbal Retrieval Problems and the Experience of Defective Memory.* The experience of defective memory differs from actual memory problems in that these patients interpret defective recall of past information and present events as due to poor memory, when their memory system is actually functioning reasonably well. Rather than difficulty learning, they have difficulty retrieving stored information reliably and rapidly – a difficulty most people experience at times and particularly under stress, but which is greatly heightened for many TBI patients (Goodglass 1980). The experience of poor memory may also result from missing out on passing events or conversations because of slowed processing with reduced span of apprehension, distractibility, and inability to take in more than one thing at a time. Again, appropriate counseling and treatment depends on accurate appraisal of the patient's complaints, including assessment of verbal retrieval along with the in-depth examination of attentional functions.

## Problems Occurring in Moderately to Severely Injured Patients

Some problems occur to a significant degree only in patients who have sustained moderate to severe brain damage. TBI patients who had little or no loss of consciousness and a relatively brief period of posttraumatic amnesia present these problems infrequently and then they tend to be quite subtle (Stuss et al. 1985).

*Extensive Retrograde Amnesia and Learning Deficits.* Unlike the experience of memory deficit, amnesia and learning deficits implicate the memory system directly (Bond 1986; Levin et al. 1982). When they are observed or suspected, a comprehensive assessment of learning and retrieval is called for (Brooks 1989). This must include a review of both rote learning and the learning of meaningful material in both verbal and visual modalities. It should also include tests of incidental learning, remote memory, and retrieval efficiency for both modalities and types of material.

*Deficient Drive States and Motivational Capacity.* When drive states and motivational capacity are compromised by brain damage, personality alterations also occur; the more severe the deficits, the more radical the personality change. These deficits are among the greatest obstacles to rehabilitation as these patients give evidence of little if any felt need to change, or to do very much of anything (Wood 1984). For these reasons, when the problem is more than mild, these patients are unlikely to achieve full social independence, even with the best rehabilitation efforts.

When the problems are severe, the flattened affect, absence of interests, and passive disposition are usually very evident. Formal assessment will not only provide information about specific areas of cognitive functioning, but should document the personality characteristics – such as passivity, anergia, and docility – which indicate the presence of a serious motivational problem occurring on an organic basis (Bond 1984; Walsh 1985). When drives are only moderately reduced and most cognitive abilities remain relatively intact, the patient's passivity and anergic tendencies may not show up in the usual well-structured clinical assessment. These problems then can be best examined by observation of the patient, ideally in a relatively unstructured setting. Often, the first clues that a motivational problem exists comes from the clinical diagnostic interview: sometimes these patients' acknowledgement of inactivity reveals their loss of drive; usually their families' reports will contain the critical information leading the examiner to suspect motivational problems (Lezak 1989). Thus it is important, wherever possible, to interview the family as part of the neuropsychological assessment.

*Reduced Executive Capacities.* Like motivational capacity, planning, self-control and self-regulation, goal-direction and initiation are central to the potential for rehabilitation and independent living (Lezak 1987, 1989). Compromise of these capacities is why so many TBI patients need rehabilitation. More than simply identifying the presence of executive dysfunction, the examiner needs to describe its nature and severity when evaluating rehabilitation potential and designing the rehabilitation program. These problems will show up under close observation. In the formal examination they can be identified by means of tests which put the burden of making structure on the patient, and also in many of the qualitative aspects of the patient's responses to more structured examination procedures.

*Impaired Judgment.* Impaired judgment, which includes loss of the abstract attitude (concrete-mindedness) and diminished self-awareness and social sensitivity, is usually documented by observation and reports from the family or other caregivers. Problems in these areas may also be elicited by tests of commonsense judgment as well as some tests of personal awareness.

## The Importance of a General Assessment of Cognitive Abilities

In addition to the intensive assessment of the most vulnerable areas of neuropsychological functioning, there are important reasons to perform a general review of the TBI patient's cognitive status. Not least of these is the need to ascertain the level at which the patient had been functioning before the accident as this will give some idea of the patient's self-expectations as well as the amount of cognitive loss that was suffered: both self-expectations and experiences of loss will contribute to the patient's ability to use rehabilitation and to accommodate to the new deficits. It is also important to document the patient's residual competencies, again both to aid in the rehabilitation process and to facilitate the patient's adaptation to an altered mental status and experience of self. Most TBI patients experience themselves as not as good as they were, as more or less defective, as inadequate and less than worthwhile people. The reassurance that many capacities and skills are still intact – as is often the case for the mildly and moderately damaged patients – can materially help to counteract discouragement and despair.

Severely injured patients require a general review of cognitive functions because some of them suffer a wide-spread loss of mental competency. Some TBI patients have also sustained focal deficits involving specific cognitive abilities or sensory or motor dysfunctions as a result of events peculiar to their injury (e.g., a penetrating skull fracture, a subdural hemorrhage). In these latter cases, when an area of cognitive deficiency is identified the examiner must then conduct an intensive evaluation of the impaired function and related abilities so that the full range of deficits is known.

## Some Specific Assessment Problems Presented by TBI Patients

*Identifying the Nature of Apparent Learning Problems.* The experience of defective memory due to either retrieval problems or attentional deficits probably accounts for most TBI patient complaints of poor memory when the memory system is essentially intact. Most of these patients have sustained only a mild or at worst a moderate degree of brain damage. A third apparent learning problem can be seen in some moderately to severely injured patients who learn effectively but *it does not occur to them* to retrieve the stored information because of compromised executive functions associated with frontal lobe damage. When these patients have also sustained damage to the memory system, this retrieval problem further compounds the primary memory defects. The determination of whether apparent memory problems are due to problems of frontal dysfunction such as inertia or inability "to remember to remember," typically relies on cuing techniques when the patient has failed to make an appropriate response.

*Misinterpretations of Organically Based Emotional and Behavioral Disorders.* The organically based emotional and behavioral disorders presented by TBI patients can be misinterpreted as psychiatric conditions by naive examiners. The nature of the apathy and anergia associated with very severe frontal damage is almost always quite evident. Diagnostic problems are likely to occur with less severely impaired patients who can carry out routine and habitual activities with little or no prompting, and who may seem reasonably bright and competent in a formal psychometric examination, yet who no longer enter spontaneously into non-routine vocational, leisure, or household activities. The most usual diagnostic error made about these patients is to call them depressed. They may then be treated for depression with little success when what they need is a rehabilitation program which includes counseling help for the family. Patients with mildly compromised motivational and affective capacity who are able to continue working at a familiar job but who no longer initiate new activities, or even old ones that are not routine (such as planning a family outing or an evening at the theatre), are also liable to be misdiagnosed, often as depressed; sometimes they are called lazy or "unmotivated" (which latter label is true, but not in the usual psychiatric or common parlance sense).

TBI patients whose injuries compromised capacities for self-control and appropriate social inhibitions may be misdiagnosed as having a character disorder such as sociopathy. This is particularly likely to happen with young patients whose reckless behavior resulted in their head injury, but whose present impulsivity or temper outbursts are more symptoms of the brain damage than an immature or poorly formed personality. Of course, premorbid predispositions to wild or acting-out behavior will exacerbate their organically based disorder. However, even disinhibited or tantrum-prone persons with premorbid histories of being well-socialized may be tagged with a psychiatrically biased label rather than understood and treated as TBI patients.

Evidence of executive dysfunction in the neuropsychological examination can bring attention to the organic basis of the TBI patient's disordered behavior. Evaluation of the executive functions through testing and diagnostic interviews will help clarify the nature of the disorder and thus contribute to a rational rehabilitation program, and to providing the family with a realistic appreciation of the patient's problems.

*Misinterpretations of Appropriate Patient Reactions to the Experiences of Mental Inefficiency with Mild TBI.* The attentional deficits associated with the slowed mental processing resulting from diffuse damage are experienced by many patients as mental dullness and susceptibility to confusion. In the first few months after a mild concussion, many patients (of whom few were informed that they might have some mental changes) become anxious and depressed due to the unexpected mental inefficiency and accompanying fatigue and heightened irritability. This response pattern may be mistaken for a neurotic personality disorder or for depression, and then inappropriately treated.

In time many of these patients acquire techniques to compensate for their mental inefficiency. Many also undergo a change in what had been their normal activity patterns because of inability to cope with high levels of stimulation, avoiding, for example, noisy restaurants or taverns, large social gatherings, shopping in crowded malls or supermarkets. Some engage in a general social withdrawal because of their problems in conversing with more than one person at a time, or their feelings of confusion when overstimulated. Many mild TBI patients develop compulsive behaviors, such as checking and rechecking themselves for accuracy, or working out rigid systems for putting things away.

This became evident in the response patterns to an inventory of symptoms of emotional/behavioral disturbances (the Symptom Check List-90 [SCL-90]: Derogatis 1983) of 58 TBI patients with injuries of mild to moderate severity (i.e., all were ambulatory, none were living in care facilities, most were working or managing households. Of the 44 patients with available records, 21 had no or questionable loss of consciousness [LOC], and LOC duration for 11 was less than an hour, making a total of 73% meeting one common criterion for mild TBI [Alves and Jane 1985; Bond 1986]. Of the remaining 12 patients with available records, LOC duration for 5 was less than a week and 7 had LOC durations from 1 to 6 weeks). All but 8 had been injured a year or more before taking the SCL-90. Forty-two patients (72%) received T-scores in the clinical range ≥70) on one or more of the nine clinical scales. Of the three scales on which each patient scored highest, 39 patients (93%) had reported an abnormal number of symptoms on the Obsessive/Compulsive scale; 50% described themselves as depressed; and 12 (29%) acknowledged symptoms on the Interpersonal Sensitivity (IPS) scale. Moreover, of the 16 patients whose symptom acknowledgements did not reach T-scores of 70 or more, 11 had one or more scale T-scores in the 60–69 range; for 10 of them, the Obsessive/Compulsive Scale was among the top three; Depression and Interpersonal Sensitivity were in the 60–69 T-score range for the eleventh. Thus, whether suffering mild symptoms of emotional distress or more severe ones, almost all these TBI patients reported an abnormal number of obsessive-compulsive traits such as being "Worried about sloppiness or carelessness," "Feeling blocked in getting things done," and "Having to do things very slowly to insure correctness"; behaviors and concerns that reflect both experiences of mental inefficiency and compensatory techniques.

Superficially these behaviors may appear abnormal and the patient in need of psychotherapy or psychiatric intervention for an emotional disturbance or stress reaction. When the presence of attentional deficits can be demonstrated by a neuropsychological examination, then the newly emerged behaviors can be understood in a meaningful context and supported as useful means of coping with mental inefficiencies rather than as psychiatric symptoms that should be rooted out.

## The Role of Neuropsychological Assessment in the Diagnosis and Treatment of TBI Patients

Sensitive neuropsychological assessment is necessary for the understanding and treatment of many different aspects of TBI patients's cognitive, emotional, and behavioral problems. Information derived from neuropsychological assessment is a prerequisite for good rehabilitation work. It can be used to facilitate the patient's self-understanding and to aid with family relationship and management problems. It should provide the foundation for planning for the patient's future after rehabilitation work has been completed.

## References

Adams JH, Graham DI, Gennarelli TA (1985) Contemporary neuropathological considerations regarding brain damage in head injury. In: Becker DP, Povlishock JT (eds) Central nervous system trauma status report. National Institute of Neurological and Communicative Disorders and Stroke, National Institutes of Health, Public Health Service, Washington, pp 65–78

Alves WM, Jane JA (1985) Mild brain injury: damage and outcome. In: Becker DP, Povlishock JR (eds) Central nervous system trauma status report. National Institute of Neurological and Communicative Disorders and Stroke, National Institutes of Health, Public Health Service, Washington, pp 255–270

Bond M (1984) The psychiatry of closed head injury. In: Brooks DN (ed) Closed head injury. Oxford University Press, New York, pp 148–178

Bond M (1986) Neurobehavioral sequelae of closed head injury. In: Grant I, Adams KM (eds) Neuropsychological assessment of neuropsychiatric disorders. Oxford University Press, New York, pp 347–373

Brooks DN (1989) Closed head trauma: assessing the common cognitive problems. In: Lezak M (ed) Assessment of the behavioral consequences of head injury. Liss, New York

Derogatis LR (1983) SCL-90-R: manual-II. Clinical Psychometric Research, Towson, Maryland

Eisenberg HM, Levin HS (1989) Computed tomography and magnetic resonance imaging in mild to moderate head injury. In: Levin HS, Eisenberg HM, Benton AL (eds) Mild head injury. Oxford University Press, New York, pp 133–141

Goodglass H (1980) Disorders of naming following brain injury. Am Sci 68:647–655

Gronwall D (1989) Cumulative and persisting effects of concussion on attention and cognition. In: Levin HS, Eisenberg HM, Benton AL (eds) Mild head injury. Oxford University Press, New York, pp 153–162

Kay T (1986) Minor head injury: introduction for professionals. National Head Injury Foundation, Framingham, Massachusetts

Levin HS, Benton AL, Grossman RG (1982) Neurobehavioral consequences of closed head injury. Oxford University Press, New York

Lezak MD (1983) Neuropsychological assessment, 2nd edn. Oxford University Press, New York

Lezak MD (1987) Assessment for rehabilitation planning. In: Meier MJ, Benton AL, Diller L (eds) Neuropsychological rehabilitation. Churchill Livingstone, New York, pp 41–58

Lezak MD (1989) Assessing the psychosocial dysfunctions resulting from head trauma. In: Lezak MD (ed) Assessment of the behavioral consequences of head injury. Liss, New York

Pang D (1989) Physics and pathophysiology of closed head injury. In: Lezak MD (ed) Assessment of the behavioral consequences of head injury. Liss, New York

Rimel RW, Giordani B, Barth JT et al. (1981) Disability caused by a minor head injury. Neurosurgery 9:221–228

Rutherford WH (1989) Postconcussion symptoms: relationship to acute neurological indices, individual differences, and circumstances of injury. In: Levin HS, Eisenberg HM, Benton AL (eds) Mild head injury. Oxford University Press, New York, pp 217–228

Stuss DT, Ely P, Hugenholtz H (1985) Neurosurgery 17:41–47

Teasdale G, Mendelow D (1984) Pathophysiology of head injuries. In: Brooks DN (ed) Closed head injury. Oxford University Press, New York, pp 4–36

Walsh KW (1985) Understanding brain damage. Churchill Livingstone, Edinburgh

Wood RL (1984) Behavior disorders following severe brain injury: their presentation and psychological management. In: Brooks DN (ed) Closed head injury. Oxford University Press, New York, pp 195–219

# The Amsterdam – Nijmegen Everyday Language Test (ANELT)

*L. Blomert*

## Introduction

One of the main interests of scientific research in the pathology of language is to analyse language problems in terms of possible linguistic disturbances. Diagnostic investigation of the aphasic patient aims at an estimation of the language deficit, i.e., which modality is disturbed and how severely. This gives an impression of a patient's formal linguistic deficit, but it is not possible to evaluate how successfully an aphasic individual can use these more or less limited linguistic resources in verbal communication. Standard measures, therefore, do not account for the functional dimension of performance (Sarno 1984; Ulatowska et al. 1983).

Knowledge about these pragmatic aspects of language behaviour of aphasic patients is theoretically relevant for several reasons. First and foremost, it can reveal something about the nature and processes involved in what we call "verbal communication". Secondly, it possibly can give insight into the nature and processes involved in the time course of recovery processes. Independent of these theoretical interests, it is of the utmost importance to establish how well a patient can get along in communicative situations in daily living. Therefore, a test was developed to measure verbal communicative behavior in aphasics.

A description of the first test version and the results of the pilot research were reported in Blomert et al. (1987). Since then, the test underwent several fundamental changes; the definite test version. The Amsterdam – Nijmegen Everyday Language Test (ANELT) has now been standardized on a sample of 125 Dutch patients (Blomert et al. 1988).

## Construction Principles of the Amsterdam – Nijmegen Everyday Language Test

The theoretical construct "verbal communication" has been defined as follows (Guttman 1981):

"Verbal communication is a function of the understandability of the message and the intelligibility of the utterance and for each facet five levels of ability are defined ranging from very badly to very well."

This description leads to two rating scales for the defined facets of verbal communication:

*Scale A: Understandability of the message*
*Scale B: Intelligibility of the utterance*

(intelligibility is judged of the utterance per se independent of the meaning of the utterance).

The response of a patient for each item is thus rated on two 5-point scales. The verbal communicative ability level is expressed in the total score for Scale A. and B.

The test consists of two parallel versions, thus providing an excellent research tool for the scientist as well as for the therapist to evaluate different aspects of recovery processes. Each parallel test consists of ten items and takes about 15 min to administer. Because the ANELT is specifically designed to measure verbal communicative skills, the test items are constructed as scenarios of familiar daily life situations, e.g., calling a doctor or talking to a sales clerk. These situations have a strong conventional character and a well-defined structure. Each situation involves two persons, the tester and the patient. The tester explains the situation to the patient, who then responds. The testing is such that the patient is the one who must do the talking: the tester is the interested listener. In this way, it is possible to have a short communicative situation which has a realistic quality and is still basically a monologue. A complete description of the ANELT is given in Blomert et al. (in preparation).

Testing normal control subjects showed that for every scenario all subjects had a maximum or nearly maximum score for both facets. The homogeneous and highly consistent results imply that an absolute criterion has been established for measuring deviations in verbal communicative behaviour. Every score less than maximum is indicative of disturbances in verbal communicative abilities.

## German Adaptation of the ANELT

In cooperation with the Neuropsychology Department of the Bezirkskrankenhaus in Erlangen, FRG, a preliminary German adaptation of the ANELT has been established. Counting on cultural and linguistic similarities, it was expected that only a few items had to be replaced or adapted.

The script-like character of the items and the very homogeneous responses of the Dutch control subjects formed another rationale for this expectation. First, a translation of the Dutch items was made. It was possible to provide a translation that hardly deviates from the Dutch version. Second, a pilot study with 15 normal subjects showed that 18 scenarios presented no problems for German subjects and were recognised as common daily-life situations. Although only two scenarios had to be adapted, this could be done without changing the nature of the script underlying the situation. A preliminary analysis of the normal controls show them to be very homogeneous and that they do not seem to deviate much from the Dutch controls.

Because of the unique scaling properties found for both facets on a Dutch aphasic population (par. 6), it can be predicted that the sample needed for the German standardization probably can be kept relatively small.

## Standardization of the ANELT–Dutch Version

The sample consisted of 125 patients, 58% male, 42% female, median age: 60 (range 20–85). A description of the sample shows that all main syndromes are sufficiently represented. All patients were also tested with the Aachen Aphasia Test and were classified according to AAT-criteria (Huber et al. 1984). Furthermore, a reasonable distribution of severity of aphasia (Token Test performance) was found for every syndrome.

## Reliability Measures

### Internal Consistency

As an estimation of the internal consistency of the test, Cronbach's alpha was calculated over items for the results of 125 patients (see Table 1).

### Stability over Time

To study stability over time, 30 patients were selected and tested in a test-retest paradigm with an interval of three months. These were chronic patients having suffered a cerebrovascular insult. On the basis of the Aachener Aphasia Test (Huber et al. 1984), patients were classified according to syndromes. All main aphasic syndromes were represented in the sample.

To estimate test stability, Product Moment Correlations (PMC) were calculated over total test scores of the patients for Scale A and Scale B of the test

**Table 1.** Summary of reliability measures

| Reliability measures | Test | Scales | | | |
|---|---|---|---|---|---|
| | | A1 | A2 | B1 | B2 |
| Consistency | Alpha | 0.94 | 0.93 | 0.96 | 0.97 |
| Stability | PMC | 0.75 | 0.84 | 0.69 | 0.75 |

PMC, Product Moment Correlations

**Table 2.** Interjudge reliability

| Scale | Median (PMC) | Min. (PMC) | Max. (PMC) |
|---|---|---|---|
| A | 0.87 | 0.66 | 0.95 |
| B | 0.67 | 0.45 | 0.84 |

and retest. To test if stability could be verified on item level, mean item scores for both scales of the test and retest were compared. None of the comparisons was significant.

### Interjudge Reliability

As a third reliability measure, agreement among judges was calculated. Six judges scored 15 different patients each. Agreement among judges is expressed in PMC's for Scale A and Scale B (see Table 2). Not only did judges agree strongly in rating patterns, they also did not differ in rating level.

### Conclusion

Reliability measures for both parallel versions were very satisfactory. The ANELT fulfills the strict reliability criteria a test for individual diagnosis has to meet.

## Ecological Validity

An assumption underlying the ANELT is that the scoring pattern of a given patient is an index of his/her verbal communicative abilities. Therefore, the ecological validity of the construct "Verbal Communication" has to be established.

A validity study was carried out to test whether naive subjects are capable of rank ordering patients on the defined facets of verbal communication. The question then is: If they are able to rank order the patients systematically, does their judgement reflect the score pattern given by trained judges on the same facets?

In this study, naive subjects were shown part of the video-recorded test sessions. The video films were edited in such a way that they only saw the patient's responses.

The tester gave the subject the necessary background information for understanding the scenario context in which the patient was acting. This scenario context gives the subject a realistic perspective on the range of possible reactions. At the same time, the precise nature of the message the patient has to communicate is not revealed to the subject. After viewing each response, the subject was asked to judge the response on the two defined facets of verbal communication.

Sixty-four subjects participated, and 16 patients were selected. Every subject judged two different patients in two different sessions, providing eight observations per patient. Items and patients were completely counterbalanced across subjects.

### Results

PMC's were calculated between the scores of a given patient for Scale A and B by a trained judge and the mean scores by the naive subjects. The correlation for Scale A = 0.89 and for Scale B = 0.60. This result shows that experts judge patients in much the same way as normal subjects do.

### Conclusion

The ecological validity of the construct "verbal communication" as defined here is quite satisfying. Naive subjects can judge the verbal communicative behaviour of aphasic patients in a systematic and precise manner.

## Differences in the Level of Verbal Communicative Abilities for Different Aphasia Syndromes

To test for differences in verbal communicative ability among main syndromes, results were analysed in a multi-variate design (MANOVA). Group effects were significant for both scales, and this was true for both parallel versions (see Tables 3, 4). Post hoc comparisons: T-tests for dependent samples corrected for unequal variances.

### Conclusion

It is evident from these results that different aphasia types can be rank ordered on both scales for verbal communicative ability. According to formal linguistic criteria, one would expect a difference between the main syndromes.

However, it is interesting to note that, according to verbal communicative criteria, globals and Wernickes do not differ as far as *understandability* is concerned, and Brocas and Wernickes do not differ as far as *intelligibility* is concerned. All remaining comparisons were significant.

**Table 3.** Significance for Scale A

| | Broca | Wernicke | Anomic |
|---|---|---|---|
| Global | ** | NS | ** |
| Broca | | ** | * |
| Wernicke | | | ** |

*, 0.05; **, 0.001; NS, not significant

**Table 4.** Significance for Scale B

| | Broca | Wernicke | Anomic |
|---|---|---|---|
| Global | ** | * | ** |
| Broca | | NS | ** |
| Wernicke | | | ** |

*, 0.005; **, 0.001; NS, not significant

## Norm Construction

The construction of the norm scales led to a rather unique finding in neuropsychological test research: The scales measuring verbal communication can be interpreted as having psychometrical properties of scales at interval level, independent of sample characteristics. This was due to the fact that a nearly perfect linear fit was found between the raw scores and the cumulative frequency of patients having at least a given scale score. Based on this unique property, scale scores can be directly interpreted as norm scores.

Secondly, it could be shown that the norm scales are not biased to biographical characteristics, like age and sex.

## Conclusions and Future Research

First, it can be concluded that it is possible to measure verbal communicative abilities in a systematic way. Standardization results of the Amsterdam–Nijmegen Everyday Language Test (ANELT) have shown that this can be done in a reliable manner and on valid grounds.

From the literature, as well as from clinical experience, it is clear that recovery of language functions takes place, presumably in the first year post onset (Kean 1985; Prins 1987). Furthermore, there is sufficient evidence that aphasia tests measuring formal linguistic aspects do not adequately assess these changes in functional language recovery (Sarno 1984). Therefore, it seems worthwhile to measure recovery in terms of verbal communicative abilities.

Because the ANELT differentiates very well between individual patients, the expectation is warranted that the test is sensitive to changes over time.

In a longitudinal study (just started), the sensitivity of the ANELT for changes over time will be evaluated in the framework of a systematic description of recovery functions of verbal communicative abilities for different aphasia types.

*Acknowledgement.* The ANELT was developed in collaboration with C. Koster and M-L. Kean at the Max-Planck Institute of Psycholinguistics, Nijmegen, The Netherlands. The standardization of the ANELT was supported by grant 28-1530 of the Dutch Praeventiefounds, The Hague. The German adaptation of the ANELT is being developed in collaboration with Th. R. v. Stockert and D. Buslach, Dept. of Clinical Neuropsychology and Behaviour Neurology, Bezirkskrankenhaus Erlangen, FRG.

## References

Blomert L, Koster C, von Mier H, Kean M-L (1987) Verbal communication abilities of aphasic patients: the Everyday Language Test. Aphasiology 1(6):463 – 474

Blomert L, Kean M-L, Schaap T (1988) ANTAT-Alledaagse Taalvaardigheids Test voor afasiepatienten. Final report. Praeventiefonds. The Hague

Guttman L (1981) What is not what in theory construction. In: Borg I (ed) Multidimensional data representations: whan and why. Mathesis, Michigan

Huber W, Poeck K, Willmes K (1984) The Aachen Aphasia Test. In: Rose F (ed) Progress in aphasiology, Raven, New York (Advances in Neurology, vol 42)

Kean M-L (1985) On the efficacy of therapy in aphasia: the present state of inquiry and its implications for future research. Internal report. Max Planck Institute for Psycholinguistics, Nijmegen

Prins R (1987) Afasie, classificatie, behandeling en herstell-verloop. Thesis, University of Amsterdam

Sarno MT (1984) Functional measurement in verbal impairment secondary to brain damage. In: Granger CV, Gresham GE (eds) Functional assessment in rehabilitation medicine. Williams and Wilkins, Baltimore

Ulatowska HK, Weiss Doyel A, Freedman-Stern R, Macaluso-Haynes S, North AJ (1983) Production of procedural discourse in aphasia. Brain Lang 18:315 – 341

# Discussion: Brain Damage and Rehabilitation: A Neuropsychological Approach

*J. C. Marshall*

The arguments in favour of standardized tests are reasonably obvious so I have no particular desire to argue against them. But I do have to say that I find it a little distressing that we have not so far talked very much about the kind of theoretical motivation behind any of these standardized tests; in particular, we have not explicitly tried to relate them to current views about the functional architectures of normal cognitive systems and how they can be impaired by brain damage. It is a related point that whilst, of course, we are all in favour of standardized tests, I do think that there should be a built-in obsolescence on every single screening battery that exists. I would suggest a period of ten years after which – without wishing to support the detractors of Mr Salman Rushdie – I think a test should be publicly burnt. The reason is this: After we have used a test for ten years, and after people have been doing research on and with that test for ten years, it would seem to me extremely depressing if we had not discovered enough to improve that particular test quite dramatically. I should perhaps not put this as extremely as I did in the first place. I think we actually have a choice. If we have improved the test in those ten years the earlier versions should be burned; alternatively, if we have not improved it in ten years, then we should fire the appropriate research workers and clinicians because they *ought* to have improved it in a period of ten years. Validity is never established for eternity.

The notion of reliability is even more fleeting. Yes, of course, we want a test to be reliable as a 'one-off' assessment and we want it to measure change over time reliably. It is, however, my experience that, at least in the relatively acute stages, there is very, very considerable within-patient variability from day to day or even morning to afternoon testing. I do not wish to ignore that fact. It seems to me that is actually a rather important aspect of the patients' behaviour. I should be attempting to understand this genuine variability out there in the real world of patient care. And I must be careful to distinguish such fluctuation from the spurious variability that can obtain as a function of constructing a bad test. Now, you could say "Well, alright we should only look at patients when they are stable." Yet that may be exactly the wrong line to go down if what we are interested in is rehabilitation. I assume (or at least believe) that one should start rehabilitation as soon as is practically possible and that means, in many instances at least, starting rehabilitation when the patient is indeed intrinsically very, very variable. So one thing we should work on is how to get a better grasp of what is happening to the patient at a time when the standard notion of reliability is simply inapplicable because the patient is just not like that.

Returning to the point about why do we not pay more attention to the theoretical underpinnings of our tests, we should make a firm distinction between *level* of performance 'severity' and the *shape* of performance (or 'differential diagnostic category' if you like). Surely, level versus shape does not mean anything on its own unless we understand how there could be either independence or an interaction between shape and level. Let me just give one quick example: It is very likely that many of our patients have a disorder of short-term memory. I presume that a quantitative change in short-term memory capacity ('severity') could have qualitative effects upon the *shape* of performance on other tests (of language impairment, for example). The only way, however, that we are going to discover if I'm right or wrong is by thinking about the underlying theoretical constructs that are determining both level and shape of performance. I actually have some considerable difficulty even with the very notion 'level of performance' when it is expressed not with respect to the patient's shape (profile) but rather with respect to the test times per se. The ubiquitous presence of 'double dissociations' makes it very difficult to interpret difficulty as 'item difficulty'. Again, it seems to me it is not sufficient to do our psychometrics in such a way that we merely rank order (or better) items for their 'intrinsic' difficulty. Surely, what we need to find out is why the items are ordered in such a 'difficulty level' series for a particular patient. In the long run (perhaps even the short run) this theory-based approach will be more helpful when actually designing therapies relevant to the individual patient.

With respect to the aphasias (and one or two other areas) we have at least a glimpse of theory, in the sense of functional architectures for cognition. When we turn to Dr. Lezak's paper we seem to be in a totally different ballpark. Her observations concern fascinating and vital phenomena that can all be observed clinically and that can, in some sense, be measured by test: decreased attention, emotional reactions to situations, failure to realize that you have to retrieve something, deficient drive states. Yet all these crucial phenomena that Dr. Lezak talked about have not – as far as I know – been placed within any kind of general theoretical framework within which we could understand formally the particular constellations of impairment shown by the individual patient. It does seem to me that one huge challenge for the immediate future is to try and get some shape, some pattern, to the kinds of impairment to which Dr. Lezak so forcibly drew our attention. One specific point about this which came up in the discussions and was then elaborated at great length: Like many of the questioners from the audience I was having some difficulty in understanding the difference between frontal apathy and depression, poor motivation and laziness. What is the difference between 'neurogenic' and 'psychogenic'? In terms of ordinary differential diagnosis we may know that our patient has had a closed head injury because he had been in a car crash. There may even be documented neuroradiological evidence, to say nothing of the results of the standard neurological examination. Yet I would not try *on that level* to distinguish between depression and head injury. Rather, I assume that we are all relatively strict monists and would in fact think that what is called 'depression' or 'sociopathy' in psychiatry also has an organic basis to it. And *in that sense*, it may well be that psychiatric depression is indeed frontal apathy, but frontal apathy that does not, at the moment, show up on such neuroradiological facilities as CT or MRI. I would thus hesitate to draw quite as firm a line between neurogenic and psychogenic disorder as I think Dr. Lezak is doing (and I would look long and carefully at studies of brain metabolism).

Finally, to Dr. Leo Blomert's presentation. For all our talk of the values of standardized testing it is really amazing that we have so few tests that reach out into the community in which the patient has to operate (namely the doctor, the grocer, the shoemaker etc.) and actually try to find out how the patient copes in those situations. I was interested to know the relationship between test scores on the Aachener battery and test scores on the Everyday Language Test. I think it would be extremely valuable to discuss in more detail with Leo the correlations and double-dissociations that one might see there.

And taking up a point, again made in discussion, by Dr. Claus Wallesch. I think it would be pertinent to follow up the notion that he was invoking about roles and play acting. There is a difference between a role acting situation and doing it in genuine life where you *really* have to go to the market and buy the food for dinner. I presume that there must be quasi-objective ways in which we could indeed follow our patients around to the market and see if they do come home with the fish and vegetables; that would provide a nice control – in a sense the ultimate control – on the validity of play acting situation in both diagnosis and therapy. And now genuinely in conclusion: Since Leo has brought the current topic up with respect to language performance: Why is it that – correct me if I'm wrong – we have so few tests that are remotely realistic for other important domains of cognitive processing? What do we actually know about how our apraxic patients perform in the home (with the can-opener) as opposed to on the test battery. What do we know about how our agnosic patients recognize knives and forks in the home as opposed to on the test battery? Leo's presentation should open our eyes to the desirability, indeed the necessity, of constructing equivalent tests for domains of cognitive functioning other than language. Thank you.

# Various Approaches for Treatment

# Early Treatment of Stroke in Man

*C. Fieschi, C. Argentino, C. Pozzilli, M. Rasura, C. Buttinelli, C. Gasperini, and M. Frontoni*

According to data from the Rochester study, both stroke incidence and mortality had declined more than 50%, and long-term survival had improved over 70% from 1945–1949 to 1970–1974 (Whisnant 1983). However, no change in survival up to three days and a very slight decrease of the 30-day death rate were recorded in the same years (Garraway et al. 1979, 1983). In other words, prevention of cerebral infarction and care for associated diseases have been increasingly effective through the past three decades, whereas stroke mortality in the acute phase has not significantly changed. Moreover, data pertaining to the same population are consistent with the end of the decline in the incidence of stroke in the early 1980s (Broderick et al. 1989).

Therefore, while prevention still remains a main goal of research, new guidelines for treatment of acute brain ischemia are also needed.

Critically evaluating the failure of traditional trials of medical therapy, a few years ago Caplan and Stein (1986) hypothesized that it could be basically related to an inhomogeneous grouping of patients. In fact, published studies had always been planned without considering the peculiar and different pathophysiological problems underlying analogous clinical events.

In the same period, studies on animal models indicated the presence and limits of a possible therapeutic window: early revascularization (within 4–8 h after the experimental occlusion) was demonstrated as necessary to minimize the ischemic damage (Plum 1986; Weinstein et al. 1986).

Functional studies on cerebral blood flow in cerebral ischemia, made possible on humans by PET and SPECT, have demonstrated the existence of an area of ischemic "penumbra" located around the infarcted area, in which an increased extraction of nutrients partially balances the decrease of blood supply (Burke et al. 1986; Lenzi et al. 1982; Vorstrup et al. 1986; Wise et al. 1983). Over a limited period of time, neurons in that area can be maintained in a state of functional deficit liable to complete recovery if the blood flow is promptly restored (Lenzi et al. 1981). Therefore, a counterpart of the experimentally demonstrated therapeutic window does exist, even if its limits still remain to be clearly defined (Fieschi et al. 1988).

Considering the above-mentioned criticisms of previous trials as well as more recent experimental knowledge, one can conclude that a modern study on pharmacological treatment of acute ischemic stroke should be carried out on the basis of early clinical observation and thorough evaluation. Both the limits of the therapeutic window and the specific pathophysiological correlates which "functional" studies (PET and SPECT) can provide should be taken into account. Furthermore, the perfusion state should be studied with neuroimaging techniques as soon as possible after the onset of cerebral ischemia. Monitoring by means of noninvasive exams, possibly supported by angiography, is also advisable since the role of collateral circulation is fundamental in the evolution of ischemic damage (Bozzao et al. 1989).

Indeed, when hypoperfusion lasts long enough to cause ischemia, tissue damage may be reasonably minimized only if "good" collateral circulation takes place very soon.

With these guidelines, a study was undertaken in which all patients admitted to the emergency room were promptly examined by a neurologist (Fieschi et al. 1989).

As soon as a diagnosis of probable focal cerebral ischemia was established, the patient was considered as eligible. Subjects older than 80 years of age, patients in coma or evaluated later than 4 h after the onset of their symptoms, and those with subtentorial clinical findings, previous ischemic stroke, other invalidating diseases, or regression of symptoms within the recruitment period were excluded.

Eligible patients had immediate brain CT scan to rule out any further cause of exclusion, like hemorrhages, tumors, or other conditions mimicking stroke.

The patients thus selected underwent a complete evaluation including: neurological and cardiovascular history and examination, pertinent laboratory tests; 12-lead EKG, grading of neurological deficit according to the Canadian Neurological Scale transcranial and neck vessel Doppler sonography and Digital Subtraction Angiography of the cerebral arteries. An assessment of cerebral blood flow was also obtained in 32 patients using $Tc^{99m}$-PAO as tracer and SPECT technique.

Further exams were performed over the 30-day follow-up period, including repeated head CT scan and daily monitoring of angiographically documented intracranial occlusions by Transcranial Doppler (TCD).

Patients with angiographically documented occlusion of the internal or middle cerebral artery were considered to have good collateral circulation only if the vessels distal to the occlusion were fully visualized within 5 s after the end of contrast injection.

Eighty out of 417 consecutively observed patients (19% of the eligible patients) were included in the study and prospectively followed.

CT scan was performed within an average of 3 h and angiography within 4 h following the onset of symptoms, with a maximum delay of 6 h.

Eighty-four percent of the patients had a normal CT head scan on admission; 9% showed an early congruous hypodensity, and 6%, indirect signs of focal brain edema.

In 8 cases (10%), the angiogram was normal, and in 11 (14%), it showed an isolated plaque at the origin of the ICA. The remaining 61 patients (76%) had complete occlusive arterial disease.

The patency of the intracranial arteries was monitored during follow up with TCD in patients with MCA mainstem occlusion, 8 of whom had repeated angiography. An overall correlation between TCD and angiography was demonstrated in 90% of MCA mainstem occlusions (Zanette et al. 1989).

Reperfusion occurred within 24 h in four and within a week in seven additional patients. None of these patients showed significant improvement following recanalization, and, remarkably, patients with documented intracranial occlusion and poor or absent collateral filling at early angiography had the worst clinical outcome.

The presence of a good collateral supply was correlated to a lesser degree of both interhemispheric and regional asymmetry index at SPECT. This neuroimaging technique could prove useful to differentiate subgroups of stroke patients according to the severity of both clinical progression and tissue damage. It could also be able to demonstrate an early perfusional deficit when CT scan was still negative.

Complete arterial occlusions in the symptomatic arteries, possibly embolic in nature and spontaneously reversible, were frequent (66%). This confirms other results from studies on early angiography in patients with cerebrovascular insult (Dalal 1965; Fieschi and Bozzao 1969), and, in contrast to previous data in less acute patients, indicates a strong prevalence of atherosclerotic extracranial carotid lesions in ischemic stroke (Bauer et al. 1962; Fields et al. 1968; Gurdjian et al. 1961).

The incidence of embolism reported in our series also exceeds the 40% of the Harvard Stroke Registry (Mohr et al. 1978) and the 50% of an autopsy study (Fisher 1954).

The interval from the onset of stroke may provide an explanation for these differences: the shorter the latency, the higher the probability of detecting a complete occlusion.

If this is true, embolic cerebral ischemia is much more common than we previously believed. These data and the results obtained with fibrinolytics in myocardial infarction (Gissi 1986, 1987) strongly support the interest in studies with kineases and r-TPA (Sloan 1987; TPA-Acute Stroke Study Group 1988).

In terms of therapeutic management, the administration of streptokinase and urokinase involves a significant risk of hemorrhagic complications because of their systemic anticoagulant action. Selective thrombolysis, due to higher affinity with fibrin-bound than with free plasminogen, may encourage the use of r-TPA or r-prourokinase in new trials. Identifying the subgroup of stroke patients suitable for fibrinolytic treatment might just represent the right attempt to exploit a therapeutic window of partially reversible ischemic damage to achieve the prompt regional perfusion essential for good recovery.

Vasodilating agents have been used with the same goal. Nimodipine, a calcium-channel blocker, limited ischemic damage by improving CBF in animals after MCA occlusion (Mohamed et al. 1985) and produced interesting results in the clinical trial of Gelmers et al. (1988). Recently, CBF measurement by SPECT in patients treated with Nimodipine within 6 h from onset has demonstrated an increased flow at the periphery of the ischemic area (Pozzilli et al. 1989).

Over the past few years, research on the pathogenesis of irreversible ischemic brain damage has shown that an increase in the intracellular calcium concentration may induce important metabolic disturbances. Calcium dependent proteases and the activation of phospholipases with the consequent release of toxic products appears responsible for cytoskeletal disruption (Siesjo 1981).

Calcium antagonists, with their properties of Ca-influx modulators, can therefore play a further role in protection against cerebral ischemia in addition to perfusional increase. Current research on animals focuses on newer calcium entry blockers with particular characteristics, as Nilvadipine (Kuwaki et al. 1989) and Emopamil (Nakayama et al. 1988) to be potentially evaluāted in future clinical trials.

The mainstream of brain protection, however, also takes into account knowledge on the role of neuromodulators like glutamate, whose accumulation in the ischemic area is believed to be responsible for neurotoxicity. A specific glutamatergic receptor activated by N-methyl-D-aspartate (NMDA) is linked to an excessive Ca-influx; thus, blocking the receptor with competitive and non-competitive NMDA-antagonists should be attempted in experimental studies.

Membrane failure is also a major phenomenon characterizing irreversible ischemic injury (Astrup 1982). Gangliosides, which interact with cerebral membranes by various metabolic processes (Davis and Daly 1980; Leon et al. 1981), have been tested in animals for their possible protection in the acute phase (Greenberg et al. 1986).

Moreover, considering the recently demonstrated existence of growth factors stimulating CNS plasticity (Freed et al. 1985), gangliosides have been also considered in the enhancement of neuronal "regeneration" (Doherty et al. 1985).

On the basis of these data, an international multicentric study on early treatment of ischemic stroke with monosialoganglioside (GMI) has been undertaken in six European countries and the USA. Up to July 1989, the stroke registry has reported over 7000 patients, 680 of whom were eligible (9.6%) and 659, randomly treated.

In conclusion, carefully planning a study on pharmacological treatment for acute ischemic stroke is certainly a difficult task. It is necessary to be aware of logistical problems which can be solved only in highly qualified centers offering different facilities, such as a neuro intensive care unit, neuroradiology, nuclear medicine, and Doppler sonography, have to work in a well-organized, cooperative system.

We strongly feel that the prospective of successfully dealing with a disease which ranks third among causes of death in industrialized countries and is the prime cause of severe disability is definitely worth the effort involved.

However, only well-designed, protected, and sufficiently extensive trials will provide clinically reliable and convincing evidence.

## References

Astrup J (1982) Energy-requiring cell functions in the ischemic brain. J Neurosurg 56:482–497

Bauer RB, Sheean S, Wechsler N, Meyer JS (1962) Arteriographic study of sites, incidence, and treatment of arteriosclerotic cerebrovascular lesion. Neurology (Minneap) 12:698–711

Bozzao L, Fantozzi LM, Bastianello S, Bozzao A, Fieschi C (1989) Early collateral blood supply and late parenchymal brain damage in patients with middle cerebral artery occlusion. Stroke 20:735–740

Broderick JP, Phillips SJ, Whisnant JP, O'Fallon WM, Bergstralh EJ (1989) Incidence rate of stroke in the eighties: the end of the decline of stroke? Stroke 20:577–588

Burke AM, Younkin D, Gordon J, Goldberg H, Graham T, Kushner M, Obrist W, Jaygi J, Rosen M, Reivich M (1986) Stroke 17:173–178

Caplan LR, Stein RW (1986) Stroke. A clinical approach. Butterworth, London

Dalal PM (1965) Angiographic observation on spontaneous clot lysis. Lancet 1:61–64

Davis CW, Daly JW (1980) Activation of rat cerebral cortical 3′,5′-cyclic nucleotide phosphodiesterase activity by gangliosides. Mol Pharmacol 17:206–211

Doherty P, Dickson JG, Flanigan TP, Walsh FS (1985) Ganglioside GM1 does not initiate, but enhances neurite regeneration of nerve growth-factor-dependent sensory neurones. J Neurochem 44:1259–1265

Fields WS, North RR, Hass WK, Galbraith JG, Wylie EJ, Ratinov G, Burns MH, Macdonald MC, Meyer JC (1968) Joint study of extracranial arterial occlusion as a cause of stroke. I. Organization of study and survery of patient population. JAMA 203:153–158

Fieschi C, Bozzao L (1969) Transient embolic occlusion of the middle cerebral artery and internal carotid arteries in cerebral apoplexy. J Neurol Neurosurg Psychiatry 32:236–240

Fieschi C, Argentino C, Lenzi GL, Fantozzi L, Sacchetti ML, Pace A, Rasura M, Bastianello S, Bozzao L, Zanette E, Buttinelli C, Giubilei F, Pantano P (1988) Therapeutic window for pharmacological treatment in acute focal cerebral ischemia. Ann NY Acad Sci 522:662–666

Fieschi C, Argentino C, Lenzi GL, Sacchetti ML, Toni D, Bozzao L (1989) Clinical and instrumental evaluation of patients with ischemic stroke within the first six hours. J Neurol Sci 91:311–322

Fisher M (1954) Occlusion of the carotid arteries. Further experiences. Arch Neurol Psychiatry 72:187–204

Freed WJ, de Medinaceli L, Wyatt RJ (1985) Promoting functional plasticity in the damaged nervous system. Science 227:1544–1552

Garraway WM, Whisnant JH, Furlan AJ, Phillips LH, Kurland LT, O'Fallon WM (1979) The declining incidence of stroke. N Engl J Med 300:449–452

Garraway WM, Whisnant JP, Drury I (1983) The changing pattern of survival following stroke. Stroke 14:699–702

Gelmers HJ, Gorter K, de Weerdt CJ, Wiezer HJA (1988) A controlled trial of nimodipine in acute ischemic stroke. N Engl J Med 318:203–207

GISSI (1986) Effectiveness of intravenous thrombolytic treatment in acute myocardial infarction. Lancet 1:397–402

GISSI (1987) Long-term effects of intravenous thrombolysis in acute myocardial infarction: final report. Lancet 1:871–874

Greenberg JH, Reivich M, Urbanics R, Tanaka K, Dora E, Toffano G (1986) The effect of GM1 on cerebral metabolism, microcirculation and histology in focal ischemia. In: Tettamanti G, Ledeen RW, Sadhoff K, Nagay Y, Toffano G (eds) Gangliosides and neuronal plasticity. Liviana, Padova, pp 397–405 (Fidia research series, vol 6)

Gurdjian ES, Lindner DW, Hardy WG, Thomas LM (1961) Completed stroke due to occlussive cerebrovascular disease. An analysis of 409 cases. Neurology (Minneap) 11:724–733

Holmes RA, Chaplin SB, Rayston FG et al. (1985) Cerebral uptake and retention of Tc-99m hexamethilpropyleneamine oxime (Tc-99m HM-PAO). Nucl Med Commun 6:443–447

Kuwaki T, Satoh H, Ono T, Shibayama F, Yamashita T, Nishimura T (1989) Nilvadipine attenuates ischemic degradation of gerbil brain cytoskeletal proteins. Stroke 20:78–83

Lenzi GLL, Frackowiack RSJ, Jones T, Heather JD, Lammertsma AA, Rhodes CG, Pozzilli C (1981) CMRO2 and CBF by oxygen-15 inhalation technique: results in normal volunteers and cerebrovascular patients. Eur Neurol 20:285–290

Lenzi GLL, Frackowiack RSJ, Jones T (1982) Cerebral oxygen metabolism and blood flow in human cerebral ischemic infarction. J Cereb Blood Flow Metab 2:321–335

Leon A, Tettamanti G, Toffano G (1981) Changes in functional properties of neuron membranes by insertion of exogenous ganglioside. In: Rapport MM, Gorio A (eds) Gangliosides in neurological and neuromuscular function, development and repair. Raven, New York, pp 45–54

Mohamed AA, Gotoh O, Graham DI, Osborne KA, McCulloch J, Mendelow AD, Teasdale GM, Harper MH (1985) Effect of pretreatment with the calcium antagonist nimodipine on local cerebral blood flow and histopathology after middle cerebral artery occlusion. Ann Neurol 18:705–711

Mohr KP, Caplan LR, Melski JW, Goldstein RJ, Duncan GW, Kistler JP, Pessin MS, Blech HL (1978) The Harvard Cooperative Stroke Registry: a prospective registry. Neurology (Minneap) 28:574–762

Nakayama H, Ginsberg MD, Dietrich WD (1988) (S)-Emopamil, a novel calcium channel blocker and serotonin S2 antagonist, markedly reduces infarct size following middle cerebral artery occlusion in the rat. Neurology 38:1667–1673

Plum F (1986) Conference closing remarks. In: Battistini N, Fiorani P, Courbier R, Plum F, Fieschi C (eds) Acute brain ischemia medical and surgical therapy. Raven, New York, pp 353–363 (Serono symposium publications, vol 32)

Pozzilli C, Di Piero V, Pantano P, Rasura M, Lenzi GL (1989) Influence of nimodipine on cerebral blood flow in human cerebral ischaemia. J Neurol 236:199–202

Siesjo BK (1981) Cell damage in the brain. A speculative synthesis. J Cereb Blood Flow Metab 1:155–185

Sloan MA (1987) Thrombolysis and stroke. Past and future. Arch Neurol 44:748–768

TPA-Acute Stroke Study Group (1988) An open multicenter study of the safety and efficacy of various doses of r-TPA in patients with acute stroke: preliminary results. Stroke 19:9

Vorstrup S, Paulson OB, Lasson NA (1986) Cerebral blood flow in acute and chronic ischemic stroke using Xenon-133 inhalation tomography. Acta Neurol Scand 74:439–451

Weinstein PR, Anderson GG, Telles DA (1986) Neurological deficit and cerebral infarction after temporary middle cerebral artery occlusion in unanesthetized cats. Stroke 17:318–324

Whisnant JP (1983) The role of the neurologist in the decline of stroke. Ann Neurol 14:1–7

Wise RSJ, Bernardi S, Frackowiack RSJ, Legg NJ, Jones T (1983) Serial observations on the pathophysiology of acute stroke. Brain 106:197–222

Zanette EM, Fieschi C, Bozzao L, Roberti C, Toni D, Argentino C, Lenzi GLL (1989) Comparison of cerebral angiography and transcerial Doppler sonography in acute stroke. Stroke 20:899–903

# Minimising Brain Damage from Head Injury by Appropriate Early Management

*B. Jennett*

## Introduction

In most Westernised countries injury is the leasing cause not only of death under the age of 45, but also of years of life lost between the ages 1 and 65 years. By these measures injury is ahead of heart disease, stroke and cancer in the UK, West Germany, France, the US and Japan. The proportion of all deaths that are due to accidents varies considerably between countries, higher in Australia and Canada than in the USA and West Germany, and less common in the UK. Road accidents account for about a half of accidental deaths in North America, Australia and West Germany but for only a third in England and Scotland. Road accident deaths per 100000 population vary from 30 in West Germany, Australia, and Canada, through 22 for the USA, to only about 15 in the UK (WHO 1987).

Head injury deaths per 100000 are about 25 for the US nationally (with considerable regional variations), 28 in Australia, 22 in France but only 9 in the UK (Jennett and Frankowski 1990). Head injuries account for only a quarter to a third of all trauma deaths, but they make up two-thirds of trauma deaths in hospital. They are by far the commonest cause of lifelong disability after trauma, at least 40 times more frequent than spinal cord injuries. Head injury admissions who survive are 10–30 times more common than all the deaths, and these are the source of those who are left with disability (Jennet and Teasdale 1992). The average age of disabled survivors is on average 27 years – and many face 40 years or more of disability.

## Brain Damage at Autopsy after Hospital Admission

Much of the permanent brain damage that affects survivors after head injury results from secondary pathophysiological processes that began after the impact damage had been sustained. Discovering the exact nature and distribution of this secondary brain damage requires careful histological examination of brains that have been in fixative for some 2–3 weeks before being cut. In most countries it has been difficult to undertake detailed neuropathological examination of traumatised brains, because of the medico-legal or forensic requirements that the fresh brain be sliced so that an immediate opinion could be given for legal purposes based on gross appearances. An agreement with the legal authorities in Glasgow has made it possible to secure for detailed dissection the brains of virtually all head injured patients dying in hospital. Neuropathological study of some 800 such brains has led to the realisation that the lesions in patients who survive to be admitted to hospital are quite different from those that have been reported by forensic pathologists on the basis of victims who died before reaching hospital (Adams and Graham 1988).

The two common types of impact damage are diffuse axonal injury in the white matter of the cerebral hemispheres and the brain stem, and cortical contusions. Secondary brain damage is usually the result of raised intracranial pressure, itself a consequence either of an acute haematoma, or of brain swelling around contusions, or of brain oedema. However, modern radiological imaging techniques and detailed neuropathological studies have revealed that brain oedema is less common and severe than was previously believed. Many patients who die in hospital have widespread ischaemic brain damage, affecting the cerebral cortex, the hippocampus, the basal ganglia and the cerebellum. Sometimes ischaemic damage is in the distribution of major cerebral arteries, in particular medial occipital infarction related to posterior cerebral occlusion as a consequence of tentorial herniation. Most of the hypoxic ischaemic damage, however, appears to be related to the combination of raised intracranial pressure and systemic hypotension and hypoxia, usually associated with extracranial injuries (Adams and Graham 1988).

The majority of these pathological studies have been on patients who died within the first week or so after injury. Of 35 patients who had survived for long periods, either in a vegetative state or with severe disability, almost two-thirds had severe diffuse axonal injury; half had ischaemic brain damage and less than a third had secondary brain stem damage (Graham et al. 1983). Combinations of these types of damage were common but secondary brain stem injury was never the only lesion. The lesson for those concerned with devising rehabilitation programmes for disabled survivors of head injury is that the damage is almost always widespread throughout the brain.

About 80% of head injuries who are admitted to hospital in the UK and US are not severely injured. Of those who reach neurosurgical units only a minority have a Glasgow Coma Score of 8 or less, and more than half are mild, as defined by a Glasgow Coma Score of 13 or more (Jennett 1988a). However, injuries that were initially only mild or moderate account for some 80% of patients with compound depressed fractures, and about half of the patients who require surgical evacuation of an acute intracranial haematoma (within 14 days of injury). Of more than 1000 patients operated on for acute intracranial haematoma in Glasgow fewer than 30% were in coma from the time of injury. More than half had talked, and a quarter had been recorded as totally lucid immediately after injury, this being twice as common in children as in adults (Miller and Teasdale 1990; Bullack and Teasdale 1990).

In 1975 we coined the phrase "head injuries who talk and die". The implication was that if an injured patient had talked then he probably should not have died – because he clearly had not sustained overwhelming impact brain damage. The aim of early management should be to prevent or minimise avoidable secondary brain damage, as reflected in the proportions of patients who talk and die, and also those who talk and deteriorate – many of whom survive with permanent brain damage. Over the years in Glasgow we have succeeded in reducing the proportions of patients who talked and deteriorated, and of those who talked and died (Miller et al. 1991). However, the mortality in those who arrive at the neurosurgical unit in coma is similar whether they have previously talked or not.

More recent American studies of patients who talked and deteriorated show a smaller proportion than in Scotland (Marshall et al. 1983; Rockswold et al. 1987). In both the Scottish and the US series acute haematomas were found in over 70% for those who talked and deteriorated, and in over 80% of those who talked and died (Jennett 1990, 1991). Many of these data were collected since the introduction of CT scanning; clearly this technology has failed to eliminate the risks of this life-threatening but potentially remediable complication. In patients who talk and in whom there is no haematoma, other pathologies found include swollen contusions, ischaemic damage, meningitis and diffuse swelling.

The risk of a haematoma is considerably greater in patients who are severely injured, but in them there is no difficulty deciding on admission and CT scanning. The real problem lies in the mild and moderate injuries, who might be sent home. There are large numbers of such injuries presenting to hospitals of whom only a very small proportion develop a haematoma. We have carried out extensive studies to develop predictive criteria to guide doctors who have to deal with this large number of less severely injured patients in general hospitals, and who must select those who are to be observed, and those to be referred for CT scanning (Teasdale et al. 1990).

The risk of a haematoma in a patient attending hospital after a head injury is about six times greater in adults than in children (<15 years). However, the risk factors are similar for children and adults, impairment of consciousness and the presence of skull fracture. In a patient who is fully conscious the presence of a skull fracture increases the risk of a haematoma by more than 100 times. That means that a skull fracture is an extremely good predictor of haematoma. In patients without a fracture impaired consciousness (short of coma) increases the risk of a haematoma by much less. On the basis of these figures we have devised guidelines to assist doctors in non-specialist units to decide which patients should be admitted and which should be referred for CT scanning or neurosurgical consultation, because of the risk of a haematoma (Group of Neurosurgeons 1984). The result of such policies has been to double the number of head injured patients who come to the regional neurosurgical unit each year, and to considerably increase the number of haematomas detected. Moreover the outcome is improved both for extradural and intradural haematomas (Bullock and Teasdale 1990). Nonetheless there is still an appreciable mortality and many disabled survivors in those who are operated on.

## Avoidable Mortality and Morbidity

Audit of the service provided for head injuries should analyse the number of patients who suffer avoidable factors in their hospital course that may have contributed to death or to increased disability in survivors. Some years ago we found that avoidable factors had occurred in some two-thirds of survivors after intracranial haematoma that had progressed to coma: in over 40% of these they had certainly contributed to the residual disability. Among those who died there was a higher incidence of avoidable factors in those who had talked than in those who were always in coma (Rose et al. 1977; Jennett and Carlin 1978).

Avoidable factors can be classified as intracranial and extracranial. Common intracranial events are delayed, inappropriate or inadequate treatment of acute intracranial haematoma, early traumatic epilepsy or of meningitis. The extracranial causes were airway obstruction, hypotension and hypoxia, and inadequate recognition and treatment of haemorrhage. Reducing the risk of complications of this kind depends on prediction and anticipation, on prevention where possible, and on early recognition and expeditious treatment when they do occur.

## Treatment of Severe Injuries

Many therapies have been devised over the last 30 years for the treatment of severe injuries, those who are already in coma. The first claim that mortality could be reduced by respiratory care and tracheostomy combined with sedative drugs and cooling were made by neurosurgeons in Newcastle-on-Tyne in England in 1958 (MacIver et al. 1958). Since then many modalities of care have been tried in intensive care units. These include steroids, hyperventilation, intracranial pressure monitoring, surgical decompression, the use of hypnotics and, most recently the use of calcium antagonists and other chemical agents. The impact of these on outcome has been very limited, when careful comparisons are made between patients whose ages and severity of injury have been well-matched (Jennett 1988 b). Few claims for improvement have stood the test of randomised controlled trials, and when the many trials of steroids were reviewed recently the claims for benefit all disappeared when a statistical correction for small numbers was applied (Todd and Teasdale 1989).

Barbiturates have been evaluated in several trials, but in the most up-to-date and largest trial, from the US Data Bank, only very modest improvement was discovered (Eisenberg et al. 1988). Perhaps the most important finding of this trial was that only 12% of 925 patients available qualified for entry to the trial. As a result the original target number of 120 had to be abandoned, and only 73 cases were randomised. These workers emphasised that this treatment was hazardous and required specially trained doctors and nurses to be always available. According to the figures in this study, the average busy unit would encounter a patient who might be eligible for treatment with barbiturates only once every 2–3 months, making it unlikely that the necessary skills for safe administration of hypnotics could be developed.

The international Data Bank of severe head injuries began in Glasgow 20 years ago, and it has been useful in indicating how much variation there is between the way severe head injuries are treated in different places, even within one country (Jennett et al. 1980; Jennett 1984). In spite of this the mortality did not vary significantly between these different places. Nor has there been any significant change in mortality over several years. In Glasgow we have considerably reduced the frequency of use of several therapies without mortality changing. It seems that the severity of injury and the age of the patient often predict what the outcome will be (Murray et al. 1986). That is not to say that intensive care is a waste of time. That a significant number of these severely injured patients become independent, making a good recovery, is a tribute to good nursing care and often to the expeditious recognition and removal of intracranial haematomas.

## Reducing Overall Mortality and Morbidity from Head Injury

It seems likely that an overall reduction in mortality and in the frequency of persisting brain damage is most likely to come from paying due attention to the less severe injuries. Striking evidence of this comes from a report this year of mortality in 41 US hospitals in nearly 8000 head injured patients (Klauber et al. 1989). As in our own studies almost 70% of the injuries were not severe; they were classified as "low risk", because the expected mortality was less than 10%. The worst hospital had 52% higher mortality than was expected, whereas the best hospital had 43% less than was expected. However, the outcome of high risk patients was hardly any greater in the worst hospital than was expected, indicating that the outcome in such cases is difficult to alter. By contrast there was a striking difference in the outcome for low risk patients in the two hospitals. In the worst hospital they were eight times *more* likely to die than was expected, and in the best hospital were nine times *less* likely to die than was expected.

There seems no doubt that the best hope for reducing the frequency of occurrence of persisting brain damage after head injuries lies in focusing more attention than hitherto on the management of less severe injuries (Jennett 1990a, b, 1991). The gradual recognition of this can be traced from the 1975 paper on head injuries who talk and die, through several other publications to this most recent comparison of hospital mortalities from the United States. How best to tackle this problem will depend on local circumstances, in particular on the number and availability of CT scanners and of neurosurgeons. Neurosurgeons should be involved in drawing up guidelines for the management of the injuries in other hospitals. They should make it clear what the risk factors are, and which cases should be referred for further observation or investigation, and under what circumstances neurosurgeons should be involved. There should be continuing audit of the detection rate of haematomas and the outcome of operating on these, using the catchment population as the denominator and not simply the number of cases admitted to the neurosurgical unit. Only in this way will it become clear whether an adequate service is being provided for the community as a whole.

## References

Adams JH, Graham DI (1988) An introduction to neuropathology. Livingstone, Edinburgh

Bullack R, Teasdale G (1990) Acute intracranial haematoma. In: Vinken PJ, Bruyn GW, Klowans HL (eds) Handbook of clinical neurology. Elsevier, Amsterdam

Graham DI, McLellan D, Adams JH et al. (1983) The neuropathology of the vegetative state and severe disability after non-missile head injury. Acta Neurochir [Suppl] (Wien) 32:65–67

Group of Neurosurgeons (1984) Guidelines for initial management after head injury in adults. Br Med J 288:983

Eisenberg HM, Frankowski RF, Constant CF et al. (1988) High-dose barbiturate control of elevated intracranial pressure in patients with severe head injury. J Neurosurg 69:15–23

Jennett B (1984) Outcome of intensive therapy for severe head injuries: an inter-center comparison. In: Parillo JE, Ayres SM (eds) Major issues in critical care medicine. Williams and Wilkins, Baltimore

Jennett B (1988a) Mild injuries: international comparisons. In: Levin H (ed) Mild head injuries. Oxford University Press, New York

Jennett B (1988b) Treatment of severe head injuries. J Int Care Med 3:284–286

Jennett B (1990a) Providing services for head injured patients and auditing their effectiveness. In: Vinken PJ, Bruyn (eds) Handbook of clinical neurology, vol 13. Elsevier, Amsterdam, pp 431–432

Jennett B (1990b) Epidemiology of severe head injury: socio-economic consequences of avoidable mortality and morbidity. In: Scriabine A, Teasdale G, Young W, Tettenborn D (eds) Nimodipine. Pharmacological and clinical results in cerebral ischemia. Springer, Berlin Heidelberg New York

Jennett B (1991) Diagnosis and management of head trauma. J Neurotrauma 8:515–519

Jennett B, Carlin J (1978) Preventable mortality and morbidity after head injury. Injury 10:31–39

Jennett B, Frankowski R (1990) Epidemiology of head injuries. In: Vinken PJ, Bruyn GW, Klowans HL (eds) Handbook of clinical neurology. Elsevier, Amsterdam

Jennett B, Teasdale G (1992) Management of head injuries, 2nd edn. Davis, Philadelphia

Jennett B, Teasdale G, Fry J et al. (1980) Treatment for severe head injury. J Neurol Neurosurg Psychiatry 43:289–295

Klauber MR, Marshall LF, Luerssen TG et al. (1989) Determinants of head injury mortality: importance of the low risk patient. Neurosurgery 24:31–36

MacIver IN, Frew JC, Matheson JG (1958) The role of respiratory insufficiency in the mortality of severe head injuries. Lancet 1:390–392

Marshall LF, Toole BM, Bowers SA (1983) The National Traumatic Coma Data Bank. II. Patients who talk and deteriorate: implications for treatment. Neurosurg 59:285–288

Murray LS (1990) Development of a traumatic intracranial haematoma after minor head injury. Neurosurgery 27

Murray GD, Murray LS, Barlow P et al. (1986) Assessing the performance and clinical impact of a computerized prognostic system in severe head injury. Stat Med 5:403–410

Rockswold GL, Leonard PR, Nagib MG (1987) Analysis of management in thirty-three closed head injury patients who "talked and deteriorated". Neurosurgery 21:51–55

Rose J, Valtonen S, Jennett B (1977) Avoidable factors contributing to death after head injury. Br Med J 2:615–618

Teasdale GM, Murray G, Anderson E et al. (1990) Risks of a traumatic intracranial haematoma in children and adults: implications for the management of head injuries. Br Med J 300:363–366

Todd NV, Teasdale GM (1989) Steroids in human head injury: clinical studies. In: Capildeo R (ed) Steroids in diseases of the central nervous system. Wiley, New York

WHO (1987) Demographic year book 1985: mortality statistics. United Nations, New York

# Cognitive Neuropsychology and Rehabilitation

*D. Howard*

## Introduction

It is now more than a hundred years since the first serious attempts at rehabilitation by a neuropsychologist. Broca described in 1865 how he attempted in daily sessions to improve the word retrieval and reading abilities of an aphasic patient. Since 1945 there has been substantial increase in formal rehabilitation particularly in Europe and North America, where a high proportion of stroke survivors now receive some formal re-education (see Howard and Hatfield 1987). Yet even now there is little agreement about which treatment methods are appropriate and effective.

Some neurologists and psychologists have even questioned whether any attempts at re-education are effective. The have wondered whether the improvements that patients show during the process of re-education might not represent the results of the (ill-understood) process of spontaneous recovery, rather than any direct result of the re-education process itself. Evidence concerning this comes from a series of randomised controlled trials of aphasia therapy. These compare the outcome for two groups of patients to which subjects are randomly assigned; one group receive formal treatment, while the second control group either receive no formal treatment or some kind of general language stimulation. Some of the trials appear to demonstrate significant effects of treatment (e.g. Wertz et al. 1988) while others find no significant differences in outcome between the treated and control groups of subjects (e.g. Lincoln et al. 1984).

In this paper I shall argue that randomised controlled trials of this kind do not address the right question. I shall argue instead that we need to investigate some much more specific questions about the effects of treatment, and I will suggest that an approach based on cognitive neuropsychological theory provides an appropriate way of addressing these questions. I shall consider briefly how theoretical accounts of patients' problems may relate to the process of therapy, and finally some examples of this approach will be outlined. These examples will be drawn from the field of aphasia therapy; this is because this is the area of neuropsychological rehabilitation that has had the most serious investigation, and where the issues have been most sharply focused. Furthermore this is the area in which the theories of cognitive neuropsychology are best developed and thus where they are most likely to be applied in treatment.

## The Case for an Effectiveness Matrix

Three simple propositions, which, when taken separately, are not controversial, can be used to demonstrate that randomised controlled trials cannot be the appropriate way to study neuropsychological therapy:

1. Patients are not homogeneous. It is universally accepted among those that study aphasia that aphasic patients do not form a qualitatively homogeneous group. That is, different patients have qualitatively different disorders of language processing. Within the Wernicke-Lichtheim model, for instance, Broca's aphasics have a primary deficit in the motor images of spoken words, while Wernicke's aphasics are impaired in auditory word images.
2. Therapy is not homogeneous. While different schools advocate different therapeutic approaches (basing these on very different views of the nature of neuropsychological therapy), they all agree that there are a number of very different kinds of things that can be done in rehabilitation.
3. Only some treatments will be appropriate for a patient of a particular type. Given that a patient has a disorder of a particular qualitative type, the effectiveness of different types of therapy will vary. Of course, for some subjects it may be the case that no discoverable kind of treatment could ever be effective; for others it may be that any kind of treatment will work irrespective of its content. But typically, for each subject with a disorder of a particular type, the different types of treatment will vary in effectiveness.

Thus one can conceive of an 'effectiveness matrix' where the treatment types ($T_1$, $T_2$ ... $T_n$) are arranged down on side, and the types of patient ($P_1$, $P_2$ ... $P_n$) are arranged along the top (see Table 1). The cells contain numbers representing how effective each particular treatment type is with each type of patient – in this example arbitrarily scaled from 1–10.

In a group study of treatment, there will be a variety of qualitatively different types of patient receiving a number of qualitatively different kinds of treatment. For each individual subject the outcome will depend on how effective the treatment s/he receives is for his/her type of impairment. Over a whole group of subjects the mean outcome will depend both on the form of the effec-

**Table 1.** Effectiveness matrix for the treatment of aphasic patients

| Treatment types | Patient types | | | | | |
|---|---|---|---|---|---|---|
| | $P_1$ | $P_2$ | $P_3$ | $P_4$ | ... | $P_n$ |
| $T_1$ | 8 | 3 | 6 | 4 | ... | 0 |
| $T_2$ | 0 | 2 | 0 | 4 | ... | 1 |
| $T_3$ | 4 | 9 | 2 | 1 | ... | 0 |
| ⋮ | ⋮ | ⋮ | ⋮ | ⋮ | ⋮ | ⋮ |
| $T_n$ | 7 | 9 | 0 | 1 | ... | 0 |

tiveness matrix and the particular treatment types applied to each individual patient type. Yet no published report of any group studies of neuropsychological therapy gives any serious detail of the exact form of therapy or the qualitative kind of the disorders that they show. Without such information such studies are simply uninterpretable. Where randomised controlled trials show significant effects of treatment, we have no way of discovering which were the effective treatments that other therapists should use with patients of the same types. Where such studies show no significant effects of treatment (for the patients as a group), we have no way of deducing which were the treatments which when applied to patients of a particular type were ineffective. Thus, such studies cannot in principle be used to improve the practice of neuropsychological rehabilitation.

Note that the argument presented here depends only on the three propositions: that patients are not qualitatively homogeneous; that treatments are not qualitatively homogeneous; and that different treatments will work with patients of different kinds. The argument was not in any way committed to a view about the particular qualitative types of impairment or types of treatment. And, in actual practice, there is very considerable disagreement about what exactly these might be. In the next section I shall discuss how one might deal with this. The argument in this section however is simple: we have to do studies of rehabilitation which will allow us to estimate how effective treatment of a particular specified kind is for a patient with a particular specified disorder. In effect such studies will allow us to start filling in the cells of an effectiveness matrix; and that matrix is the data needed to answer the clinical question that all therapists face with each of their patients: what is the most effective kind of treatment I can use for a patient with this specific kind of disorder?

## Using the Right Theory

A medical textbook typically consists of a section describing diagnosis (that is a set of procedures needed to identify a qualitatively homogeneous group of patients), a section describing therapy (that is a set of possible treatment procedures), and a section on prognosis (that is information about the effectiveness of the various treatment procedures). Note that diagnosis typically consists of identifying the category a patient falls into where that category is homogeneous with respect to treatment. As a result we can only know what the categories are when we know what the treatment outcomes are; the result, historically has been a bootstrap process: diagnosis becomes more precise and differentiated as the treatment methods are developed which are able to make use of the distinctions that the diagnostic procedures can draw. That is, there is no point in making a differential diagnosis any more precise than will make a difference to the outcome of treatment.

In terms of neuropsychological rehabilitation, this presents a problem. We do not know in advance which aspects of a patient's pattern of impairment will be relevant to the outcome of treatment. There remains very little agreement about whether one can identify qualitatively homogeneous groups of subjects.

Modern adherents of the Wernicke-Lichtheim school (e.g. Goodglass and Kaplan 1972) tend to study groups of subjects defined in terms of diagnostic categories as if they were homogeneous groups – that is, each patient in a group has the same underlying disorder that differs only in severity. The assumption that such diagnostic groups are homogeneous has recently been widely challenged (e.g. Caramazza 1984; Ellis 1987; Shallice 1989) in two different ways. The empirical challenge comes from the demonstration that there are qualitative differences in the type of impairment between patients who fall within a single diagnostic group. The theoretical challenge has come from authors who have argued that the patients' underlying impairments are unknown a priori; it is not therefore permissible to argue that patients should be grouped together.

If there are no widely accepted diagnoses, how can we do studies of treatment? Clearly we cannot simply describe our subject as say a 'Broca's aphasic'. In ten years time, the category may no longer be accepted, or it may be subdivided into five varieties, or the meaning of 'Broca's aphasia' may change. Diagnostic labels are creatures of their time, and only make sense within the theoretical schema of the moment. Readers who doubt this should simply reflect on what has happened to Goldstein's 'central aphasia' or Head's 'semantic aphasia', and remember that Broca's original aphasic subject Tan would now not even be described as a 'Broca's aphasic'. The answer must be to describe the patient's behaviour in as much detail as possible, without assuming that any particular syndrome label will provide a description.

In terms of designing the right therapy one needs to know not only what the patient's behaviour is, but one also needs a theory about which information processing functions are impaired and which are not affected. Treatment which is aimed at the functions that are impaired, and treatment which builds upon the functions that remain intact, will have the greatest probability of being successful.

None of this necessarily requires any particular theoretical perspective. Over the last few years neuropsychologists have been applying cognitive theories of information processing to understand the patterns of performance of neuropsychologically impaired patients; this approach, which has been called 'cognitive neuropsychology', first developed in the study of disorders of reading and writing, and more recently the approach has been extended to other areas of language and other kinds of neuropsychological impairment (see Marshall 1986; Coltheart et al. 1987; Ellis and Young 1988; Shallice 1989). As Beauvois and Derouesné (1982) argue, this approach is ideally suited to the design of therapy procedures because cognitive neuropsychologists have developed sophisticated ways for identifying information processing systems that are intact and those that are impaired. Furthermore, cognitive neuropsychological theories are phrased in terms of information processing, and thus they deal directly with the kinds of techniques that therapists can use. In contrast, theories which are framed, for example, in terms of neuroanatomical structures are not useful to therapists; an analysis that tells one that a patient's problem is due to a lesion in the parietal lobe is not useful to the therapist who has no direct way of affecting the function of parts of the brain. A cognitive neuropsychological account, however, is likely to say that a patient's difficulty is due to an impairment in, say, the processes of word identification at a lexical level. It is, then, possible for a therapist to devise techniques to improve lexical word recognition: cognitive neuropsychological analyses of a patient's behaviour are at exactly the level which therapists can use to devise appropriate treatments.

To summarise: to do studies of treatment that are of lasting value, therapists neeed to avoid describing their patients in terms of syndrome labels. Instead, they need to describe the patient's behaviour in sufficient detail that other therapists can decide whether their patients resemble the original subject. Assessment has a second purpose: one needs to know the impaired and intact information processing systems, in order to devise treatments that are rationally related to a patient's difficulties. A cognitive neuropsychological approach provides a suitable technique for patient assessment which fulfils both these criteria. It would, of course, be foolish to claim that modern cognitive neuropsychological theory is the best possible basis for rehabilitation; these theories will develop and improve, but also they will ultimately be superceded by other more satisfactory perspectives. But a description of the outcome of therapy based on a detailed assessment of a patient's processing abilities and impairments should be amenable to reinterpretation in terms of another better theory at some time in the future.

## Doing the Right Therapy

With the effectiveness matrix, and a set of diagnostic procedures for establishing the patient type into which any individual subject can be categorised, therapists could always guarantee to provide the best possible treatment for each subject. However, the effectiveness matrix remains an idealisation; our current problem is to try to attempt to establish which approaches to treatment are effective. An analysis of a patient's problems does not necessarilly tell us anything directly about what to do about it. In this neuropsychological rehabilitation is exactly the same as any other kind of remedial intervention. In medicine, for instance, one can understand a considerable amount about the nature of a disease process without that determining what to do about it.

Treatments in neuropsychological rehabilitation have, in general, taken one of three different approaches. In *facilitation* approaches, the therapist tries to improve the functioning of impaired access routines to knowledge which is itself intact; this was, for instance, the approach used by Schuell in her treatment approaches (e.g., Schuell et al. 1964). Where information is itself lost as a consequence of the brain damage, therapists have tried to help their patients *relearn* the damaged information or procedures; this is the approach on which many of the traditional didactic approaches to rehabilitation are based, as well as being the foundation of behaviour therapy approaches to treatment. The third approach was popularised by Luria (1963) and his colleagues in the Soviet Union: *reconstitution of function* aims to use intact processes to perform a task in an unusual way avoiding the involvement of processes which are impaired.

Clearly the choice between these approaches depends partly on precise knowledge of the information processing functions that are impaired or intact. Deciding between *relearning* and *facilitation* techniques depends on accurate assessment of whether, for each individual patient, information or procedures are themselves lost or it is simply access or output routines which are damaged, while the information itself remains intact. Shallice (1987) suggests some criteria for distinguishing between access and storage deficits. Treatments based on *reconstitution of function* depend critically on knowledge of exactly the processes that are impaired and on knowledge of how these can be reorganised to perform the desired task. Beauvois and Derouesné (1982) provide some very clear examples of how this can be achieved.

Thus correct assessment places constraints on the types of treatment that may be addressed to a particular problem: however, within these constraints, there is a great deal of scope for devising treatments. One approach to this is the argument that we must start to devise a theory of therapy – that is a metatheory describing how therapy procedures relate to a deficit assessment (see Howard and Hatfield 1987). This is not a trivial problem: in part this is because most contemporary information processing theories of cognitive function have no specification of how the system can develop or change – in classic Saussurian terms they are *synchronic* theories. But it is also a fault of therapists: few practitioners engaged in rehabilitation have considered and explicitly discussed the links between assessment and therapy – in general it is taken as obvious that with a particular problem a specific kind of therapy is necessary. The best option currently available to the therapist is to make the set of decisions involved in deducing the form of treatment explicit and open so that these may become a part of the domain of scientific enquiry.

There are two further obligations on the therapist. The treatment itself must be described in sufficient detail that another therapist could carry out the same set of treatment procedures with another patient – that is the description must be, as Coltheart (1983) argues, in 'cookbook' detail. And, so as to establish whether or not the treatment used was effective with a specified patient, the therapist needs to adopt an experimental design which can discriminate between the effects of treatment and the results of spontaneous improvement or non-specific placebo effects of treatment. A number of experimental designs are available for studying the effects of treatment procedures with single subjects; discussion of them is beyond the scope of this paper (see McReynolds and Kearns 1983; Howard 1986; Howard and Patterson 1989).

## Some Examples of Cognitive Neuropsychological Approaches to Treatment

It follows from the arguments presented above that cognitive neuropsychologists have to (a) describe the nature of the patient's deficits (and intact abilities) in some detail; (b) describe in detail the treatment used; (c) describe why the treatment should be expected to change the patient's impairments, and (d) demonstrate whether or not the treatment is effective. Because treatment procedures will probably have to be different for problems of each qualitatively different kind, generalisations are not available. In this paper it would be impossible to describe any treatment procedures in the kind of detail which I have argued is required. A variety of examples of case studies applying cognitive neuropsychological methods to neuropsychological rehabilitation may be found in Seron and Deloche (1989) and the articles referred to by the papers in that book; a rather briefer review of cognitive neuropsychology and aphasia therapy is in Howard and Hatfield (1987, pp. 97–105). In this section I will briefly mention one study following each of the approaches of facilitation, relearning and reconstitution of function; these studies will concern the treatment of word retrieval deficits in aphasia. However, I should emphasise that studies of many other areas including disorders of memory, calculation, reading, sentence comprehension and production are available.

When an aphasic subject fails to name a picture or object, information from a prompt, such as a cue of the first sound of the word, can frequently help the subject to produce the correct word. In such cases the phonological representation of the sought for word cannot be lost, and the difficulty is then most likely to be in the process of access to phonological word forms from the semantic system. In this case it seems logical to attempt facilitation of the processes of access. In a study of the facilitative effects of single treatment events on word retrieval, Howard et al. (1985) found that techniques that required a patient to access the semantic representation corresponding to a word that could not be retrieved significantly improved word retrieval, and this effect lasted for at least 24 hours even for a single treatment event. Examples of such techniques are pointing to a picture of the object on auditory command, or verifying a spoken sentence involving the meaning of the word which could not be found as a name. In contrast, techniques which provide subjects with information about the phonological form of a word, such as cueing with its first sound, or repeating the word had very short lived effects, lasting for only a few minutes. In a treatment study which contrasted these two types of facilitation, Howard et al. (1985) demonstrated that they both resulted in significant improvements in word retrieval, and improvement with the semantically-based techniques showed greater generalisation to other words that had not themselves been involved in treatment.

Scott (1987) adopted a relearning approach with her subject, AB. She argued that a loss of information in verbal semantic representations was responsible for the patient's difficulties in word comprehension and in word retrieval.

His treatment therefore concentrated on teaching him to draw ever finer semantic distinctions on a set of treatment words. The early tasks involved simple categorisation of pictures and words into living and non-living, progressing towards more complex discriminations. As a result of this, AB's comprehension improved as well as his naming of the pictures from the set involved in treatment. Other tasks, unrelated to this therapy programme, in contrast showed no change, demonstrating that the improvement was a specific consequence of the treatment.

Prompts from a therapist can help patients to retrieve words, but depend on having a therapist available; attempts have therefore been made to find ways to enable patients to generate their own cues. Aphasic patients who benefit from cueing with the first sound of a word and who can recall its first letter will be able to generate their own cues if they can generate the sound from the letter. In a study of 20 patients, Bruce and Howard (1987) could not find any subject with all three of these abilities. Four subjects who benefitted from phonemic cues and who knew about first letters, were taught to use a microcomputer-based prosthesis which converts letters into sounds to generate their own phonemic cues. Once patients had learned to use the prosthesis, they were significantly better at naming than when they had no help. Here an external prosthesis is used to reconstitute the operations involved in word retrieval.

## Conclusion

Modern cognitive neuropsychology has developed only over the last 20 years. As an approach it first developed in the study of disorders of reading and it has gradually extended into other areas of processing. It is therefore natural that most of the treatment studies concern reading and other areas of language breakdown. The argument of this paper has been that a cognitive neuropsychological approach allows therapists to identify problems with the level of detail that they need, and that this assessment provides information at exactly the level at which therapists can aim their interventions – that is the level of information processing. No theoretical approach can ever encapsulate the whole truth, but I have argued that cognitive neuropsychology can allow us to approach the questions of rehabilitation with the precision needed to develop a truly scientific theory of therapy. That is our most urgent need.

## References

Beauvois M-F, Derouesné J (1982) Recherche en neuropsychologie et rééducation: quels rapports? In: Seron X, Laterre C (eds) Rééduquer le cerveau. Mardaga, Brussels

Bruce C, Howard D (1987) Computer-generated phonemic cues: an effective aid for naming in aphasia. Br J Dis Commun 22:191–201

Caramazza A (1984) The logic of neuropsychological research and the problem of patient classification in aphasia. Brain and Language 21:9–20

Coltheart M (1983) Aphasia therapy research: a single case study approach. In: Code C, Muller D (eds) Aphasia therapy. Arnold, London

Coltheart M, Sartori G, Job R (eds) (1987) The cognitive neuropsychology of language. Erlbaum, London

Ellis AW (1987) Intimations of modularity or the modelarity of mind; doing cognitive neuropsychology without syndromes. In: Coltheart M, Sartori G, Job R (eds) The cognitive neuropsychology of language. Erlbaum, London

Ellis AW, Young AW (1988) Human cognitive neuropsychology. Erlbaum, London

Goodglass H, Kaplan E (1972) The assessment of aphasia and related disorders. Lea and Febiger, Philadelphia

Howard D (1986) Beyond randomised controlled trials: the case for effective case studies of the effects of treatment in aphasia. Br J Dis Commun 21:89–102

Howard D, Hatfield FM (1987) Aphasia therapy: historical and contemporary issues. Erlbaum, London

Howard D, Patterson KE (1989) Models for therapy. In: Seron X, Deloche G (eds) Cognitive neuropsychology and rehabilitation. Erlbaum, Hillsdale

Howard D, Patterson KE, Franklin S, Orchard-Lisle VM, Morton J (1986) Treatment of word retrieval deficits in aphasia: a comparison of two therapy methods. Brain 108:817–829

Lincoln NB, McGuirk E, Mulley GP, Lendrem W, Jones AC, Mitchell JRA (1984) Effectiveness of speech therapy for aphasic stroke patients: a randomised controlled trial. Lancet 1:1197–1200

Luria AR (1963) Restoration of function after brain injury. Pergamon, Oxford

Marshall JC (1986) Description and interpretation of aphasic language disorder. Neuropsychologia 24:5–24

McReynolds LV, Kearns KP (1983) Single subject experimental designs in communicative disorders. University Park Press, Baltimore

Schuell H, Jenkins JJ, Jimenez-Pabon E (1964) Aphasia in adults: diagnosis, prognosis, and treatment. Harper and Row, New York

Scott C (1987) Cognitive neuropsychological remediation of acquired language disorders. MSc Thesis, City University, London

Seron X, Deloche G (eds) (1989) Cognitive neuropsychology, and rehabilitation. Erlbaum, Hillsdale

Shallice T (1987) Impairments of semantic processing: multiple dissociations. In: Coltheart M, Sartori G, Job R (eds) The cognitive neuropsychology of language. Erlbaum, London

Shallice T (1989) From neuropsychology to mental structure. Cambridge University Press, Cambridge

Wertz RT, Weiss DG, Aten JL, et al (1988) Comparison of clinic, home and deferred language treatment for aphasia. Arch Neurology 43:653–658

# The Personal Level in Cognitive Rehabilitation

*A.J. Marcel*

This essay focuses on the "Stimulation" approach to recovery of cognitive function. Data will be reviewed which suggest that intentional, social and emotional factors are relevant to elicitation and rehabilitation of function. This implies that we need to invoke the 'personal' level to achieve success at the 'subpersonal' or functional level. However, in terms of the personal level, a problem still remains in certain impairments if the patient does not become an independent agent or if they have a deficit in phenomenal experience.

## Introduction

In Philosophy of Mind and in Psychology a distinction is made between the personal level and the subpersonal level of analysis and discourse (Dennett 1969). The Personal level involves (a) beliefs, desires and intentions (i.e., propositional attitudes), (b) the intentionality of mental states – their referentiality, content or 'aboutness', (c) phenomenal experience and subjectivity, i.e., not only pain and other qualia (qualitative properties of sensations) but also agency, and (d) an implied unity, of personhood and of point of view. The personal level is not, however, synonymous with consciousness, since we may attribute to someone beliefs, desires and other intentional states of which the subject is not aware and which have no qualia. The subpersonal level refers to the functional or physical. It is causal or mechanical rather than rational. It does not involve a point of view, phenomenology or subjectivity. It does not imply unity and can be segmented into constituent, modular parts. It is the language of brain science and of information-processing. Psychology, to the extent that it is anxious to become a natural science, explaining by causes and mechanisms, deals at the subpersonal level, while neurology could not do otherwise. It is quite natural that neuroscientists should turn to this kind or level of psychology when they seek to give functional accounts of parts of the central nervous system. It is also easy to see why diagnosticians should avail themselves of this type of neuropsychology, and why subpersonal psychology should look to brain damage to aid its componential analysis. Indeed this union has proved fruitful both in refining psychological theory and in refining diagnosis. But this level of discourse has its drawbacks. It cannot deal comfortably with certain legitimate areas of psychology which exist at the personal level. Nor, it will be argued below, does it tell a therapist what to do in so far as therapeutic interactions involve the personal level.

This essay is addressed to only one approach to cognitive rehabilitation, the "Stimulation" approach; and it is so addressed in the context of the two levels of discourse outlined above. How that context informs my remarks will become clearer later. But it may help if I make certain introductory remarks which make explicit some of the themes of what follows.

1. In the kind of rehabilitation to which this essay is addressed appropriate intervention does not necessarily follow in any simple way from diagnosis of the problem. Indeed it has been argued (Caramazza 1989; Marcel 1978) that hardly any intervention follows from the types of subpersonal theories currently available. In fact theoretical justification tends to depend on the success of the intervention and is post hoc. Obviously valid theory-based diagnosis should and can constrain the goals and methods of the therapist. But such subpersonal theories cannot tell one anything about pedagogy or about the personal-level factors which may influence rehabilitation, or about problems which are best characterised at that level.

2. In current information-processing approaches cognition is treated as separate from (though perhaps influenced by) the conative, affective and social-personal domains. In contrast, it may be suggested by some of the data reviewed below that certain aspects of cognition are inseparable from and hierarchically embedded in these other domains, and that rehabilitation needs to take account of this embedding.

3. Characterizing what a person is doing may be entirely different when considered (a) in terms of what is actually going on at the level of "implementation", e.g., the hardware, (b) as an external third-person account or functionalist algorithm, and (c) from the viewpoint of the subject's experience or the agent's intention. Any one account may be only nominal in terms of the others. It is my contention that as regards therapy, the first type of account is largely irrelevant, the second is a starting point and criterion, but it is the third which determines how rehabilitation is conducted, especially for certain types of deficit and for certain types of therapy. (Hardware is by no means completely irrelevant; for a good illustration of its relevance, see Jenkins and Merzenich, this volume.)

4. In the spirit of a disclaimer, the factors which will be discussed are most relevant to the type of therapy on which I will focus, and that type of therapy is probably suited only to certain kinds of problem.

## Rehabilitation and Recovery of Function

There are a large number of approaches to rehabilitation of function after brain damage. Each approach reflects underlying assumptions. Thus in one approach, if a function or way of carrying out that function is impaired or lost, it is assumed that little or nothing can be done about it. In this case the therapist attempts to find a substitute. The analogy here would seem to be if someone loses both legs there are either given artificial legs or an alternative method of moving, e.g., a wheelchair. The approach associated with Luria makes the slightly less pessimistic assumption that there is a degree of plasticity in the way brains implement function. Thus the aim of the therapist is to produce a reorganisation or reconstitution of function, usually by means of appropriate mediating steps. In a third type of approach it is assumed that certain abilities can be relearnt, i.e., competence is preserved but instantiation is lost. The therapist may attempt to help the patient recover the function by concentrating explicitly and directly on training (often by repeated trials) of instances of that function. Dysarthric or articulatory apraxic patients may be drilled in trying to produce a target phoneme. A variant of this approach and its assumptions is evident in attempts to use techniques of behaviour modification.

Apart from a variety of other interventionist schemes, there is also what is sometimes called the "Stimulation" approach. Here the assumption is that the impaired function or mechanism is not completely lost, but rather is inaccessible. If one can find the appropriate method of elicitation, the patient might be able to recover, rather than relearn, the function in question.

The work of Weigl on aphasics is of particular relevance to the Stimulation approach. He discovered a method of facilitation which he called "deblocking" (Weigl 1961). Use of a word or syntactic structure in a task or modality that is unimpaired in a particular patient (e.g., reading) could make it temporarily available for use in an impaired task or modality for that patient (e.g., object-naming). Although this cross-mode facilitation was short-lived, once the behaviour had been produced in the impaired mode, it was found to remain available in that mode for a long time, even up to 2 years (Weigl and Kreindler 1960). It is significant for what follows that the most efficacious deblockers depended on the individual patient. (See Howard and Hatfield 1987, for further discussion.) Patterson, Purell and Morton (1983) suggest from their findings that Stimulation techniques are less likely to work if only relatively peripheral processes are involved (phonemic cueing), and probably depend for success on the involvement of meaning and a rich set of elicitation cues (gestures, synonyms). This supports what is argued later in the present paper.

It is to this last approach, that of Stimulation, that what follows is addressed. This is for several reasons. In the cases for which it is suitable it appears to offer a hope of genuine recovery. Those cases which are appropriate would be ones where it is access to a function that is impaired. These types of case are of special interest to me not only because I am concerned with consciousness, but because most assessments of cognition are decontextualized and far too little attention is paid to situational and personal context. The question arises as to what factors might be relevant to elicitation of an impaired function. The most obvious domain to turn to is that of intentions. However, since most real-life intentions themselves are normally embedded in a person's persisting goal-structures (their personal needs and aims) it may be relevant to examine what the impaired functions represent to the patient in social and personal terms. I will therefore first cite evidence on the dependence of performance on intention and then discuss the effect of social and personal significance.

## The Role of Intention

There are several domains where the functional deficit or objective performance seems to depend on the nature of the intention underlying the behaviour, on the patient's "attitude", or on situational or social factors. While the question will remain of changing this dependence, nonetheless utilization of these factors offers a means to *elicit* the behaviours in question which can then be worked on or serve in a bootstrapping strategy.

The first example concerns some current research of my own. The initial objective of the work was to document the extent to which phenomena observed in ideomotor apraxia occur in a range of motor-impaired neurological patients who are not necessarily classified as apraxic, and to explore Leontiev's techniques of rehabilitation. In ideomotor apraxics, who are otherwise unimpaired in perception, comprehension or performance, actions which cannot be produced on request or by imitation are often produced or improved when performed in the course of normal activities of which such actions are a part. Leontiev and Zaporozhets (1960) report that when hand functioning is impaired (even by relatively peripheral damage), it is often more effectively rehabilitated by the patient's performance of the impaired behaviour as a meaningful activity than by exercise of the behaviour as an isolated movement. While this is to be found as unwritten lore among occupational therapists, its profound implications seem largely unnoticed by consultants and academics. In the current work, ten patients, not classed as ideomotor apraxics but who showed such phenomena, were identified and filmed in a variety of situations. As an example, one woman who had difficulty in grasping, in lifting and in fluency in moving an object, showed clear improvement when drinking during a meal than when asked to lift a cylinder of the same weight and size as the glass of liquid and to move it to or from her. One hypothesis was that of "over-attention" to the required movements. This is derived from William James's observation that motor coordination breaks down when we attend to our movements. To test this idea, dual-task conditions were designed, appropriate to the relevant behaviour in each individual, to divert attention from the action in question. In only one case did this procedure lead to some improvement in the relevant motor performance. By contrast, when an activity was induced of which the relevant behaviour was a component, or was indeed a lower-level decontextualized description, improvement was obtained in all cases.

An unexpected but important finding was that in all but one patient, a further significant improvement in performance was found under certain other conditions. This third level of performance was discovered by chance, sometimes only when we visited the patients at their homes, but was then tested by

**Table 1.** Four examples of improvement of motor control according to situation and intention

| Patient and deficit | Level of performance | Actions | Supposed intention |
|---|---|---|---|
| A. Grasping, lifting, fluency in lifting and placing (woman) | 1 | Lifting cylinder and moving to/from self | As instructed |
| | 2 | Drinking during meal | Drinking |
| | 3 | Passing tea cups at home | Offering hospitality |
| B. Coordination, timing, and sequencing in finger control (woman) | 1 | Copying letterlike forms | As instructed |
| | 2 | Writing words to dictation | Transcribing lexical entries |
| | 3 | Writing appointments and achievements in diary | Self-management |
| C. Grip and release, adduction/abduction of elbow, tremor (man) | 1 | Laying out blank cards | As instructed |
| | 2 | Matching suits of playing cards | Matching and ordering patterns |
| | 3 | Dealing poker hands | Playing a game/conviviality |
| D. Grip combined with shoulder protraction and elbow extension (woman) | 1 | Moving a rod back and forth | As instructed |
| | 2 | Cutting while eating | Eating |
| | 3 | Cutting food for a meal | Fulfilling family role (self-validation) |

finding individually relevant real-world situations. It appears that the crucial common feature for this further improvement is when the action has personal or social significance. Four examples are illustrated in Table 1. Consider two of them. A patient who had grasping, lifting and fluency impairments (level 1) showed clear improvement when drinking during a meal (level 2), and showed further improvement when giving us cups of tea at her home (level 3), but not when clearing up the cups (level 2). Another patient who had coordination, timing and sequencing problems in finger control was very poor in copying letterlike Gibson-figures (level 1), was improved when writing words to dictation (level 2), and further improved when writing appointments and achievements in her diary (level 3). To summarise the examples in Table 1, the initial improvement from level 1 to level 2 seems to be due to contextualization into an activity and meaningfulness of the intention. That is, having a drink or writing words already exist as intentions embedded in the goal structures of people's everyday scripts, whereas lifting cylinders and copying meaningless patterns do so far less. What matters is the description under which an action is encoded. As regards the further improvement to level 3, the only well-characterized explanations we can offer are that in the first case the intention is the specific realization of a broader intention "to offer hospitality", while in the second case the larger intention is in terms of self-management. The improvements to a third level of performance found in the other patients all fit an explanation in terms of a characterization of the intention at the social-personal level. Analysis of such intentions involves their 'significance', something which involves how a culture categorizes what activities represent, and how such activities signify states of the self in relation to others (for elaboration, see Marcel 1988a, pp. 179–188). To the extent that our interpretations are valid, the data suggest that motor control is subject to the nature of the generating intention. Not only are motor structures more accessible as realizations of real-life dynamically unfolding activities, but such activities themselves may be realized more effectively when they signify at a personal level. This can be capitalized on by therapists.

Other related examples exist in different domains of function. In a recent (as yet unpublished) case, I tested a Conduction Aphasic patient in Grenoble with Annik Charnallet and Serge Carbonnel. The patient was presented auditorily with single 3-syllable (CVCVCV) nonwords (e.g., miladu) and asked to repeat them. The best she could manage was to repeat a single syllable, sometimes combining the consonant and vowel of different syllables, sometimes making phonemic paraphasias. However, dramatically contrasting results were achieved when she was given a different task: "I know you dislike these nonsense words. All I want you to do is to listen to three of them and tell me which one you prefer or dislike least". The patient was then presented auditorily with three stimuli (e.g., miladu, rabeli, potina). On 28 out of 30 trials she succeeded perfectly in saying one of the words, choosing the first, second and third roughly equally. Was the patient not repeating one of the stimuli? Well, no! She was telling us which she preferred. But this *involved* repetition. Indeed, to perform the task, on many trials she must have remembered more than one of the stimuli. The question arises as to whether her short-term auditory-verbal memory was impaired or whether it was the access to and use of her memory which was the problem. (How many other cases of conduction aphasia are similar to this?) Again, the patient could not repeat under the intention "to repeat", but could do so under the intention "to say which is preferred".

While the above cases illustrate the efficacy of a "higher level" intention, others indicate the effect of different "types" of intention. Brouchon et al. (1986) have shown, in both Optic Ataxic patients and in normal subjects, that perceptual-motor coordination in what is "objectively" the same movement is qualitatively influenced by whether the instruction is "to reach for and touch" or "to indicate" whichever light-emitting diode of an array is illuminated. Indeed, Brouchon has suggested that the functional organization of perceptual-motor space itself (near/far, allocentric/egocentric) depends upon the nature of the current intention: prehension is self-related, while deixis always implies another person. Two further dramatic examples come from congenitally deaf users of American Sign Language (ASL) who have brain damage in adulthood. The first example involves signers with aphasia and those with apraxia. In ASL certain signs are exactly the same movements as used in conventional pantomime gestures; for example the *sign* for the gerund of the verb to drink (drinking) is the same as the *mime* for drinking (hand holding a vessel raised to lips and lowered). The aphasic patients could neither produce nor comprehend such movements as linguistic entities, but they could do both when the movements were under the description of the mime. The apraxic patients showed exactly the reverse pattern (Poizner et al. 1984). This rather neatly illustrates that in the mental domain both production of action and recognition are always "under a description". The other example concerns deaf signers with unilateral spatial neglect. In ASL (a) syntax makes use of space and (b) when entities are introduced in a discourse they are each assigned a spatial location around the signer which is returned to for anaphoric (especially pronominal) reference. Patients with left neglect had little or no trouble with either of these uses of left hemispace in discourse. However, when asked to describe spatial layouts or given conventional tests of neglect they neglected those very same spaces (Poizner et al. 1987; Chaps. 7 and 8). It appears that space is a medium which can be used to represent either langugage or itself. A disorder of space turns out to be a disorder of *represented space*, evident only when the subject so intends.

All of the above examples illustrate how the availability and execution of behaviour is influenced by the intention under which such behaviour is generated. They also relate to the difference between the Nominal and the Functional, i.e., the characterization of the action by the theorist as opposed to the agent's intention. There is a very good example of this distinction from therapy itself. De Partz (1986) devised a successful treatment programme for a Deep Dyslexic patient. De Partz's diagnosis of the patient's problem relied on a particular theory of oral reading (Coltheart 1980) and specified the problem as a loss of grapheme-phoneme correspondences. De Partz characterized her treatment as an attempt to re-teach such correspondences. But a close examination of the training procedures employed reveals that this was exactly what was *not* done. In fact what was done was (a) to teach the association of letters with real meaningful words chosen by the patient which started with those letters (M for Mother), and (b) to teach phonemic segmentation of such real words. Interestingly, certain theories (Marcel 1980; Bertelson and De Gelder 1985) suggest that in normal readers of alphabetic scripts, nonword, or phonological, reading is achieved not by grapheme-phoneme translation but by orthographic and phonological segmentation of lexical entries, and that reading acquisition is highly related to awareness of words as segmentable phonological strings. But, more importantly for our present purposes, that patient in question did *not* learn to transcode graphemes to phonemes; but rather he reachieved an analytic process by mediation of and recourse to knowledge of meaningful entities (words).

## The Social and Personal

In the examples discussed above the type and level of intentional description under which mental acts are performed seem to influence the efficacy of the realization of those acts. Social and personal aspects of intentions may play a similar role. It was suggested that this is so in the cases of motor control that I have been investigating. Indeed our personal goals and motives plausibly provide the energizing mechanism which transforms intentions into action. However, social factors may play other roles. They may even determine the nature and form of a deficit. In one case I have seen of an agrammatic patient, the severity of the aphasia seemed much greater in the presence of the patient's wife, becoming at times almost a global aphasia. It was as though in the wife's presence if the man could not fill the desired male role through language, the only alternative was to become a total dependent (a baby?) in his language. In another case (Margolin et al. 1985), RF started out as a global aphasic; but with therapy appeared to switch between being either mainly agrammatic or mainly anomic, *according to the social pragmatics of the situation.* Both of these types of phenomena have been reported to me by speech therapists, but they do not seem to have been studied and written up in academic journals.

An exception to this silence is Lebrun's (1976) review of aphasia in polyglots. Lebrun reports a number of cases of aphasia in multi-lingual speakers where either one language is relatively spared or one language is recovered (spontaneously or under therapy) to a much greater extent than the others. The important point is that in the cases reviewed the advantage of the privileged language could not be attributed either to linguistic factors such as syntactic or morphological complexity nor to acquisition factors such as first or last language learnt. Sociolinguistic factors such as the linguistic environment of the patient at the time of or after trauma (especially the language of individuals close to the patient) do seem to play a part. However, in several cases the only explanation seems to be what the language represents in social or emotional terms to the individual. One case was that of a Swiss man whose mother-tongue and usual vernacular was Schwyzer Dütsch, but who had learned High German at school and continued to use it frequently in every day life, and who had learned French as a young man during a stay in France. After a stroke at 44 years old some comprehension of all languages returned but the patient could only produce French. It turns out that the years in France were regarded as the happiest in his life and he had fallen passionately in love with a French woman. In another case a man's native language was Dutch, he learnt German as a teenager when his family moved to Germany and later learnt English, Spanish and French, settling in Brussels. After a severe head injury at 68 years old English was the best recovered language. Although the patient could not explain this, it turned out that he had been a fervent Christian Scientist. The official documents of that Church are in English and English was to him a sacred language (as Latin for many Catholics and Hebrew for many Jews).

Social and personal factors can also play roles that are quite different from the above. A neurologically caused deficit may deprive a patient of an ability which gives them a desired social role or a desired self-image. It is easy to see how professional roles may be undermined both specifically and generally (agraphia in a writer, frontal problems for almost any responsible job). But more than that, language and memory constitute our very selves and self-expression. Further, language, memory and agnosic disorders (especially prosopagnosia) turn the patient into a stigmatized social freak. One might think that the patient would be highly motivated to recover or compensate for such losses, and I am sure that is so in many cases. But such losses can also bring about a catastrophic reaction, profound depression and loss of the sense of self, removing the patient's will to rehabilitation (see Gainotti, pp. 215). In all such cases the therapist needs to place the cognitive rehabilitation in the context of psychotherapy for it to be effective.

As the converse of the preceding, a deficit may itself serve a positive functional purpose for the patient. Sensitivity to psychodynamics is also required in such cases. Several physiotherapists and speech therapists have plausibly explained their difficulties by suggesting that the impairment gains care and attention for the patient or releases the patient from responsibility. The patient may not even be aware of this problem or of their ambivalence to rehabilitation. Cognitive psychologists may be ready to see such factors as genuine problems but view them as quite external to the cognitive deficit itself and its therapy. However in everyday life outside the laboratory our cognitive abilities do not merely support our biological existence. They are almost always the instruments of our personal and social goals and constitute us as competent individuals. The social-personal and the cognitive are not just mutually dependent, they are inseparable. The role of motivation, social relationships and the significance of learning is a first principle of education. Just so in neurological rehabilitation.

The role of motivation and social relations in neurological rehabilitation is illustrated by a study by Parsons and Stewart (1966). They examined perceptual-motor learning over three testing sessions in 20 brain-damaged and 20 neurotic individuals. They also compared two interviewing styles during testing: one disinterested/factual and the other emotionally supportive. The neurotic group showed no effect of interview type on performance. But the brain-damaged group whose testers were supportive showed significantly greater learning than those with disinterested testers.

Finally, several characteristics of neurological disorders may be adjustments to or compensations for the primary impairment. It has been argued by Butterworth (1979) that the neologisms in jargon aphasia are an attempt to obey conversational pragmatics by filling word-finding pauses with whatever phonology is available. Confabulation in certain cases (but not all) of amnesia or of bodily neglect with anosognosia may be attempts to save a sense of rationality or to save face. In surface dyslexia, where people have a problem reading lexically, patients commonly orally lexicalize what would otherwise be phonological nonwords (Marcel 1980). Interestingly the only cases reported where they do not do so (i.e., they only produce regularizations of the printed letter-string) are those where the patients are dementing and are probably unable to monitor their utterances with regard to presuppositions and goals (Shallice et al. 1983). Goldstein (1948) gives many other suggestions in a similar vein to those above. The importance of this for rehabilitation is that in many cases therapy cannot proceed until the patient can be persuaded to desist from a compensation. Thus the therapist cannot help the Wernicke's aphasic in word finding until the production of jargon stops, spontaneously or otherwise. In other cases the primary problem cannot be aided unless an adjustment to it which is maladaptive is removed. If the adjustment serves some personal goal, consciously or not, then the therapist needs to be aware of this to get the patient to desist.

## Cognitive Models and Therapy

The discussion above suggests one reason why information-processing models of cognition, which are in terms of the sub-personal level of discourse, have so little to say about what the therapist should actually do and how it should be done. The problem is that while deficits tend to be diagnosed and characterized at the subpersonal level, therapy necessarily involves the personal level. Let me illustrate what this statement means in a couple of ways. If an electrician diagnoses the problem in a circuit as the lack of a connection between two terminals, he can simply wire the two terminals together. His diagnosis is prescriptive because there is no disparity between his diagnostic description and the nature of his intervention. But the case is quite different for neuropsychology. It is not just that we cannot open up the head and join or insert bits. (In any case, would that constitute donating knowledge or neurons?) We cannot *directly* repair short-term memory or grow a lexicon, etc. Our interventions are of necessity *indirect.* (We have to get the person to do x in order for them to acquire y). Furthermore they involve interactions between *persons.* No doubt much learning is possible automatically and by mere exposure. But in practical terms what goes on in rehabilitation requires communication, and if the patient is to do anything it requires compliance and intentions. This involves the personal level and illustrates how current models of cognition, with one or two exceptions, are radically incomplete. For such models do not deal with how beliefs and desires are either arrived at or get translated into action or the processing underlying it. As I have discussed elsewhere (Marcel 1988b), models that start with a stimulus and end with a response are inadequate, if not self-contradictory. Such models are derived from performance of tasks (tasks that are often used in neuropsychological diagnosis); yet there is nothing in such models which explains how it is that one task rather than another gets performed (i.e., how it is that a subject, given a written word, reads it rather than copies it, classifies it or attends to its typeface). To provide such an explanation, as well as to deal with neurological cases where the problem involves access to a function, we need a psychology of intention.

All of the factors reviewed above (intentional, social and personal) have important implications for psychological theories of control of function, for assessment, for elicitation of function or behaviour, and for rehabilitation. It may be argued that, as regards the latter two issues, there is no necessity to alter current practice in the theoretical characterization of specific brain damage. But, at least for practical purposes, such functional impairments do not exist in isolation. In practice, therapists usually are sensitive to the relevant factors and do what is being suggested. However, it is not clear that they do so in a principled fashion, nor do they explicitly characterize their practice in such a way.

There are, of course, limitations on the applicability and implications of what has so far been raised. First, and most simply, there are many deficits to which principles of intentionality and attitude, and the social dimension do not apply. Besides the more peripheral sensory and motor problems, there are clearly many cognitive deficits where the function, representation, or "implementation" really is lost. Degenerative cases would also seem to fall into this category. Second, the type of rehabilitative approach which is most appropriate will depend on several factors. What has been discussed, while having general implications, is applicable mostly to approaches which aim to elicit behaviour, to "stimulate" it or to "deblock" it. There are a whole set of training procedures discussed in this volume as well as in others (Howard and Hatfield 1987; Seron and Deloche 1989) to which the factors discussed here are relevant but genuinely marginal. However, where a deficit is to be considered one of access or intention or consciousness, of which we are discovering a growing number, then such factors can be seen to be of great potential relevance.

This issue of the existence of deficits of *access* to a function, however, raises a paradox which questions the very goal of therapy and may place severe limitations on what can be hoped for. It is to this that I will now turn.

## Problems of Agency and Experience

Neuropsychological research over the last 10 years seems to be revealing a growing number of the type of cognitive impairments which can take two forms. One form is where function itself is impaired or lost; the other is where the deficit is one either of domain-specific consciousness or of intentional access to the function. Candidates include forms of amnesic syndrome, cortical blindness (c.f. blindsight), associative agnosias, prosopagnosia, neglect and sensory loss, Wernicke's aphasia, some acquired dyslexias (especially pure alexia), and certain apraxias. In all these disorders cases can be found which appear to show preservation of (a) unconscious (or "implicit") processing of the kind that is supposedly impaired, or of (b) processing which the patient cannot initiate at will (although in other apparently similar patients such preservation is absent). It is just such cases which might seem to offer the best hopes for some kind of rehabilitation. At the very least, one might hope to construct an appropriate environment, or find ways to evoke implicit or automatic processing, or help the patient to utilize substitute strategies. Further, in cases where the type of deficit seems to be subject to intention and contextualization, one might even hope that the function or behaviour could be recovered and made accessible if certain conditions or attitudes can be realised by the Stimulation approach. But there remains a problem, a problem which concerns the paradoxical contrast between functional analysis and the agent's viewpoint. The normal person can decide to do all the relevant things *at will*, largely independently of attitude or context, and behave at least adequately. If the patient will still have to find the right intention or the appropriate eliciting situation, they will not be independent agents. That is, if the patient wants to do x, she will have to change the desire to "wanting to do y" in order to achieve x. In fact, it is not entirely true that normal people are free of the effect of intention and situation. But they are so to a far greater degree than neurological patients. In this sense I can see nothing that will offer the patient (in a principled fashion) full rehabilitation. However, this is not a cause for despair but rather a challenge.

There is a second, related, problem which illustrates the contrast between subpersonal, third-person analysis and the personal-level or agent's viewpoint. Consider problems that may well be ones mainly of conscious experience. For example, if it is the case in Anterograde Amnesia and Blindsight that much memory and visual function is intact, as opposed to loss of the corresponding phenomenology, then it may be possible to find ways that the intact functions can be accessed and put to use. In fact, some examples already exist, including the use of an amnesic's procedural memory for the patient to learn to use a microcomputer (Glisky et al. 1986). However, as both Weiskrantz (1988) and myself (Marcel 1988b) have recently emphasised, this would have little effect on the major problem. If the patients remain unconscious (in the first-person sense of phenomenal experience) of their memory or vision, they will remain unwilling to behave *as if* they can remember or see and so still remain impaired.

Could such patients be induced to behave as if they knew their (tacit) abilities? In the case of Blindsight, it remains a possibility that by the use of feedback and knowledge of results two effects could be achieved. First, the patients might gain confidence in relying on nonconscious vision. Second, biofeedback techniques might give them knowledge by other sensory modalities of what they were 'seeing' via the blind field. In fact, in certain special cases feedback from eye movements to lights in the region of the scotoma has produced a small shrinkage of the edges of the blind regions, as measured by perimetry (Zihl 1981). However, such effects are so far only slight. But the main point is that, quite apart from functional aspects of behaviour, for patients with these types of deficit and who are not anosognosic, their impairments of consciousness concerning memory, perception or understanding, constitute the major part of their mental suffering. In terms of the subpersonal level (e.g., an information-processing approach), rehabilitation of experience is not even a logical possibility. For the patient it is the central problem: to live in the present, to be unable to consciously recognize people, to be unable to feel that one understands or communicates. Unfortunately, as an empirical issue, rehabilitation of experience remains a problem to which there is little answer at present.

## Concluding Remarks

Currently the dominant approach of psychologists who are concerned with cognitive activities with regard to neurological breakdown is to treat them at a subpersonal level and as modular. As far as this is informed by Fodorian notions (Fodor 1983), the working of the underlying systems is automatic and unaffected by those factors here identified with the personal level. This may be true of adults in whom such capacities are well learned and in studies which exclude personal level factors. However, it says nothing about the acquisition of such capacities nor their status when impaired (Marcel 1990). Thus we can make no constraining inferences from such a theoretical approach to rehabilitation techniques which might utilize the personal level.

The diverse phenomena discussed in this essay concern supposedly modular, subpersonal cognitive activities. Yet these activities seem to be not independent of, but rather embedded in and realizations of personal level goal structures. Furthermore, such intentions can be seen to depend on the social domain in at least two ways. First, personal significance depends on cultural sign systems (Marcel 1988 a). Second, personal goal structures involve the self as a social entity (Oatley and Bolton 1985). It has been suggested that even if relevant deficits are analysed at a subpersonal level, rehabilitation that aims at reinstatement needs to take account of personal level factors. In addition, if rehabilitation attempts to confront neurologically caused problems of agency and phenomenal experience, it is necessarily dealing with the personal level. Even when competence may be improved by wholly subpersonal techniques such as behaviour modification, the patient is unlikely to take advantage of this unless they are reflexively aware of their ability. Anyway one of the great benefits of such techniques is that they can in turn reduce a sense of inability and increase motivation. Finally, at the risk of seeming sanctimonious, let us re-state the obvious. Earlier it was maintained that assessment itself of cognitive processes in subpersonal terms may be appropriate. However, the ultimate criterion of rehabilitation used by therapists themselves is not performance on individual decontextualized tests, but the real-life abilities and welfare of the individual.

*Acknowledgement.* I would like to thank Susan Goodrich and Ian Robertson for comments on the text.

## References

Bertelson P, De Gelder B (1985) Learning about reading from illiterates. In: Galaburda AM (ed) From reading to neurons. MIT Press, Cambridge, Mass.

Brouchon M, Joanette Y, Samson M (1986) From movement to gesture: "here" and "there" as determinants of visually guided pointing. In: Nespoulos JL, Perron A, Lecours RA (eds) Biological foundations of gesture. Erlbaum, Hillsdale, NJ

Butterworth B (1979) Hesitation and the production of verbal paraphasias and neologisms in jargon aphasia. Brain Lang 8:133–161

Caramazza A (1989) Cognitive neuropsychology and rehabilitation: an unfulfilled promise? Seron X, Deloche G (eds) Cognitive approaches in neuropsychological rehabilitation. Erlbaum, Hillsdale, NJ

Coltheart M (1980) Reading, phonological recoding and deep dyslexia. In: Coltheart M, Patterson KE, Marshall JC (eds) Deep dyslexia. Routledge and Kegan Paul, London

Dennett DC (1969) Content and consciousness. Routledge and Kegan Paul, London

De Partz M-P (1986) Re-education of a deep dyslexic patient: rationale of the method and results. Cogn Neuropsychol 3:149–177

Fodor JA (1983) The modularity of mind: an essay on faculty psychology. MIT Press, Cambridge, Mass.

Glisky EL, Schacter DL, Tulving E (1986) Computer learning by memory-impaired patients. Neuropsychologia 24:313–328

Goldstein K (1948) Language and language disturbances. Grune and Stratton, New York

Howard D, Hatfield FM (1987) Aphasie therapy. Erlbaum, London

Lebrun Y (1976) Recovery in polyglot aphasics. In: Lebrun Y, Hoop R (eds) Recovery in aphasia. Swets and Zeitlinger, Amsterdam

Leontiev AN, Zaporozhets AV (1960) Recovery of hand function. Pergamon, London

Marcel AJ (1978) Prerequisites for a more applicable psychology of reading. In: Gruneberg MM, Morris PE, Sykes RN (eds) Practical aspects of memory. Academic, London

Marcel AJ (1980) Surface dyslexia and beginning reading: a revised hypothesis of the pronunciation of print and its impairments. In: Coltheart M, Patterson KE, Marshall JC (eds) Deep dyslexia. Routledge and Kegan Paul, London

Marcel AJ (1988a) Electrophysiology and meaning in cognitive science and dynamic psychology. In: Horowitz M (ed) Psychodynamics and cognition. University of Chicago Press, Chicago

Marcel AJ (1988b) Phenomenal experience and functionalism. In: Marcel AJ Bisiach E (eds) Consciousness in contemporary science. Oxford University Press, Oxford

Marcel AJ (1990) What does is mean to ask whether cognitive skills are a prerequisite for learning to read and write? Cogn Neuropsychol 7:41–48

Margolin D, Marcel AJ, Carlson N (1985) Common mechanisms in dysnomia and post-semantic surface dyslexia: processing deficits and selective attention. In: Patterson KE, Marshall JC, Coltheart M (eds) Surface dyslexia. Erlbaum, London

Oatley K, Bolton W (1985) A social-cognitive theory of depression in reaction to life events. Psychol Rev 92:372–388

Parsons O, Stewart K (1966) Effects of supportive versus disinterested interviews on perceptual-motor performance in brain-damaged and neurotic patients. J Consult Psychol 30:260–266

Patterson K, Purell C, Morton J (1983) Facilitation of word recognition in aphasia. In: Code C, Muller D (eds) Aphasia therapy. Edwards Arnold

Poizner H, Bellugi H, Iragui V (1984) Apraxia and aphasia for a visual-gestural language. Am J Physiol 246:R868–R883

Poizner H, Klima ES, Bellugi U (1987) What the hands reveal about the brain. MIT Press, Cambridge, Mass.

Seron X, Deloche G (eds) (1989) Cognitive approaches in neuropsychological rehabilitation. Erlbaum, Hillsdale, NJ

Shallice T, Warrington ER, McCarthy R (1983) Reading without semantics. Q J Exp Psychol 35A:111–138

Weigl E (1961) The phenomenon of temporary deblocking in aphasia. Z Phonetik, Sprachwiss Kommunikationsforsch 14:337–364

Weigl E, Kreindler A (1960) Beiträge zur Auffassung gewisser aphasischer Störungen als Blockierungserscheinungen. Arch Psychiat Z Gesamte Neurol 200:306–323

Weiskrantz L (1986) Blindsight. Oxford University Press, Oxford

Weiskrantz L (1988) Some contributions of neuropsychology of vision and memory to the problem of consciousness. In: Marcel AJ, Bisiach E (eds) Consciousness in contemporary science. Oxford University Press, Oxford

Zihl J (1981) Recovery of visual functions in patients with cerebral blindness. Exp Brain Res 44:159–169

# A Family-System Approach to Brain Damage

*Ch. Rüger, J. Vollmann, and M. Wirsching*

## Introduction

Family dynamic research and family therapy are modern methods of psychotherapy and medicine. Although Richardson already stated the importance of family support for patients in 1948, family therapy as a new institution within psychotherapy was not developed before 1960. This early period is charcterised by an enthusiastic rise in popularity and pioneer-like improvement, whereas, in the 1970s, different schools within family therapy developed different theoretic concepts. Nowadays, we seem to be in a period of consolidation and critical reflexion of the existing concepts aiming at a pragmatic integration into practice (Gurman et al. 1986; Wirsching 1986). In what follows, basic notions of the family-dynamic approaches are outlined. As there exists at present only limited knowledge with respect to the application of the family-dynamic approach to patients with brain injury, our reasoning is of a more general nature and focuses only at the end on problems with patients who have suffered brain injuries.

## Theoretical Concepts

To understand the new concept of psychotherapy in family dynamics, we have to state that dynamic family therapy is not just a new method of established psychotherapy, but a new approach and view towards disease itself.

Developing from system theory in biology, cybernetics, and sociology, psychic disease is understood as a multidimensional process. We try to approach a patient's problem not only as a singular somatic or intrapsychic conflict, but also as a part of his family background. If we do so, the doctor's life becomes easier in recognition, diagnosis, and therapy (ecosystemic theory of disease, Willi 1985 a, b). From the family-dynamic point of view, we emphasize the important interaction between formation and effect of psychopathological symptoms. To acknowledge the momentum of complex living systems, we have to extend the traditional linear thinking in reasons and consequences with a systemic theoretical approach. Another new aspect of psychodynamic family therapy is the interpretation of psychopathological symptoms as an intrapsychic conflict as well as a problem of human relations. As we realize these two sides of psychotherapy, the family therapy focuses on resources available within the family rather than psychologizing the already stressful situation. The following examples emphasize the importance of interpersonal conflicts in psychosomatic and chronic disease. If a family member suffers from a severe or chronic disease, the consequences of therapy are not restricted to the patient but influence his whole family surrounding as well. This is particularly important for chronic and life threatening diseases. A diabetic child, for example, changes the whole life of his family. To treat the diabetes well, insulin input, nutrition, and daily life have to be organized and well controlled. This has a strong impact on different aspects of daily living and family activities (meals, school, sports, holidays, etc.). Bronchial asthma or neurodermitis are typical psychosomatic problems with a strong interaction between origin of the disease itself and impact on the family. Anorexia nervosa, ulcerative colitis, morbus crohn, myocardial infarction, and malignant diseases are other common examples of the importance of family dynamic processes connected with somatic symptoms. In 1977, Weakland described the importance of family relations for initiation and reinforcement of psychosomatic disease in his concept of "family psychosomatics". In 1978, Minuchin et al. coined the term "psychosomatic family". From a modern integrative system-analytic point of view (Olson 1983), these families are characterised by three typical variants.

In psychosomatic families or families with members who suffer from chronic diseases, we find typical close relationships among the family members. In recent publications, this has been described as "enmeshment" (Minuchin et al. 1978) and "bounded families" (Wirsching and Stierlin 1982). Typically we find an overprotecting anxiety between the family members for each other. Towards outside observers, for example psychotherapists, the family emphasize their close and well-working relationships. The intrafamiliar boundings are blurred; the family appears as a closed unit, and the surrounding is watched sceptically. In a stressful situation like the disease of one family member, the family cohesion increases to cope with the impending danger. With mutual consideration and maintenance of the status quo, the family tries to solve the new problem.

As the family focuses on its ill member, necessary evolution and adaptation processes in the new challenging situation become impossible. Jackson (1959) described this behavior as maintenance of "family homoeostasis", whereas Yalom called them "restricted families", (Jackson and Yalom 1966) and Minuchin et al. (1978) "rigid families". These strategies might be helpful in the short run, but they don't stabilize the family for a longer period of time, because they neglect the new reality.

In the long run, this artificial harmony in the family, which does not take into account the new situation, becomes a problem itself (Minuchin et al. 1978; Nemiah and Sifneos 1970). Defense mechanisms, like avoidance of conflicts, denial of own interests, and repression of aggressive feelings, ruin the chance of adaptation and future development in the new reality. The family gets into a vicious cycle of denial and worry or, in the end, in a breakdown.

## Therapeutic Approach

We have tried to describe the typical family-dynamic aspects by three variants:

1. Close connections within the family, blurred intrafamiliar boundings, and strong demarcation from the environment isolate the family
2. The abilities to adapt or to develop according to the new situation are restricted because the family tries to avoid any sort of alterations
3. Defence mechnisms, like rationalization, suppression of personal interests, and denial of aggressive emotions, result in a stressful atmosphere

From these three variants, we point out the following therapeutic aims:

1. The family needs more autonomy and independence to experience new strategies and to develop and find new forms of human relations.
2. We try to alter the tendencies to neglect conflicts by emancipation and support to help the family members towards a better understanding of their conflicts.

In family therapy we already have the problem of how to weigh to exposition of intrapsychic conflict versus a supportive approach. On the one hand, we can't obtain any development within the family without psychologizing the intrafamiliar and intrapsychic conflicts. On the other hand, the family therapist should not focus too early on these conflicts because many families react strictly defensively and may break up the therapeutic setting. In practice, it has proven advantageous for the family therapist to try a combination of both: He plays a neutral, impartial role, listening to the family in a supportive manner to establish a trustful relationship. Later, when a closer, trustful family-therapist relation has been developed, the family and the therapist can focus more on the critical conflicts. Special methods, e.g., the paradoxical intervention or the therapeutic alliance with the family's own defence mechanisms may be helpful, although paradoxical intervention in frontal-lobe patients may appear questionable. Since important psychodynamic changes in the family take place between the circa monthly therapeutic settings, this approach seems to be particularly favourable for family therapy. Therefore, the family itself can determine the intensity and frequency of their family therapy.

## Effectiveness and Efficiency

Few empirical data exist concerning outcome and process in family therapy. Case reports and clinical experience prevail.

Gurman et al. (1986) report on meta-analyses comparing effectiveness of family therapy and other methods of treatment: In two-thirds of all cases, symptoms improved as assessed by independent raters, therapists, and families themselves. Compared to other methods, family therapy was briefer but not better. The respective types (or schools) of family therapy showed no differences. An average of six sessions was administered in monthly intervals. The most pertinent effects took place between the first and the twentieth sessions. An early onset of therapy is recommended, as chronification worsens the prognosis. Family therapy appears to be an effective and economic method for a whole variety of mainly severe psychosocial conditions.

Process research investigates developments taking place during treatment. The discrepancy between theory and actual therapist's behavior is striking. In practice, the integration of different approaches is widespread. The dogmatic delineation of schools is decreasing.

Orlinsky and Howard (1986) investigated which factors have an impact on the outcome of treatment. The strongest predictor is the quality of the therapeutic bond. Interest in succeeding, empathy, and support are the most influential variables. Moreover, the information a patient receives before treatment motivation and the treatment contact are of importance. Different methods have only a marginal impact on the results. These findings underline the widespread trend towards an integration of different approaches in practical family therapy. They are also in accordance with findings from individual and group therapy research.

## Current Research

Today research demands an awareness of complex and interacting processes (dynamics of living systems), differentiation, and individualisation of treatment processes. Problems of indications, goals, and therapeutic procedures arise, i.e., which family, suffering from which disturbances, is best treated by which therapist, applying which methods in a respective context?

Though many questions remain unanswered, the following results can be taken for granted:

- Theoretical or technical rigidity ("schools") should be avoided in favor of a pragmatical integral approach.
- An ecological (or systemic) view focusing on interactions in the surrounding field is applied in family therapy, as well as in other human sciences (philosophy, sociology, biology).

The above-mentioned results have mainly been obtained from so-called psychosomatic disorders (anorexia, asthma, colitis, Chron's disease). The circular interaction of course and effect is especially prominent in these situations. This allows for powerful interventions. In other disorders that follows predominantly biological laws (like many types of cancer), a direct impact on the course of the illness is limited. In these cases, more indirect approaches are valid: Support and counselling of those in charge of the patient (e.g., nursing and medical staff). According to Wynne et al. (1986), we speak of systems consultation.

## Current Issues

Seen from a family-therapeutic point of view in the field of neuropsychological rehabilitation of patients with brain damage, the following questions must be asked: which family-dynamic aspects are of importance, to what extent are they specifically affected by brain damage and its sequelae, and which conclusions can be drawn to ensure an appropriate therapeutic approach?

To begin with, we can state: patients suffering from brain damage are burdened with various physical and psychic sequelae, like neurological dysfunctions or complete loss of functions. In addition, neuropsychological deficiencies or psychopathological disorders occur. Beside these impairments affecting the patient as an individual, brain damage and its sequelae have a severe impact on her or his social environment, especially on the family.

So far, preliminary clinical experience from consultation/liaision work and very limited scientific literature have shown the following patterns of conflict. The site of the damage itself is of importance. Brain damage causes massive anxiety followed by insecurity concerning the patient's future development, Relatives wonder what the extent of the psychological defect will be and how to cope with it? Individual and psychosocial defense mechanisms, like denial, overrating of sequelae, or stigmatizations, may contribute to misestimation of the patient's virtual capacity. Resignation or overprotectiveness will only serve to make things worse. Particularly it may cause inadequate role casting and role taking, through which a patient's motivation and, consequently, possible improvements are hindered. To get a definitive estimation of the sequelae of a given brain damage for the family system, we have to ask: Which family member is affected to what extent?

In this context, it is of importance to take a multigenerational perspective: Does the impairment of one parent, for example, basically jeopardize the existence of the whole family? What difficulties have to be expected for the psychological and psychosocial development of the children if one parent will not longer be able to fulfill parental responsibilities as done before. If one of the children suffers from brain damage, what does this mean for her or his parents, e.g. to realize that it won't be possible for the child to come up to its parents' former expectations. Further such issues could be enumerated. However, as the family's structure of roles and responsibilities is altered within short time, the family's flexibility is challenged. Feelings of being overburdened, helplessness, and hopelessness often arise acutely.

While supporting the family to cope with traumatizing sequelae and to develop new perspectives, we should bear in mind that, in fact, each family has its own history. Conflicts of psychogentic relevance occurred to a different extent and affected the development of each family member in a specific manner. The capacity of a family system to master issues caused by the brain damage successfully depends on their conflict-solving potential. It seems obvious that a family burdened with unsolved familiar problems before the onset of the brain damage will be able to manage conflicts only in a restricted manner. Resources are limited.

Intensifying of premorbid conflicts may disrupt an already critical balance within the family system. Family members might blame each other or demand too much of one another. An ulcious cycle may arise provoking intensified defensive maneuvers. (Subsequently these may also involve the attending medical and nursing staff.) To put it briefly, these defense maneuvers might be suitable to provide short-term relief, but over the medium term, they won't really help to clarify problems.

In addition, we have to consider to what extent family members not directly affected by the brain damage will underlie specific pressure to grapple with common developmental demands at a given stage in the life-cycle. If the family's normal abilities to develop are blocked during these periods of crisis, intensive bindings appear or, as a (not so common) alternative, the family breaks away.

Regarding these exemplary family-dynamic aspects briefly presented, the family's active involvement during the process of rehabilitation appears important from the following points of view:

1. Families with a member suffering from brain damage are burdened by multidimensional conflicts: intrapsychic stress (anxiety, guilt, narcissistic trauma), a stigmatizing environment, and the breakdown of the family's accustomed defense mechanisms result in a loss of potential for development. This happens at a time when the family's capacity to make decisions under stress is extremely burdened.
2. Destructive coping mechanisms may arise. This transforms an already stressful situation into a disaster.
3. Secondary, symptomatic complications may arise in other members of the system, thus laying the foundation for the formation of a multiproblem family.

Which conclusions can now be drawn concerning the development of an appropriate therapeutic concept? A family-centered intervention has to follow basic guidelines which have proven valid in comparable problem situations:

1. Information and support are basic ingredients of a helpful alliance.
2. Cooperation among those involved in the rehabilitation program is essential. Especially in consultation/liaison services, many practical possibilities have been developed.
3. The goal is seldom to initiate family therapy in a stricter sense. More often, secondary and tertiary prevention is indicated. The therapy has to focus on resources available rather than to pathologize an already stressful situation.

To sum up, we can say: A main goal of family-centered interventions is to initiate an extended bio-psycho-social perspective; that involves taking into account the importance of interdependent relationships, especially within the family, instead of focusing exclusively on the biomedical problems. Thus, we may not only support the family's own resources and self-help potential to cope with problems. We may also even open up a necessary chance for all family members to grieve over irretrievably lost ways of life.

Looking through available publications, we can state that family systems-oriented therapy has almost completely neglected patients suffering from brain damage in research and practice. Multidisciplinary programs favorably combining assessment and controlled interventions are urgently needed.

## References


Bergerhoff B, Hertenstein B, Cierpka M (1989) Die Bedeutung der Familie für die Rehabilitation knochenmarktransplantierter Patienten. Syst Fam 2:82–89

Bloch DA (1983) Family systems medicine: the field and the journal. Fam Syst Med 1:3–11

Carley L (1986) The family loves Samy but hated eachother. Nursing 16(10):44–46

Gerhardt U, Friedrich H (1983) Familie und chronische Krankheit – Versuch einer soziologischen Standortbestimmung. In: Angermeyer M, Freyberger H (eds) Chronisch kranke Erwachsene in der Familie. Enke, Stuttgart, pp 1–25

Gurman AS, Kniskern DP, Pinsof WM (1986) Research on marital and family therapies. In: Garfield SL, Bergin AE (eds) Handbook of psychotherapy and behavior change. Wiley, New York, pp 566–624

Jackson DD (1959) Family interaction, family homeostasis and some implications for conjoint family psychotherapy. In: Hasserman J (ed) Individual and family dynamics. Grune and Stratton, New York

Jackson DD, Yalom I (1966) Family research on the problem of ulcerative colitis. Arch Gen Psych 15:410–418

Lansky MR (1984) Family psychotherapy of the patient with chronic organic brain syndrome. Psychiatr Ann 14:121–129

Lansky MR (1989) Organic brain disease in the family: illness, personality, and family system. Fam Syst Med 7:66–76

Minuchin S, Rosman BL, Baker K (1978) Psychosomatic families: anorexia nervosa in context. Harvard University Press, Cambridge

Nemiah JC, Sifneos PE (1970) Psychosomatic illness: a problem in communication. Psychother Psychosom 18:154–160

Olson DH (1983) Families – what make them work. Sage, Beverly Hills

Orlinsky DE, Howard KI (1986) Process and outcome in psychotherapy. In: Garfield SL, Bergin AE (eds) Handbook of psychotherapy and behavior change, 3rd edn. Wiley, New York, pp 311–384

Reiter L (1988) Über die Anfänge, Ziele und Zielkonflikte in der internationalen Arbeitsgemeinschaft für Familienforschung und Familientherapie. Syst Fam 1:23–32

Richardson HB (1948) Patients have families. Common Wealth Foundation, New York

Weakland JH (1977) Family somatics – a neglected edge. Fam Proc 16:263–273

Willi J (1985a) Selbstverwirklichung in einer ökologisch gesehenen Gesellschaft. Praxis Psychotherapie Psychodynamik 30:35–43

Willi J (1985b) Die Familiengeschichte als Evolution des familiären Ideengutes. In: Willi J (ed) Die Koevolution. Rowohlt, Reinbek

Wirsching M (1986) Familiendynamik und Familientherapie in der Psychosomatik. In: Adler R, Herrmann JM, Köhle K, Schonecke OW, Uexküll T v, Wesiack W (eds) Psychosomatische Medizin. 3rd edn. Urban and Schwarzenberg, Munich, pp 303–315

Wirsching M (1989a) Familientherapie bei schweren psychischen Störungen. 31st Lindauer Psychotherapiewochen, Lindau

Wirsching M (1989b) In Zukunft Familientherapie? Entwicklungshypothesen. 10. Jahrestagung der Deutschen Arbeitsgemeinschaft Familientherapie, Darmstadt

Wirsching M, Stierlin H (1982) Krankheit und Familie. Konzepte – Forschungsergebnisse – Therapie. Klett-Cotta, Stuttgart

Wirsching M, Drings P, Georg W, Riehl J, Schmidt P (1989) Familien-System-Konsultation beim Bronchialkrebs. Syst Fam 2:65–81

Wynne L, McDaniel, Weber T (1986) Systems consultation. A new perspective for family therapy. Guilford Press, New York

# Discussion: Various Approaches for Treatment

*R. Cohen*

As the title of this session indicates, there is more heterogeneity than homogeneity among the three contributions of this afternoon. Accordingly, I shall not even try to squeeze out any communality I could discover. Instead I shall pose a number of questions that occurred to me while I was reading the manuscripts or listening to the presentations. For all of these questions there are no ready made answers; the questions are posed primarily to reflect where I consider further thinking and research most urgently needed. I shall now follow the route of today's program starting at David Howard's base camp crossing over Tony Marcel's pass to Rüger's heights from where I shall return on the same road.

David Howard's state of the art report from the cognitive neuropsychology camp allowed us a wide and optimistic view of the whole rehabilitation area. As it frequently happens when competent people discuss psychological problems from the viewpoint of cognitive psychology, everything appears clear, orderly and well-groomed, perhaps slightly sterile and somewhat hygienic, but nevertheless quite promising both with respect to basic science and to applied work. I see the beauty of this approach and David Howard convincingly demonstrated the versatility of this model as a hammer whenever you interpret something as a nail. We shall come back to this paper at the end.

The second section brought us to Tony Marcel and his presentation. Suddenly everything appeared vibrant and scintillating – and probably not only because of Tony Marcel's dramatic skills. The impairments and disabilities that compel people to ask for neuropsychological help are now seen as facets of a self-conscious and social being with all kinds of intentions and motivations (whether or not psychologists can appraise them properly). This being is usually painfully aware of the changes in his physical, psychological and social identity, no matter to what extent they may provoke attention or sympathy, and to what extent the common reduction in external demands is experienced more as relief or more as humiliation.

Unexpectedly, I lost sight of this social being during the last part of this afternoon's tour when we had to climb through the mists of system theory and family dynamics frequently covering the high ground. What Christian Rüger told us about illness, conflicts and problems sounds highly plausible, but, unfortunately, he dealt with it on such a general level that I had difficulties identifying what might be specific to the problems families have to face when one of their members is brain-damaged and when his or her disabilities not only create new problems but also provoke old conflicts. What is it that system theory and family dynamics can offer us for a better handling of all the many questions that prevail in this context? To give just a few examples:

1. How can one explain the surprisingly low prevalence rate of suicides in severely handicapped traumatic patients. The rate may be somewhat higher in aphasic patients, especially in Broca aphasics, – but apparently it did not play any role in the groups Christian Rüger dealt with. Is there something special in his families that may diminish depression? Or could frontal lobe lesions and their psychopathological correlates have dampened the basic despair?
2. How do families cope with the conflicts that are likely to arise when the patient can be blamed for the trauma because he/she had been e.g. driving under alcohol? I do not know of much evidence that manifest guilt feelings and reproaches play the prominent role one might expect in these families.
3. What difference does it make whether an undesirable trait like apathy or emotional indifference can be traced to premorbid characteristics of the patient or has developed only after the brain injury?
4. How does the sex of the patient affect the acceptance of different handicaps?

There is probably general agreement that (a) the impairments of a patient and his/her recovery are an integral part of family life, that (b) certain types of family interactions can counteract the possible progress in treatment – although this is not necessarily the most likely explanation of poor recovery in treatment – while others can raise the success of rehabilitation measures to a higher power – and not simply because the relatives are trying to copy the therapists –, and that (c) the interactions within a family have to change with every progress in therapy if the situation is not to become deleterious for the family. Finally, everybody will agree – we have heard this repeatedly in this conference – that the patient and his family should have "realistic expectations". But what do we mean by "realistic expectations"? From all we know the intra- and interindividual variance in recovery is just amazing. Can we expect mothers, fathers and spouses to be better prophets than we are? First of all, they have to learn to live with an extremely high degree of uncertainty, and we should learn how to help them in this endeavor.

In psychiatry strong evidence has accumulated, thanks to the seminal work of George Brown, Julian Leff and Christine Vaughn, that even in quite different cultures the probability of a relapse in patients with schizophrenia and with other psychiatric illnesses is systematically related to the amount of overinvolvement and critical attitudes in the relatives with whom the patient is living. Moreover, if these attitudes are modified through family intervention programs the sick members of the families require less therapeutic measures. It seems plausible, and should be tested, whether the same relationship between attitudes in the family and deterioration of a patient also hold for patients in neuropsychological rehabilitation.

Let us now turn around and retrace our steps to Tony Marcel's paper. In line with a number of other speakers on this conference he distinguishes between approaches that look for substitutes for the impaired function – Barbara Wilson will give us a number of beautiful examples, approaches that aim at recovery of the original function through proper training, and finally the "stimulation" approach which he illustrated with the treatment of apractic patients. In many respects Marcel's stimulation approach corresponds closely to what Egon Weigl had in mind when he wrote about "deblocking" in the treatment of aphasics through contextualization and introducing the critical behavior as an integral part of a meaningful behavior sequence. (Obviously, this "stimulation approach" is completely different from what Ed van Zomeren will discuss as "stimulation therapy" in his presentation tomorrow.)

Tony Marcel's distinction between the three approaches of rehabilitation is not only plausible but probably also necessary from a scientific and functional point of view. Nevertheless, we should keep in mind Hans-Lukas Teuber's warning that we shall hardly ever be able to decide in a given case whether some improvement is really a case of recovery and not of substitution. So far we have no good data to tell us under which conditions which strategy is preferable; but even if we had such evidence we have to realize – and Walter Huber will present evidence from his studies – that not every patient is prepared to accept substitutes no matter how little hope there is for a retraining of the original function.

I do not think Tony Marcel wants us to believe that "intent" is a simple question of free will, independent of contextual and attitudinal restraints. Ed van Zomeren will comment on this tomorrow. Psychotherapists since Freud have often written about all the many sorts of "resistance" against behavioral and attitudinal changes during therapy. We have to acknowledge that in addition to these resistances a considerable number of brain-injured patients have impairments in executive functions that are inversely related to the integrity of the prefrontal cortex and its connectivities. Yves von Cramon will probably discuss the pertinent problems in detail. More often than not the therapist cannot simply wait for the necessary intentions to arise; if he cannot elicit them, he has to create them. In future studies it may be worthwhile to study when therapists fail to create intentions and just blame the patient.

Let us go back to where we started in David Howard's base camp. His "effectiveness matrix" tells us that we have to expect three independent sources of variance: (a) a main effect for patient type with some patients responding positively to any kind of treatment while others hardly respond to anything; (b) a main effect for treatment type; and (c) an interaction with different outcomes for different types of patients receiving the same treatment. (I wonder whether the main effect of patient type could be reduced to the same dimension that we have in mind when we talk about "spontaneous recovery".) I do not want to discuss the controversial question of how best to categorize treatments and patients (according to lesion, to behavioral handicaps, to psychological impairments ...?) for such an analysis. Instead I would like to focus on the similarity of this model with Lee Cronbach's Aptitude-Treatment-Interaction model from 1957 for studying the effects of educational programs. When he reviewed the work on this model in 1975, his outlook was extremely pessimistic: although many studies found the expected interaction effects, hardly any of them could be replicated in subsequent studies. The subjects one experimenter studies in one setting are usually systematically different from those another experimenter studies in another setting; the patients you see in a University clinic, for example, are usually not a random sample from the same population you can see in a rehabilitation centre. Apparently, most of the interactions and other effects that are found in individual studies are so closely interwoven in higherorder interactions with other significantly moderating factors (like premorbid level of functioning, duration of illness, therapeutic setting etc.) that each study can only capture a nonrepresentative segment out of a much larger and considerably more complex matrix. I am afraid we have to expect that the interactions determining the effects of different types of rehabilitation will be of about the same high order as those for educational programs and psychotherapy.

One last comment: In line with other speakers at this conference David Howard stressed that we should not only talk about the measurement, evaluation and treatment of those functions that are impaired but also about those that are not affected through the injury. David Howard is as disappointed as I am with the usefulness of categorizing the impairments according to neuropathological or diagnostic categories. He hopes a sufficiently detailed description of the patient's behavior might be more promising. For several reasons I have serious doubts that a categorization of the behaviour independent of etiology is a way out:

1. It might be misleading to think of a dichotomy between impaired and intact functions instead of a continuum.
2. We know from such phenomena as have been described as "diaschises" that neurologically "intact" functions may easily appear severely impaired.
3. Since we hardly ever have precise information about the premorbid status of a patient with respect to a certain function, clinicians are usually bound to base their judgment on inter- instead of intraindividual comparisons, as if a score above or below an interindividual mean is the same as a score above or below the individual level of performance.
4. Every bit of behaviour is ambiguous as long as we do not know the context – a low rate of speech is to be interpreted completely differently in a global aphasic, in an acutely psychotic patient or whilst making love.

To be meaningful every description of behaviour must always comprise the systematic exclusion of alternative explanations, and nearly always behavioural descriptions tacitly imply assumptions about quite a number of motivational and intentional states. What we mean by "description of behaviour" is much more than just "description of behaviour"; and that is what is needed even if it is scientifically not kosher.

I fully agree with David Howard that information-processing models can help significantly in clarifying out thinking about what happens in therapy and that these models can profit from studies about what happens in therapy. It is a mutually stimulating experience from which quite a number of further text- and cookbooks about rehabilitation may originate. What may be needed most today is research on the conditions under which therapy works best and those under which therapists and patients do not succeed in their attempts. When can we expect to get a good meal in a house with a proper cookbook? The question sounds quite simple, but to find an answer should be far from simple, especially if we were to find it by controlling every possible variable that could effect the outcome. How complex a model are we prepared to take seriously if it comes to testing. We have to find a way between the Scylla of being simple-minded and the Charybdis of being muddle-headed. Let's face it; otherwise we shall never reach our destination.

# Specific Treatment of Specific Deficits

# Impairments of Attention in Brain-Damaged Patients

*A.H. van Zomeren and L. Fasotti*

## Introduction

People who have sustained cerebral damage often complain of increased mental fatiguability, poor concentration, and an inability to divide their attention over two simultaneous tasks. These impairments seem related to a central concept of *attention.* However, it is difficult to describe the clinical phenomena in unequivocal terms. Attention is definitely not a clearcut function, as the word refers to several aspects of perceptual processes and motor responses. Moreover, the term also covers basic biological aspects of the central nervous system, such as its level of activation. This chapter is concerned with attention on task level, and hence with a psychological approach. In the next section, impairments in five aspects of attention will be discussed. The last section deals with attempts to ameliorate attentional impairments by cognitive rehabilitation.

## Attentional Impairments

### Hemi-Inattention

Hemi-inattention or one-sided neglect is the phenomenon that patients fail to respond to or report stimuli in one half of space or to one half of their bodies (Heilman et al. 1985). It can be caused by lesions in a variety of brain regions: cortical areas, such as the temporo-parietal-occipital junction; limbic areas, such as the cingulate gyrus; and subcortical areas, such as the thalamus and the reticular formation in the mesencephalon. The subcortical structures are important for mediating arousal and an adequate level of activation, but the cortical component is involved in the analysis of the behavioral significance of stimuli. In the Heilman model, hemi-inattention is viewed as an attentional-arousal disorder, caused by dysfunction of a cortico-limbic-reticular loop.

The substantial asymmetry in hemispheric lesions causing neglect suggests that the right hemisphere is more important for the monitoring of our outside world than the left. Research with both normal subjects and patients very strongly suggests that the right hemisphere has a capacity to monitor *both* halves of extrapersonal space, while the left hemisphere merely monitors the contralateral hemispace. This implies that the manifestations of hemi-inattention caused by lesions in the left hemisphere are usually masked by compensatory mechanisms stemming from the intact right hemisphere. If, however, the right hemisphere is rendered inactive by a lesion somewhere in the cortico-limbic-reticular loop, the intact left hemisphere will only attend to and act in the right hemispace.

Hemi-inattention is usually caused by focal lesions, particularly cerebrovascular accidents. Closed head injury seldom results in neglect phenomena, although their frequency may have been underestimated in this category by lack of large-scale investigations.

The *assessment* of hemi-inattention makes use of several readily available techniques. The first of these is simple observation of a patient's behaviour. Hemi-inattention also often reveals itself in drawings by the patients or in their copies of complex patterns. A more standardized approach makes use of visual search tasks. These may present either nonstructured (Albert 1973) or structured stimulus fields to the subject. Most widely used are tasks in which targets are arranged in horizontal lines (Diller and Weinberg 1977; Wade et al. 1988) or reading tests (Caplan 1987). Wilson et al. (1987) have published the Rivermead Behavioural Inattention Battery, a well-standardized series of tests with satisfactory normative information.

## Focused Attention

Focused attention is defined as selectively reacting to target stimuli in the presence of irrelevant stimuli having a distracting potential, for example, by a certain resemblance of distractors to target stimuli. In normal subjects, focusing is amazingly efficient.

Subjects who have sustained cerebral damage, be it through head injury, cerebro-vascular accident (CVA), hypoxia, or any other cause, often complain that irrelevant stimulation is unusually unpleasant to them. However, despite this subjective intolerance for irrelevant stimulation, experimental studies have shown that most patients can focus on relevant signals just as well as control subjects with a healthy brain. This has been demonstrated with verbal distractors, i.e., voices presenting irrelevant messages simultaneously with a relevant one (Dencker and Löfving 1958; Gronwall and Sampson 1974) and with the use of delayed feedback, in which subjects heard their own voice, while reading aloud, in an echo-like way (Van Zomeren and Brouwer 1987). In the visual domain, Miller and Cruzat (1980) reported that head-injured patients were not influenced by irrelevant stimuli printed on cards that had to be sorted as quickly as possible.

Finally, the Stroop effect (1935) has been used to study focusing in brain-damaged subjects. This effect is created by presenting stimuli with two dimensions: colour and verbal meaning. These dimensions are conflicting on the response level, i.e., the subject may see the word "blue" in green letters. The subject is instructed to name the colour of such words, but the highly automatized reading process guarantees that the word meaning works as a powerful distractor, causing response interference. The Stroop paradigm has failed to demonstrate impaired focusing after closed head injury (Chadwick et al. 1981; Stuss et al. 1985; van Zomeren et al. 1988). In contrast, disproportionate Stroop effects have been found in patients with neoplastic and vascular lesions in the frontal lobes (Perret 1974; Holst and Villki 1988). On the level of clinical observation, an increased distractability and a tendency to react to irrelevant aspects in a given situation has been reported frequently in patients with focal lesions of the frontal lobes (Luria 1966).

To summarize, it seems that focused attention can be normal in brain-damaged subjects, unless the frontal lobes are involved. Regarding the assessment of this aspect of attention, The Stroop Colour Word Test has some value, in addition to clinical observation.

## Divided Attention

Divided attention refers to the ability to attend to more than one source of stimulation, to more than one aspect of stimuli, or to several subtasks within a given activity. The effectiveness of divided attention is determined by two factors: processing capacity, and strategies. In this section, the emphasis lies on processing capacity, or the amount of information that can be processed in a given time unit. This capacity is largely dependent on the *speed of information processing.* If information processing is slow in a given subject, he will have "less attention to pay" per time unit.

People who have sustained brain damage may complain of mental slowness and an inability to divide their attention (van Zomeren and van den Burg 1985). In this case, the complaints can be related to empirical data: a variety of neurological conditions, from encephalitis to neoplasms, have been demonstrated to result in prolonged reaction times (Blackburn and Benton 1955; Hicks and Birren 1970). As Lezak (1983) states it, the phenomenon of mental slowness shows up in longer than average total performance times on various tasks in the absence of a specific motor disability. Benton and Joynt (1958) demonstrated that unilateral cerebral disease resulted in prolonged reaction times, even when patients were tested with the hand ipsilateral to the lesion.

Although particularly choice reaction times are quite fit to demonstrate a slowing of information processing (Miller 1971; van Zomeren and Deelman 1978), these tasks are usually not aimed at divided attention. A widely accepted test of divided attention is the Paced Auditory Serial Addition Task as devised by Gronwall and Sampson (1974). In this task, a random series of digits is presented to the subject and, after hearing each digit, he or she is supposed to add it to the preceding one and give the answer aloud. This is basically a very simple task. However, when rate of presentation is increased, subjects begin to make errors, as they are forced to divide their limited processing capacity over three subtasks: listening, calculating, and responding. Gronwall and co-workers have shown that PASAT reveals a temporary slowing of information processing after mild head injury. On the other hand, severe head injury may cause a long-lasting impairment in PASAT performance (O'Shaugnessy et al. 1984), and this is in agreement with the mental slowness as demonstrated in several follow-up studies of reaction times after severe to very severe injuries (Norrman and Svahn 1961; van Zomeren and Deelman 1978).

In the traditional arsenal of tests available to the clinical psychologist, there are many speed tests that are fit for the assessment of a slowing in information processing. In the Wechsler Adult Intelligence Scale (Wechsler 1955), the subtest Digit Symbols is useful, as this is essentially another divided attention task, including visual perception, translation of symbols into digits, and writing. In the assessment of mental slowness, one should make use of age-adjusted norms and beware of the negative influence of any visual or motor impairments.

## Sustained Attention

The word "sustained" merely indicates that some aspect of information processing is studied with a special interest for changes in performance over time. For clinical work, three phenomena may be relevant: time-on-task effects, lapses of attention, and intra-individual variability. However, only the first phenomenon has been investigated to some extent in neuropsychological research.

The term *time-on-task effects* refers to gradual changes in continuous performance. In normal subjects, negative effects have been studied in particular, such as a decrease in quality of performance or in signal detection. In the present context, the question is whether such time-on-task effects are stronger after brain damage. Goldstein (1952) suggested that performance of brain-damaged subjects would deteriorate quickly, but this has not been confirmed by later investigators (Dencker and Löfving 1958; Greber and Perret 1985; van Zomeren and Brouwer 1987). Various groups of neurologic patients appeared to perform poorly on tasks of sustained attention, such as vigilance tasks, continuous reaction time tasks, and even lane-tracking while driving on a highway (van Zomeren et al. 1988). Reaction times are longer, signal detection is poorer, and lane-tracking ability is weakened after brain damage, but the important point is that in all studies patients maintained their initial level of performance just as well as subjects in control groups. Therefore, the conclusion must be that no special time-on-task effects have so far been demonstrated – but a word of caution is necessary. In all these studies, patients were left free to choose their own speed of performance or rate of errors. This is unusual in tasks in daily life, for example in working situations.

For *assessment* of sustained attention, a variety of prolonged tests can be used, provided that performance can be reliably scored in time blocks, be it either in speed or accuracy. The availability of personal computers for assessment makes it easy to devise a continuous reaction-time task in which time-on-task effects might reveal themselves. Likewise, a Continuous Performance Test (Rosvold et al. 1956) can be presented by pc.

## Supervisory Attentional Control

After the development of information processing models, cognitive psychology has shown an increasing interest in *strategies of attention* that enable an efficient use of available processing capacity. Such controlling supervisory strategies form the Supervisory Attentional System (Shallice 1982) and are part of the executive functions of the brain (Luria 1966; Lezak 1982). Supervisory control becomes especially important in non-routine situations, where a subject has to react in a flexible way to changing or unusual task demands. It is, therefore, linked closely with controlled information processing as opposed to automatic processing (Shiffrin and Schneider 1977).

The concept of supervisory attentional control has so far seldom been used explicitly in neuropsychological research. Shallice (1982) studied the clinical usefulness of his theory in patients with focal brain lesions by means of a look-ahead puzzle in which problems can only be solved by suppressing apparently correct, straight-forward responses in favour of an indirect approach. On this task, called the Tower of London, patients with left frontal lesions performed significantly poorer than subjects with posterior lesions.

Another approach of flexibility was realized by Brouwer et al. (1989), who made use of a dual-task methodology. Subjects who had survived very severe head injuries 5–12 years before were trained to learn two tasks separately: lane tracking in a car simulator while an electronic "sidewind" was hindering them, and the counting of groups of dots that were projected onto the same video screen that presented the "road" in the simulator. For both tasks, the difficulty was adjusted to the patient's individual capacity (90% correct counts, 90% of time on target). In the critical stage of the experiment, the two tasks had to be carried out simultaneously. It was found that, with individual differences controlled for, the patients had no special problems in dividing their processing capacity over two tasks. The same results were found in a second study of patients who had sustained their injuries recently. These results suggest that the strategy for dealing with the combined tasks was not impaired in the head-injured groups.

## Summary

Lesions in the right hemisphere may cause hemineglect. Focused attention is usually unimpaired after brain damage. An impairment may be found in patients with frontal lesions only when distractors tend to evoke well-trained responses. Divided attention is very often impaired, obviously as a result of a slowing of information processing that renders the subject unable to deal with all relevant signals in a task situation, particularly under time pressure. In sustained attention, no deficits have been demonstrated so far: although patients often perform poorly, they usually maintain their initial level of performance. Finally, on theoretical grounds, impairments in Supervisory Attentional Control might be expected after frontal lesions.

## Rehabilitation of Attentional Impairments

The fact that deficits of attention have implications for every domain of functional independence has led to the development of various training programs. Their practical background is often reflected in a loose connection with current theories of attention, as well as in the increasing use of computers as training tools. Training programs are based on one of the following three models: stimulation therapy, strategy substitution, and behavioural conditioning (Gross and Schutz 1986).

### Stimulation Therapy

The major premise of this training model is that attentional impairments can be remediated by direct stimulation of brain structures assumed to be involved in attending or in a particular aspect of attention. Treatment is based on submitting patients to repetitive exercises and providing them with feedback about their performance. The reiterated stimulation of brain structures would facilitate neuronal growth or regeneration (Powell 1981), and attention would respond like a "mental muscle" whose function, as in the case of real muscles, could be improved by repeated exercise (Harris and Sunderland 1981). Training efficacy can be measured in three ways: at task level, at the level of task-related psychometric tests, and at the level of daily functioning.

*Task-Level Measures.* All studies in which improvement was systematically measured on trained tasks reported noticeable progress. Wood and Fussey (1987) trained very severely head-injured patients to scan moving symbols on a computer screen. They found a gradual and significant increase in number of correct responses during the first 7 days and a halving of variability in individual performances. In a case study of a radiologist with a right temporal lobectomy, Rao and Bieliauskas (1983) noted a considerable training effect in a Symbol Cancellation Task. Ben-Yishay et al. (1987) applied the Orientation Remedial Module, a computerized series of five tasks forming an overlapping hierarchy in complexity of reception/response demands. In severely head-injured patients, the training resulted in a progression from initially impaired performance to the average normal range.

*Psychometric Measures.* Stimulation studies often make use of psychometric tests to find any generalization effect of training. Results have been somewhat conflicting. In the Wood and Fussey (1978) study, psychomotor measures and vigilance measures did not reveal significant changes after training on the scanning task. Malec et al. (1984) employed video games to improve sustained attention in patients with traumatic brain injury. Three tests of sustained attention and a reaction-time task were used as dependent variables. The only measure that approached significance (without reaching it) was the reaction-time task. Ponsford and Kinsella (1988) also trained a group of severely head-injured patients who had to respond rapidly and selectively to information presented on a computer screen. Progress on psychometric measures of information-processing speed did not exceed spontaneous recovery level.

However, a few studies report training effects that were visible in psychometric evaluations. Ben-Yishay et al. (1987) trained a very severely head-injured subject with the Orientation Remedial Module and found significant improvements in visual reaction times, auditory digits, and the WAIS verbal IQ. Sturm et al. (1983) employed a series of 16 psychometric tests for the evaluation of training with reaction times and memory-search tasks. Improvement was most evident in the tests that resembled the training tasks. Two studies in which head-injured patients were trained with various visuomotor, visual search, and reaction-time tasks (Sivak et al. 1984a, b) reported better performance after training on a variety of psychological tests, including several WAIS-subtests.

Sohlberg and Mateer (1983) designed Attention Process Training, a hierarchical, multilevel computer program that should remediate various aspects of attention. Four brain-damaged subjects underwent 5–10 weeks training, and all of them showed significant and stable gains in PASAT performance. Gray et al. (1989) reported that a group of traumatic and non-traumatic brain-damaged patients improved more than a control group on PASAT, Backward Digit Span, and the WAIS subtests Block Design, Arithmetic and Picture Completion.

In view of this conflicting evidence, it is difficult to formulate a conclusion. About half of the studies described do not report progress on psychometric measures after stimulation therapy, while some of the remaining studies are either based on a single case, poorly controlled for spontaneous recovery, or find effects only in psychometric measures resembling the trained tasks.

*Effects on Daily Functioning.* Three studies have evaluated effects of stimulation therapy on daily-life functioning. Wood and Fussey (1987) recorded "attention to task" during patients' therapy activities. This measure produced significant differences between baseline and post-treatment assessment. The training of perceptual skills given by Sivak et al. (1984b) resulted in improved driving performance. The degree of improvement in driving quality was related to the degree of improvement in trained perceptual skills. Finally, Ponsford and Kinsella (1988) used a rating scale for day-to-day attentional behaviour. Improvements on this rating scale were mainly due to spontaneous recovery. On the basis of this scarce evidence, the effects of stimulation therapy on daily-life attentional behaviour seem as yet unconvincing.

## Strategy Substitution

This therapy model is based on the assumption that patients can be helped by providing them with compensatory strategies, either in the form of external aids (e.g., a checklist) or as internal procedures like self-instruction. Frequently used compensatory strategies are *verbal mediation* techniques. These are based on Luria's idea (1966) that the regulation of attention is largely dependent on subvocal or inner speech. Webster and Scott (1983) trained a construction worker to use self-instructional statements to focus attention during reading or listening, two years after a severe head injury. Results suggested that not only attention, but also recall of information improved significantly. Barry and Riley (1987) introduced verbal mediation while teaching hand-movement patterns to a young woman with a severe closed head injury. Significant improvements were found, which could be partially attributed to the assimilation of the verbal strategy. In the study by Rao and Bieliauskas (1983), stimulation therapy was combined with verbal mediation techniques. The patient-radiologist was encouraged to use his verbal skills to solve non-verbal tasks and to write verbal summaries immediately after seeing movies. After training, improvement was noted in several areas. Most relevant was the improvement in the patient's professional skills: his accuracy rate in reading radionuclide scans increased from 80% to 100%.

In addition to these case studies, Robertson et al. (1989) studied the effect of computerised scanning and attentional training in 20 patients with left-sided visual neglect. The method was partially aimed at habit formation by verbal mediation ("look left – touch left"). A blind evaluation at the end of training and at six months follow-up revealed no significant results, in comparison with a control group.

Although the three case studies seem to indicate that strategy substitution can be effective, further research on groups is needed to confirm the benefits of this training model. However, two advantages of strategy substitution are undeniable: the model is explicitly based on a theoretical idea, and the exercises are directly aimed at problem behaviours and consequently avoid the generalization problems that are so prominent in stimulation therapy.

## Behavioural Conditioning

One study only addressed the use of behavioural techniques for training attention. Wood (1987) used contingent reinforcement, in the form of tokens, to improve focused and divided attention during therapy tasks. In two out of three patients with very severe head injuries, the method resulted in significant changes in attention to task performance.

Behavioural-conditioning techniques presumably will be most appropriate for patients with very severe brain damage whose extensive cognitive impairments impede the application of strategy substitution.

## Summary

Stimulation methods and the use of computers do not seem to hold great promise for the rehabilitation of attentional impairments. Strategy substitution and behavioural methods might be more efficient as treatment methods. Moreover, they are based on firm theoretical grounds, and their generalization problems are less prominent. From a theoretical point of view, it is interesting to note that the model of strategy substitution is linked with the concept of Supervisory Attentional Control, as new strategies have to be learned on the basis of controlled processing.

## References

Albert ML (1973) A simple test of visual neglect. Neurology (Minneap) 23:658–664

Barry P, Riley JM (1987) Adult norms for the Kaufman Hand Movement Test and a single-subject design for acute brain injury rehabilitation. J Clin Exp Neuropsychol 9:449–455

Ben-Yishay Y, Piasetsky EB, Rattock J (1987) A systematic method for ameliorating disorders in basic attention. In: Meyer MJ, Benton AL, Diller L (eds) Neuropsychological rehabilitation. Livingstone, Edinburgh

Blackburn HL, Benton AL (1955) Simple and choice reaction time in cerebral disease. Confin Neurol 15:327–338

Benton AL, Joynt RJ (1958) Reaction time in unilateral cerebral disease. Confin Neurol 19:247–256

Brouwer WH, Ponds RWHM, van Wolffelaar PC, van Zomeren AH (1989) Divided attention 5 to 10 years after closed head injury. Cortex 25:219–230

Caplan B (1987) Assessment of unilateral neglect: a new reading test. J Clin Exp Neuropsychol 9:359–364

Chadwick O, Rutter M, Brown G, Shaffer D, Traub M (1981) A prospective study of children with head injuries. II. Cognitive sequelae. Psychol Med 11:49–61

Dencker SJ, Löfving B (1958) A psychometric study of identical twins discordant for closed head injury. Acta Psychiatr Neurol Scand [Suppl 122] 33

Diller L, Weinberg J (1977) Hemi-inattention in rehabilitation: the evolution of a rational remediation program. In: Weinstein EA, Friedland RP (eds) Advances in neurology vol 10. Raven, New York

Goldstein K (1952) The effects of brain damage on personality. Psychiatry 15:245–260

Gray JM, Robertson I, Pentland B, Smith S (1992) Microcomputer-based attentional retraining after brain damage: a randomised group controlled trial. Neuropsych Rehabil (in press)

Greber R, Perret E (1985) Attention and short-term memory disorders after brain stem lesions. EBBS Workshop, Zurich

Gronwall D, Sampson H (1974) The psychological effects of concussion. Auckland University Press, Auckland

Gross Y, Schutz LE (1986) Intervention models in neuropsychology. In: Uzzell BP, Gross Y (eds) Clinical neuropsychology of intervention. Nijhoff, Boston

Harris JE, Sunderland A (1981) A brief survey of the management of memory disorders in rehabilitation units in Britain. Int Rehabil Med 3:206–209

Heilman KM, Watson RT, Valenstein E (1985) Neglect and related disorders. In: Heilman KM, Valenstein E (eds) Clinical neuropsychology. Oxford University Press, New York

Hicks L, Birren JE (1970) Aging, brain damage and psychomotor slowing. Psychol Bull 74:377–396

Holst P, Villki J (1988) Effect of frontalmedial lesions on performance on the Stroop test and word fluency tasks. J Clin Exp Neuropsychol 10:79–80

Lezak MD (1982) The problems of assessing executive functions. Int J Psychol 17:281–297
Lezak MD (1983) Neuropsychological assessment. Oxford University Press, New York
Luria AR (1966) Higher cortical functions in man. Tavistock, London
Malec J, Rao N, Jones R, Stubbs K (1984) Video game practice effects on sustained attention in patients with craniocerebral trauma. Cogn Rehabil 2:18–23
Miller E (1971) Simple and choice reaction time following severe head injury. Cortex 6:121–127
Miller E, Cruzat A (1981) A note on the effects of irrelevant information on task performance after mild and severe head injury. Br J Soc Clin Psychol 20:69–70
Norrman B, Svahn K (1961) A follow-up study of severe brain injuries. Acta Psychiatr Scand 37:236–264
O'Shaugnessy EJ, Fowler RS, Reid V (1984) Sequelae of mild closed head injuries. J Fam Pract 18:391–394
Perret E (1974) The left frontal lobe in man and the suppression of habitual responses in verbal categorical behavior. Neuropsychologia 12:323–330
Ponsford JL, Kinsella G (1988) Evaluation of a remedial programme for attentional deficits following closed head injury. J Clin Exp Neuropsychol 10:693–708
Powell GE (1981) Brain function therapy. Gower-Aldershot, Hants
Rao SM, Bieliauskas LA (1983) Cognitive rehabilitation two-and- one-half years post right temporal lobectomy. J Clin Neuropsychol 5:313–320
Robertson I, Gray JM, Pentland B, Waite LJ (1990) A randomised controlled trial of microcomputer-based rehabilitation for unilateral left visual neglect. Arch Phys Med Rehabil 71:663–668
Rosvold HE, Mirsky AF, Sarason I, Bransome ED, Beck LH (1956) A Continuous Performance Test of brain damage. J Consult Psychol 20:343–350
Shallice T (1982) Specific impairments of planning. In: Broadbent DE, Weiskrantz L (eds) The neuropsychology of cognitive function. Royal Society, London, pp 199–209
Shiffrin RM, Schneider W (1977) Controlled and automatic human information processing. II. Perceptual learning, automatic attending and a general theory. Psychol Rev 84:127–190
Sivak M, Hill CS, Olson PL (1984a) Computerized video tasks as training techniques for driving-related perceptual deficits of persons with brain damage: a pilot evaluation. Int J Rehabil Res 7:389–398
Sivak M, Hill CS, Henson DL, Butler BP, Silber SM, Olson PL (1984b) Improved driving performance following perceptual training in persons with brain damage. Arch Phys Med Rehabil 65:163–167
Sohlberg MM, Mateer CA (1987) Effectiveness of an attention training program. J Clin Exp Neuropsychol 9:117–130
Stroop JR (1935) Studies of interference in serial verbal reactions. J Exp Psychol 18:643–662
Sturm W, Dahmen W, Hartje W, Willmes K (1983) Ergebnisse eines Trainingsprogramms zur Verbesserung der visuellen Auffassungsschnelligkeit und Konzentrationsfähigkeit bei Hirngeschädigten. Arch Psychiatr Nervenkr 233:9–22
Stuss DT, Ely P, Hugenholtz H, Richard MT, Larochelle S, Poirier CA, Bell I (1985) Subtle neuropsychological deficits in patients with good recovery after closed head injury. Neurosurgery 17:41–47
Wade DT, Wood VA, Langton Hewer R (1988) Recovery of cognitive function soon after stroke: a study of visual neglect, attention span and verbal recall. J Neurol Neurosurg Psychiatry 51:10–13
Webster JS, Scott RR (1983) The effects of self-instructional training on attentional deficits following head injury. Clin Neuropsychol 5:69–74
Wechsler D (1955) The measurement of adult intelligence. Williams and Wilkins, Baltimore
Wilson BA, Cockburn J, Halligan P (1987) The development of a behavioral test of visuospatial neglect. Arch Phys Med Rehabil 68:98–102
Wood RL (1987) Brain injury rehabilitation: a neurobehavioral approach. Croon Helm, London
Wood RL, Fussey I (1987) Computer-based cognitive retraining: a controlled study. Int Disabil Stud 9:149–153

Van Zomeren AH, Brouwer WH (1987) Head injury and concepts of attention. In: Levin HS, Grafman J, Eisenberg HM (eds) Neurobehavioral recovery from head injury. Oxford University Press, New York

Van Zomeren AH, Deelman BG (1978) Long-term recovery of visual reaction time after closed head injury. J Neurol Neurosurg Psychiatry 41:452–457

Van Zomeren AH, van den Burg W (1985) Residual complaints of patients two years after severe closed head injury. J Neurol Neurosurg Psychiatry 48:21–28

Van Zomeren AH, Brouwer WH, Rothengatter JA, Snoek JW (1988) Fitness to drive a car after recovery from severe head injury. Arch Phys Med Rehabil 69:90–96

# Assessment and Management of Memory Problems

*B. Wilson*

## Assessment

Assessments are carried out to answer questions and the nature of these questions determines assessment procedure. Thus questions about theoretical issues require a different approach to assessment than do questions about treatment issues. For example, if we want to know whether implicit memory is a unitary concept we should assess as many different aspects of implicit memory as possible and also assess a large number of people in an attempt to find dissociations between subjects. If, on the other hand, we want to know which memory problems are causing most distress for a particular patient, we should interview that patient and perhaps other family members. We may need to observe the patient in a number of different settings and refer to rating scales, checklists, questionnaires and/or self report measures.

In rehabilitation we need answers to questions about general intellectual functioning and about specific cognitive functions such as perception, memory, attention and language. For example, we may need to find out whether a patient has visual agnosia or unilateral neglect, whether memory deficits are global or restricted to certain kinds of material, whether processing of information is unduly slow, and what the particular cognitive strengths of a patient might be. All these questions can be answered by neuropsychological tests.

In addition, we need answers to questions relating to treatment or management. For example, we may need to know how many times a patient repeats a particular question each day, whether s/he remembers to put on the wheelchair brakes when transferring to the toilet, whether s/he can learn information if we present it in a certain way, and what understanding the patient has of his or her memory deficits.

Such questions are unlikely to be answered by neuropsychological tests. Instead we have to resort to behavioural assessment procedures such as rating scales, checklists, questionnaires and direct observation. A summary of behavioural assessment procedures can be found in Wilson (1987), and a dicussion of the advantages and disadvantages of self report measures is presented in Wilson et al. (1989a).

Good management or rehabilitation of memory problems requires appropriate assessment. Appropriate assessment involves testing of cognitive functioning and assessing everyday aspects of memory. We need to know, for example, whether a person is impaired on a paired-associate learning task, but we would not wish to treat poor performance on this task. Impaired performance might indicate organic memory impairment and predict poor performance at work but it would not in, and of, itself greatly affect everyday life. Memory impaired people and their families are more likely to be concerned about the loss of personal belongings, whether a task has been completed, forgetting people's names, getting lost on a journey and inability to learn new skills. Behavioural assessments allow us to identify and measure these aspects. In order to design and evaluate treatment programmes we must combine neuropsychological and behavioural assessments.

## Recovery

Having assessed a memory impaired person, what are we going to do with the information? Should be do anything? Will some patients recover without help?

There is no doubt that some memory impaired patients show considerable improvement over time, which could be regarded as recovery or partial recovery. However, it is not clear whether this improvement can be enhanced or accelerated by intervention procedures. Furthermore, the term "recovery" is open to a number of interpretations. Almli and Finger (1988) list seven definitions of recovery:

1. Resumption of normal life even though there may be minor neurological and psychological deficits (Jennett and Bond 1975)
2. Achievement of a goal (Laurence and Stein 1978)
3. A return to normal or near normal levels of performance following the initially disruptive effects of an injury to the nervous system (Laurence and Stein 1978)
4. Impairments in behavioural or physiological functions that abate as time since injury increases (Marshall 1985)
5. When persistent behavioural deficits are reduced by special training or by pharmacological, surgical or other independent manipulations (Braun 1978)
6. Recovery is the post lesion reinstatement of the specific behaviours that were disrupted by the brain injury (LeVere 1980)
7. Recovery is a theoretical construct that implies a complete regaining of the identical functions that were lost or impaired after brain injury (Almli and Finger 1988)

One might find memory impaired people who fit into each of the above definitions but it might be wiser to avoid the use of the term "recovery" of memory functioning. Perhaps more reasonable terms would be "improvement" and "compensation". Thus we can ask whether brain injured people show improvements in their memory functioning over time and do they learn to compensate for their deficits?

A long-term follow-up study of 54 memory impaired people who were offered memory therapy between 1980–1985 is currently underway in Britian. The 54 patients comprise 29 with traumatic head injury. 7 with sub-arachnoid haemorrhage, 3 with strokes (other than SAH), 3 with Korsakoff Syndrome, 2 who had attempted suicide with carbon monoxide poisoning, 4 with encephalitis, 2 with cerebral tumor, 2 with severe epilepsy, 1 with anoxia following a near drowning, and 1 with both a stroke and a headinjury; one patient refused to take part in the study. Seven had died at follow-up and 6 could not be contacted. Of the 38 currently being seen, about 33% have shown marked improvement in memory functioning as measured by the Rivermead Behavioural Memory Test (Wilson et al. 1989b), although some still have significant memory problems. One encouraging sign is that most are making more use of external memory aids (such as notebooks and tape-recorders) than they were before the onset of their memory problems or during the rehabilitation period. External aids were introduced, discussed and practised during rehabilitation, but not used a great deal then. This finding suggests that these ex-patients are compensating more now.

Almost 40% of the sample are in some kind of employment, although only two people are in jobs comparable to those held before the onset of the memory problems. Nearly 20% are living at home with no regular attendance elsewhere. Thirteen per cent are attending day centres, 13% are in long term care and just under 11% are in full time education.

It is not possible to say from this follow-up study how far the improvements are due to the earlier provision of rehabilitation, but the study does tell us that a considerable percentage show improvement over time, particularly those with traumatic head injury. Also, relatively few are in long term care. Of those who are unable to live at home, most are suffering from cerebral vascular disorder or encephalitis.

Despite the knowledge that improvement is likely to occur over time for 30% or more of memory impaired people without a deteriorating condition, a great deal needs to be done to help families and patients cope with and understand memory difficulties. This is true not only for those who do not improve, but also for those who improve but whose memory functioning remains impaired. There are a number of strategies we can use to help reduce, by-pass or overcome poor memory functioning.

## Memory Rehabilitation Strategies

### Environmental Adaptations

One of the simplest ways of managing severe memory problems is to structure the environment in order to reduce the memory load on the individual. This is the principle of avoiding or by-passing the problem. Labels, signposts, colour coding, positioning material so that it cannot easily be missed, or even changing the wording used when speaking to memory impaired people, are examples of changing the environment. One young man, for example, when asked "Are you ready Martin?", always replied, "Ready, willing and disabled". Although this was mildly amusing at first, several repetitions of this phrase led to great irritation in those around him. The simple solution was to stop saying, "Are you ready Martin?", substituting this with, "We are going to start now Martin".

For those with very severe intellectual handicap, or those with progessive deterioration, environmental change may be the best we can do to enable people to cope and reduce some of their confusion and frustration. Few studies have discussed ways in which environments can be designed to help severely amnesic people, although it would seem a fruitful area for architects, typographers and psychologists to join forces.

## External Aids

External aids attempt to help people remember by using systems to access or record information. Harris (1984) says there are two major kinds of external memory aids. The first are those which enable us to access internally stored information. An example would be a timer to remind us to take something out of the oven. These aids are not very helpful for people with severe memory impairment, as they cannot remember what it is they are supposed to remember. The second major group of external memory aids according to Harris (1984) includes aids which record information externally. These are widely used by nonmemory impaired people and include diaries, (appointment schedules) memos, lists, writing on one's hand, ringing or writing on a calendar, asking someone to remind you and putting something in a special place in order not to miss it. Memory impaired people, on the other hand, frequently use fewer external aids than the general population. There are probably several reasons for this. Some people feel it is cheating in some way to use such aids, and they may make such statements as, "I don't want to rely on such things, I want my memory to get better by itself". There is in fact no evidence to suggest that using aids will prevent return of memory. Indeed the opposite is likely to be true. Others simply forget to use the aids or forget to refer to them when they have recorded information. Some patients, because they live in protected environments, do not have to rely on their own resources to cope with memory demands of everyday life. Those who feel it is cheating to use external aids should be made aware that it is quite normal for non-memory impaired people to use external aids, their use will not slow down recovery of memory, and that it is sensible to use anything which will improve the ability to remember. For those who cannot remember to use certain external aids, it may be worth exploring alternatives. There is such a wide range available, that it should be possible to find one or two suitable for each individual. In addition, it may be necessary to use a behaviour programme to teach or encourage people in the use of external aids.

In addition to the better known external aids such as diaries, notebooks, lists, alarm clocks, wall charts and calendars, a number of external aids have been devised to cope with particular problems. Davies and Binks (1983), for example, used a small card (the size of a credit card) for a Korsakoff patient. On one side of the card was the man's name and address and on the other side was a statement explaining that the man had memory difficulties and needed information written down. The man could show the card to strangers he met in his everyday life. Other patients have been taught to check their notebooks when a timer on their watch sounds; some units catering for patients with Alzheimer's Disease use special bracelets which cause an alarm to ring when the patient wanders off the ward. In one such case, the alarm began to act as a cue for the patient to turn around and walk back into the ward by himself. Repeat alarms which can be set to ring at whatever is the appropriate interval have been used successfully to remind patients with poor sensation to life regularly, and for patients with dysarthria to swallow regularly. It is worth remembering too, that external aids can be pictorial for use with severely dysphasic patients who cannot read. Wilson (1984), for example, described a pictorial aid used to help a dysphasic woman remember how to transfer from her wheelchair to an ordinary chair, and Wilson (1991) describes how a globally aphasic man used visual symbol systems in order to refer to the past and the future.

External aids appear to work because they enable people to remember by an alternative route, i.e. people who have difficulty in remembering through their own efforts are able to remember by making use of other systems.

## Computer-Based Interventions

A few years ago there was considerable excitement about the use of microcomputers in rehabilitation. People hoped and expected memory training programmes would revolutionise rehabilitation and enhance the memory functioning of brain injured people. Skilbeck (1984), for example, believed that microcomputers could assist in the management of memory disorders through assessment, monitoring treatment effectiveness, and in the retraining procedures themselves. Numerous software programs have appeared in the 1980s. However, as Robertson et al. (1988) point out, "the role of microcomputers in cognitive rehabilitation has not been subjected to controlled investigation until recently" (p. 151).

There are some encouraging reports about computers in cognitive rehabilitation. Sohlberg and Mateer (1987, 1988), for example, demonstrated improved attention functioning in head injured people. The three patients of Robertson et al. (1988) showed less visual neglect after a computer training program. On the whole, however, computer training programs have not been evaluated. Given the huge increase in the use of computers in rehabilitation centres around the world, demonstrations of their effectiveness have been negligible. Even the few success stories tend to report changes in test scores rather than changes in real life situations. Furthermore, several studies have reported the non-effectiveness of computer programs (e.g. Ponsford and Kinsella 1988; Robertson 1988).

It is, perhaps, not surprising that computers have had little effect in cognitive rehabilitation programmes. As Harris and Sunderland (1981) pointed out, memory is not like a muscle which improves or strengthens with exercise. Practice at a particular task or activity may well improve performance on that task, but will not improve functioning in other areas, or will not improve general memory functioning. The classic experiments of Ericsson et al. (1980) demonstrated that students could increase their digit span from the normal 7 (plus or minus 2) to a phenomenal 80 or more with constant drilling and practice. Post training assessment, however, on a similar letter span task, revealed normal scores of 7 (plus or minus 2). Thus no improvement of memory functioning per se had occurred.

Computers can, of course, be of great help in rehabilitation. Computer assessment procedures may be time saving and efficient, computers as feedback devices are also useful (see Mackey 1989) and training in the use of computers has led to some exciting results from Schacter and Glisky (1986) and Glisky and Schacter (1987). The Glisky and Schacter studies are probably the best to date in the field of computers in memory rehabilitation. The authors taught a number of amnesic patients computer terminology using 'The Method of Vanishing Cues'. (This method is identical to the forward and backward chaining used in behaviour modification.) One of Glisky and Schacter's patients was able to obtain employment as a computer programmer following several months of training.

## Internal Strategies or Mnemonics

Most people will have occasion to use mnemonics. In Britain, for example, when we need to remember how many days there are in a given month, we use a rhyme which begins:

"30 days hath September,
April, June and November..."

We also learn the names of musical notes by employing sentences such as "Every good boy deserves fruit", to remind us that the notes of a stave are EGBDF. Medical students learn a rhyme to help them learn the names of cranial nerves and pilots use another mnemonic system when learning how to fly an aircraft. Such rhymes and first letter mnemonics can be employed to teach memory impaired people some new information. Gardner (1977), for example, describes how a severely disabled amnesic man was able to learn some personal details by incorporating them into a song. Moffat (1984) and Wilson (1987) describe a number of verbal and visual mnemonic systems.

Mnemonics probably work through enabling people to use their residual memory skills and learning ability to better advantage. When using mnemonics in rehabilitation, however, it is unrealistic to expect memory impaired people to use these systems spontaneously. The value of mnemonics is that they aid learning, i.e. people learn information quicker with mnemonics than without. Although amnesic people are unlikely to rely upon mnemonics to assist their remembering, therapists and relatives can employ them as teaching strategies.

### Rehearsal and Study Techniques

Two methods are particularly useful here. One is PQRST from the field of study techniques, and first described by Robinson (1970). PQRST is an acronym which stands for Preview, Question, Read, State and Test and describes a series of steps to work through when trying to retain verbal material. It probably works because it encourages deeper processing of the material to be remembered, i.e. it follows the levels-of-processing principle of Craik and Lockhart (1972). Wilson (1987) describes a series of experiments evaluating PQRST.

The second method is expanding rehearsal (Landauer and Bjork 1978) in which the information to be remembered is presented then tested immediately, tested again after a short delay, tested again after a slightly longer delay, and so forth. Rote rehearsal or repetitive practice is usually less helpful.

### Memory Games and Exercises

Providing memory impaired people with memory exercises or memory games is the most widely used therapeutic strategy in Britain (Harris and Sunderland 1981). There is, however, no evidence that playing games and engaging in memory exercises improves memory generally. These activities will probably not do any harm but we should not expect them to bring about improvement in memory skills. They may nevertheless have an indirect therapeutic value. For example, many memory impaired people and their relatives think such games and exercises will help and thus they are likely to believe that something is being done. Secondly, memory games and exercises can be designed so that even the most severely memory impaired person will succeed on some occasions. For people who are used to failure, success can be rewarding. Thirdly, the games and exercises can be fun, and again memory impaired people may be limited in the amount of fun they experience in therapeutic situations.

## Generalisation

We can provide aids or strategies for memory impaired people but we cannot guarantee that patients will use them. Furthermore, a patient may use a strategy for one problem but not for others, or a patient may use a strategy in one situation but not in others. This does not mean that the strategies are no good; after all, if a patient needs glasses but refuses to wear them this is not a criticism of the glasses themselves. Given such circumstances, we must ask ourselves how we can improve generalisation.

We should never assume that generalisation will occur automatically. If it should happen it is a bonus which rarely occurs with severely memory impaired people. We have to plan for and teach generalisation. In the case of a patient who will not use a strategy, e.g. using a dictaphone to record important information, we are unlikely to achieve our goal by simply giving the patient the dictaphone and demonstrating its use. Perhaps the first step here would be to teach the patient how to load the tape, record information, play back information and change the battery. This might require considerable effort and use of verbal instructions, demonstrations, practice and encouragement. Meanwhile we must prompt the patient to record important information about his or her day. Again this might require a specifically designed programme. The patient may not be able to select relevant from irrelevant information. He or she may need frequent reminders. Use of a timer on a watch, clock or calculator could prompt the patient to refer to the machine and play back the recently recorded messages.

The patient who uses a strategy for one problem but not another, e.g. uses the dictaphone to record information about therapy but not family or social life, should be taught its use in a range of situations. The method employed to teach use of the machine in the first place can be employed to teach use of the machine for recording other kinds of information.

Psychologists working with people with a mental handicap would never expect generalisation to occur from one problem to another or one situation to another without a specifically designed programme. The same should be true for memory impaired people. If these people have difficulty learning, then it is the responsibility of professionals and relatives to devise ways to help them learn or bypass their problems or manage their everyday lives. Although memory impaired people may not be able to expect much in the way of general memory improvement, this does not mean that nothing can be done to help them in their everyday life.

## References

Almli CR, Finger S (1988) Toward a definition of recovery of function. In: Finger S, LeVere TE, Almli CR, Stein DG (eds) Brain injury and recovery. Plenum, New York, pp 1–14

Braun JJ (1978) Time and recovery from brain damage. In: Finger S (ed) Recovery from brain damage: research and theory. Plenum, New York, pp 165–197

Craik FIM, Lockhart RS (1972) Levels of processing: a framework for memory research. J Verb Learn Verb Behav 11:671–684

Davies ADM, Binks MG (1983) Supporting the residual memory of a Korsakoff patient. Behav Psychother 11:62–74

Ericsson KA, Chase WG, Falcon S (1980) Acquisition of a memory skill. Science 208:1181–1182
Gardner H (1977) The shattered mind: the person after brain damage. Routledge and Kegan Paul, London
Glisky EL, Schacter DL (1987) Acquisition of domain-specific knowledge in organic amnesia: training for computer-related work. Neuropsychologia 25:893–906
Harris JE (1984) Ways of improving memory. In: Wilson BA, Moffat N (eds) Clinical management of memory problems. Croom Helm, London
Harris JE, Sunderland A (1981) A brief survey of the management of memory disorders in rehabilitation units in Britain. Int Rehabil Med 3:206–209
Jennett B, Bond M (1975) Assessment of outcome after severe brain damage. Lancet 1:480–484
Landauer TK, Bjork RA (1978) Optimum rehearsal patterns and name learning. In: Gruneberg MM, Morris PE, Sykes RN (eds) Practical aspects of memory. Academic, London
Laurence S, Stein DG (1978) Recovery after brain damage and the concept of localization of function. In: Finger S (ed) Recovery from brain damage: research and theory. Plenum, New York
LeVere TE (1980) Recovery of function after brain damage: a theory of the behavioral deficit. Physiol Psychol 8:297–308
Mackey S (1989) The use of computer-assisted feedback in a motor-control task for cerebral palsied children. Physiotherapy 75:143–148
Marshall JF (1985) Neural plasticity and recovery of function after brain injury. Int Rev Neurol 26:201–247
Moffat N (1984) Strategies of memory therapy. In: Wilson BA, Moffat N (eds) Clinical management of memory problems. Croom Helm, London
Ponsford JL, Kinsella G (1988) Evaluation of a remedial programme for attentional deficits following closed head injury. J Clin Exp Psychol 10:693–708
Robertson I (1988) Unilateral visual neglect. PhD Thesis, University of London
Robertson I, Gray J, McKenzie S (1988) Microcomputer-based cognitive rehabilitation of visual neglect: 3 multiple-baseline single-case studies. Brain Injury 2:151–164
Robinson FP (1970) Effective study. Harper and Row, New York
Schacter DL, Glisky EL (1986) Memory remediation: restoration, alleviation and the acquisition of domain-specific knowledge. In: Uzzell BP, Cross Y (eds) Clinical neuropsychology of intervention. Nijhoff, Boston, pp 257–282
Skilbeck C (1984) Computer assistance in the management of memory and cognitive impairment. In: Wilson BA, Moffat N (eds) Clinical management of memory problems. Croom Helm, London, pp 112–131
Sohlberg MM, Mateer CA (1987) Effectiveness of an attention-training program. J Clin Exp Neuropsychol 9:117–130
Sohlberg MM, Mateer CA (1988) Introduction to cognitive, rehabilitation. Guilford, New York
Wilson BA (1984) Memory therapy in practice. In: Wilson BA, Moffat N (eds) Clinical management of memory problems. Croom Helm, London
Wilson BA (1987) Rehabilitation of memory. Guilford, New York
Wilson BA (1991) Cognitive rehabilitation for brain injured adults. In: Deelman BG, Saan RJ, van Zomeren AH (eds) Traumatic brain injury. Swets and Zeitlinger, Lisse, pp 121–143
Wilson BA, Cockburn J, Baddeley AD (1989a) Assessment of everyday memory following brain injury. In: Mines ME, Wagner KA (eds) Neurotrauma: treatment, rehabilitation and related issues, vol 3. Butterworth, London, pp 83–99
Wilson BA, Cockburn J, Baddeley AD, Hiorns R (1989b) The development and validation of a test battery for detecting and monitoring everyday memory problems. J Clin Exp Neuropsychol 11:855–870

# The Influence of a Cognitive Remediation Programme on Associated Behavioural Disturbances in Patients with Frontal Lobe Dysfunction

*D. Y. von Cramon, G. Matthes-von Cramon and N. Mai*

## Introduction

Human problem-solving performance (i.e., the challenge to accomplish a specified result, often under prescribed conditions; cf. Oxford English Dictionary) is very often disturbed in brain-injured people. However, the term "impaired problem solving" is very broad and so indefinite that it does not really help to explain what is wrong with the complex cognitive process after brain damage.

Problem-solving performance in brain-damaged patients has been evaluated in most studies by the use of psychometric (intelligence) tests which were developed primarily for personnel decisions in normal subjects. Such tests usually lack sufficient sensitivity to distinguish between various degrees of disturbance because they are constructed to differentiate maximally at average levels of normal performance. However, a more important shortcoming of most problem-solving tests is their restriction to abstract problems. A performance deficit in such a test provides very little information about the particular aspects disturbed and is, therefore, of no help in devising a specific treatment regimen to improve the problem-solving behaviour in a brain-injured patient. Such psychometric intelligence tests are of little use in evaluating the specific effect of a behavioural-training procedure.

Discussions concerning discrepancies between the results of psychometric evaluation and team observations of a patient's performance of problem solving in daily life activities are a familiar part of many team conferences in a rehabilitation center. Surprisingly, no studies have yet tried to exploit such observational data in a more standardized format.

As a first step, we introduced a formal procedure for the rating of problem-solving behaviour and behavioural components which might contribute to a performance deficit. The behaviour of each patient has to be rated by several staff members.

The rating format probably most familiar to staff members is a direct comparison of patients, i.e., a ranking of patients on the specific aspect of performance under discussion. A ranking procedure might be feasible within small patient groups, but is impossible in large groups. Another problem of ranking procedures emerges when rankings of several raters have to be combined in a single ranking. According to Arrow's impossibility theorem (Arrow 1966;

Schwartz 1970), there exists no acceptable way to transform the individual rankings into a common group ranking.

Instead of direct ranking of a patient's performance, evaluation criteria for each aspect may be defined. This enables an "absolute" judgment of each patient at the expense of fine details which resist reliable description.

In a multidisciplinary clinical team, raters cannot be thought of as independent in their judgments due to the joint many discussions about a given patient. However, raters who are not part of the acting staff have only a poor chance to assess reliably the patients' behaviour because they have not seen them in a sufficiently large number of relevant situations. In the evaluation study of a neuropsychological training programme reported below, individual ratings were reconsidered in staff meetings in which rating differences were discussed, and a final group score for each patient was assigned.

## Rating Problem-Solving Behaviour

We asked raters to assess two aspects of the patient's impaired problem-solving behaviour which can be observed rather easily, considering the following operational definitions (with reference to Rowe 1985):

1. *Problem definition and formulation:* Patients are able/unable to survey information by reading and rereading directions. They are able/unable to pick out the main points discriminating between relevant and irrelevant information (i.e., between objective facts and assumptions, opinions and inferences). They are able/unable to find a way to organize complex information into a sequence of distinct chunks. They are able/unable to formulate questions (to themselves or to somebody else) for the clarification of a given problem.
2. *Solution verification:* Patients are able/unable to notice whether what is done (e.g., in a problem-solving task) works well. This includes an assessment of the appropriateness and correctness of their problem-solving activities for the purpose of accepting or rejecting, continuing or discontinuing the particular activity. They are able/unable to notice obvious discrepancies and, when they have been pointed out, to correct them themselves.

Raters were requested to assess these aspects before treatment, having observed the patients in at least three everyday activities. These standard situations were: (a) planning the next weekend, (b) running a patients' assembly, and (c) working through a newspaper article.

Impaired problem-solving behaviour was rated 0/1:

0 no problem solving deficit, if patients were inconspicuous in both problem-solving aspects;
1 problem solving deficit, if patients were impaired in at least one of the two aspects.

## Rating Behavioural Disturbances

Our Behavioural Rating Scale comprises 19 operationally defined items:

- *Unawareness:* patients are (completely) unaware of their cognitive deficits. A demonstration of their failures is not responded to at all or sometimes met with explicit denial. Occasional unawareness means that patients have a vague notion of their cognitive deficits when confronted with their failures. They do not, however, anticipate difficulties in their everyday activities.
- *Apathy (Abulia/Hypobulia):* complete (abulia) or partial (hypobulia) loss of motivation and volition. Expectancies (anticipation) and incentives (impulses) for egocentric actions are critically reduced. Patients do not complain about abulia/hypobulia.
- *Lack of ideas:* poverty of imagination (and phantasy) preventing patients from producing a sufficient number of alternatives. Even in simple, everyday tasks they depend on the ideas and proposals of others to accomplish a specified result.
- *Lack of mental effort:* actions will be immediately abandoned (without any intent to renew) when solution barriers occur and a goal cannot be attained "in the first run". Mental effort will be augmented (for a short period of time) by topical events or by any demand made with authority. (Abulic patients may have normal mental effort as long as they are stimulated sufficiently.)
- *Inflexibility:* inability to adapt to (quickly) changing tasks and situations. Concepts, plans and actions are not given up even if altered circumstances demand modifications. Subjects appear stubborn and rigid.
- *Concrete attitude:* patients stick to persons, objects and events which "catch their eyes at once". Their explorations do not go beyond the immediately given situation. Their power of imagination is critically reduced (cf., Goldstein 1971).
- *Rule breaking:* violation of rules which are indispensable for the correct execution of tasks or games. Patients tend to neglect rules when barriers occur which demand a modification of plans or hypotheses. Rule breaking is often elicited by tasks which do not offer a simple solution, where a workable solution cannot be found without a thorough search for some concealed aspects.
- *Premature actions:* illconsidered and rash actions. Patients do not wait for instructions or clarifications. Most of the time they jump to conclusions without thinking about all the relevant facts. They seem to be "forced" to realize their behavioural responses immediately.
- *Perseverations:* higher-order perseverations in which no defects in the execution of elementary acts are present. According to Sandson and Albert (1984) "stuck-in", "recurrent" and "continuous" perseverations are identified.
- *Lack of empathy:* a neutrality of attitude embracing a wide range of subjects and (inanimate) objects in the patient's environment. Interest in per-

sonal matters of friends and relatives may still be declared ("preserved cognitive component of empathy") but without deeper sympathy ("impaired affective component of empathy"; cf. Brems 1989). Anhedonia, in this context, is due to a lack of interest in gratification and pleasure.

- *Tactless behaviour:* the behaviour is dominated by indiscrete, tasteless, offending and obtrusive utterances or actions. Patients may still be aware of their rude behaviour, but mostly are not ashamed or do not feel regret. They are obviously unable to suppress this consternating behaviour.
- *Violent outbursts:* a propensity for episodic (short-lived) aggressive acts, the intensity of which is entirely disproportionate to the causative events. They mainly appear as verbal aggression and rarely as destructive rage. It is often the case that following an aggressive outburst, patients will after a certain delay admit their inappropriate behaviour and show remorse.
- *Emotional reactions to tasks:* patients express strong negative feelings (swearing, crying) about a test (task) they cannot solve and often refuse to go on with it (cf. Rowe 1985). They may claim that there is no reasonable solution to this problem or that the task is "rubbish".
- *Logorrhea:* press of speech neglecting natural pauses and turn-taking rules. One is often forced to talk "on top" of the patient in order to interrupt his/her excessive speech.
- *Reduced speech:* rare spontaneous speech utterances in the absence of any standard or nonstandard aphasic syndrome (including transcortical motor aphasia). Replies to questions are short and comprise only little information. On request, longer and more detailed utterances can be "lured out".
- *Reduced exploration of the environment:* rare spontaneous head and eye movements to actively explore the environment. Patients seem to be unaware of relevant stimuli (events), even if they are related to their personal domain. Their diminished curiosity is especially conspicuous when they find themselves in a completely unfamiliar environment (cf. Deutsch et al. 1979).
- *Action slips:* patients seem to perform actions without either conscious control or knowledge. Their prevailing errors are known as "capture errors" (cf. Norman 1981). Patients appear "preoccupied" and "distracted".
- *Utilization and imitation behaviour:* objects will be utilized according to their function even if the actual situation does not require or even excludes their utilization. Gestures and actions will be imitated, although the imitating behaviour is not requested or even explicitly forbidden (cf. Lhermitte et al. 1986).
- *Euphoria:* patients feel particulary optimistic for no particular reason. They may show excessive joking and a constant flippancy in inappropriate life contexts.

Each item was rated twice (before and after treatment) on a 3-point scale:

0 absence of any observable behavioural disturbance;
1 behavioural disturbance(s) occurred only occasionally, but more than once a day;
2 disturbed behaviour(s) occurred continuously

## Neuropsychological Rehabilitation Programme

Our primary intention was to provide patients with techniques enabling them to reduce the complexity of a multi-stage problem by breaking it down to more manageable proportions. A slowed-down, controlled and stepwise processing of a given problem should replace the unsystematic and often rash approach these patients spontaneously choose.

In our "Problem-Solving Training" (PST), groups of six to eight inpatients were seen 4 days per week, 3 h per day, for approximately 3 months. Each patient was additionally treated in an individual training format at least 1 h twice a week. Additionally, patients had to do homework daily. During the training period (of 3 months), they did participate in physical and recreational therapy but in no other cognitive or psychotherapeutic remediation programme.

We were aware of the fact that orienting patients towards a more realistic evaluation of their cognitive performance should be an essential part of our therapeutic approach. In other words, we invested much time in making patients understand that their "problem-solving disability" is relevant enough to their personal lives to cope with.

We arranged the PST either in parallel or in project groups (cf. Mosey 1986). Patients suffering from marked apathy ("abulia") or a lack of mental effort had to be treated in a parallel group setting in which the therapist was compelled to continually prompt each patient to maintain a certain mental effort. In the project group setting, two or three group members cooperated on a task as a team for a limited time.

Our therapeutic goals were oriented towards the training model D'Zurilla and Goldfried (1971) proposed for training in social problem solving: (a) problem orientation, (b) problem definition and formulation, (c) generation of alternatives, (d) decision making, and (e) solution verification.

At the problem orientation stage, patients were to recognize generally a given task or situation as a "problem" for which an obvious solution was not yet available.

At the next stage (problem definition and formulation), clients learned to survey information by reading and rereading directions and by formulating questions to augment their understanding of the "big picture". They were asked to describe the main points (in their own words), discriminating between relevant and irrelevant information (i.e., between objective facts and assumptions, opinions and inferences). Eventually, they were taught to identify problem-solving goals, restraints and circumstances which make a given task problematic.

At the third stage, patients were to generate alternatives. This implied brainstorming procedures to produce as many alternatives as possible to a given problem.

The stage of decision making involved the systematic evaluation of a range of alternative solutions and the selection of the "best" or most effective one(s). The utilities of various options were discussed by pondering the premises for their realization and by anticipating their potential positive or negative consequences.

To improve solution verification, we worked primarily on developing greater sensitivity to errors and discrepancies based on a means-end relationship. Patients learned to recognize faulty paths, to correct errors and to return to former hypotheses.

## Patient Sample and Psychometric Measures

Seventy ad-hoc admitted inpatients with traumatic brain injury (TBI), cerebrovascular accidents (CVA) and other brain damage were included in the study. The main clinical data are shown in Table 1 for the PS+ group (24 patients rated without pretreatment problem-solving deficit) and for the PS− group (46 patients rated with pretreatment problem-solving deficit). Patients were at least 4 months post onset. They were all nonaphasic. Patients with hemispatial neglect were excluded because of their obvious inability to fully explore the environment for problem-relevant information.

The classification of the patients' problem-solving impairment by our raters in PS+ and PS− corresponded to the psychometric findings displayed in Table 2.

In the lower half of this table, tests are shown that are said to examine aspects of frontal lobe dysfunction.

The patients' capacity to form concepts and to shift from one category to another was assessed by the Modified Card Sorting Test, using the version of Nelson (1976).[1] This test was given before training only. Retest results would be inconclusive because some patients could have remembered the solutions.

For an assessment of the patients' ability to learn from experience and observation, we used the Tower of Hanoi puzzle. The "Tower" comprises one of the best known transfer problems available in cognitive psychology (Kotovsky et al. 1985).[2]

We developed the "Planning Test" as a standardized instrument with high ecological validity (Stoltze 1991). The patients were to schedule several items on an agenda which they should carry out within a certain time limit. Thus, they had to organize multiple bits of information, such as various opening hours, fixed dates (appointments), time required for a certain activity, time needed to go from one place to another.[3]

---

[1] Test performance was evaluated by the number of categories reached and the "total error score", which is calculated as the percentage of perseverative errors in comparison with the total number of errors.

[2] We used a computerized version of the 4-disk problem with defined start and target positions (Matthes-von Cramon 1988). The patient optimized his/her solution strategies across five consecutive trials. The test score consisted of the added numbers of moves of the fourth and fifth trial (T4+T5).

[3] The test score was defined by the number of correctly scheduled items.

**Table 1.** Main clinical data of 70 brain-injured patients

| | PS+ ($n = 24$) | | PS− ($n = 46$) | |
|---|---|---|---|---|
| | Median | Range | Median | Range |
| Age (years) | 39 | (19–60) | 43 | (19–68) |
| Sex (m, f) | 15, 9 | | 31, 5 | |
| Education (years) | 10 | (9–18) | 9.5 | (9–18) |
| Time since lesion (months) | 6 | (4–60) | 6 | (4–99) |
| *Etiology* | | | | |
| TBI ($n = 35$) | 13 | | 22 | |
| CVA ($n = 21$) | 7 | | 14 | |
| Others ($n = 14$) | 4 | | 10 | |

PS+, Good problem solvers; PS−, poor problem solvers; TBI, traumatic brain injury; CVA, cerebro-vascular accidents

**Table 2.** Psychometric data for 24 good and 46 poor problem solvers including pre- and posttreatment data for the PS− group

| | PS+ ($n = 24$) | PS− ($n = 46$) | |
|---|---|---|---|
| | | Pretreatment | Posttreatment |
| *Intelligence tests* (T-values; median, range) | | | |
| Reasoning (LPS) | 50 (40–60) | 47 (25–60) | 47 (30–50) |
| Categorizing (IST) | 50 (41–60) | 44 (20–62) | 46 (38–68) |
| Analogies (IST) | 52 (41–59) | 46 (29–58) | 46 (30–51) |
| Similarities (IST) | 42 (33–68) | 38 (22–53) | 44 (30–56) |
| Proverbs (WIT) | 52 (45–67) | 47 (20–67) | 50 (37–51) |
| *Problem-solving tasks* (median, range) | | | |
| MCST (Nelson 1976) | | | |
| Categories | 7 (5–7) | 5 (0–7) | – |
| Total error score | 0 (0–33) | 14 (0–48) | – |
| Tower of Hanoi | | | |
| Moves (T4+T5) | 30 (30–42) | 43 (30–101) | 30 (30–106) |
| Planning test | | | |
| Raw score | 15 (13–15) | 6.5 (0–15) | 9 (0–15) |

LPS, Leistungsprüfsystem (Horn 1983); IST, Intelligenz-Struktur-Test (Amthauer 1973); WIT, Wilde-Intelligenz-Test (Jäger and Althoff 1983); MCST, Modified Card-Sorting-Test (Nelson 1976); T4+T5, added moves of the fourth and fifth trial

# Results

## Problem-Solving Ability

The selected five subtests from standardized German intelligence tests showed a monotonous decline of 4 to 5 T-values from the PS+ group to the pretreatment PS-patients (Table 2).

The pre-/posttreatment comparison within the PS− group revealed a relevant positive effect (> 5 T-values) for the "Similarities" subtest only.

Compared to the intelligence tests, the PS+ group and the pretreatment PS− group differed widely regarding the three problem-solving tasks, as Table 2 demonstrates.

After treatment, the number of moves (T4+T5) necessary to solve the Tower of Hanoi puzzle declined significantly. As for the Planning Test, the raw score rose from a median of 6.5 to 9 points (maximum 15 points).

Pre-/posttreatment in comparison of the raters' judgments on the patients' ability in problem definition and formulation and solution verification revealed a highly significant improvement (Wilcoxon Matched-pairs Signed-ranks Test: $p<0.001/2$-tailed).

## Associated Behavioural Disturbances

In Tables 3 and 4, the numbers of patients with behavioural disturbances are displayed for the 19 items in our behavioural rating scale.

In the PS+ group, only the item "inflexibility" could be observed in approximately 30% of the cases and another 5 items in more than 5% of the

**Table 3.** Frequency of behavioural disturbances in the PS+ group. Percentages of disturbances and number of patients with occasional and continuous occurrence of this disturbance

| | PS+ (no problem-solving deficit) ($n$ = 24) | | |
|---|---|---|---|
| | % | Occasional occurrence | Continuous occurrence |
| Inflexibility | 29 | 7 | – |
| Apathy (abulia) | 14 | 2 | 1 |
| Lack of ideas | 10 | 1 | 1 |
| Concrete attitude | 10 | 2 | – |
| Lack of empathy | 10 | 2 | – |
| Lack of mental effort | 10 | 1 | 1 |
| Premature actions | 5 | 1 | – |
| Reduced speech | 5 | 1 | – |
| Reduced exploration | 5 | 1 | – |
| Perseverations | 0 | – | – |
| Rule breaking | 0 | – | – |
| Unawareness | 0 | – | – |
| Tactless behaviour | 0 | – | – |
| Euphoria | 0 | – | – |
| Violent outbursts | 0 | – | – |
| Emotional reactions | 0 | – | – |
| Logorrhea | 0 | – | – |
| Action slips | 0 | – | – |
| Utilization behaviour | 0 | – | – |

**Table 4.** Frequency of behavioural disturbances in the PS− group

| | PS− (with problem-solving deficit) ($n$ = 46) | | | | | | |
|---|---|---|---|---|---|---|---|
| | Pretreatment | | | Posttreatment | | | $p^a$ |
| | % | Occasional occurrence | Continuous occurrence | % | Occasional occurrence | Continuous occurrence | |
| Inflexibility | 83 | 17 | 21 | 67 | 5 | 10 | * |
| Lack of ideas | 78 | 17 | 19 | 67 | 22 | 9 | * |
| Concrete attitude | 76 | 19 | 16 | 61 | 23 | 5 | ** |
| Unawareness | 61 | 11 | 17 | 43 | 12 | 8 | ** |
| Apathy (abulia) | 52 | 10 | 14 | 37 | 8 | 9 | ** |
| Rule breaking | 46 | 13 | 8 | 17 | 3 | 5 | ** |
| Lack of empathy | 46 | 10 | 11 | 39 | 6 | 12 | |
| Premature actions | 43 | 14 | 6 | 24 | 9 | 2 | * |
| Perseverations | 37 | 10 | 7 | 13 | 2 | 7 | ** |
| Violent outbursts | 30 | 9 | 5 | 20 | 8 | 1 | * |
| Tactless behaviour | 28 | 8 | 5 | 20 | 7 | 2 | * |
| Emotional reactions | 26 | 4 | 8 | 20 | 6 | 3 | |
| Lack of mental effort | 24 | 5 | 6 | 22 | 7 | 3 | |
| Reduced speech | 24 | 5 | 6 | 13 | 3 | 3 | |
| Action slips | 13 | 1 | 5 | 13 | 3 | 3 | |
| Reduced exploration | 20 | 5 | 4 | 13 | 3 | 3 | |
| Euphoria | 13 | 6 | – | 4 | 2 | – | |
| Logorrhea | 11 | 3 | 2 | 0 | – | – | |
| Utilization behaviour | 4 | 2 | – | 2 | 1 | – | |

[a] Pre-/posttreatment comparison (Sign-Test); * $p<0.05$; ** $p<0.01$.

cases. Very few patients in this group showed continuous behavioural disturbances (Table 3).

Compared with the PS+ group, the PS− group showed a much higher incidence of all behavioural disturbances (Table 4). Five items were observable in more than 50% of cases. Noteworthy was the great number of patients with continuous behavioural disturbances at the pretreatment rating.

A pre-/post treatment group comparison showed a significant overall decrease in impairment after treatment (Wilcoxon Matched-pairs Signed-ranks Test: $p<0.01$; 2-tailed). A significant difference was observed in patients with a post-onset time of more than 9 months. Even patients with severe initial problem-solving deficits, i.e., patients with pretreatment ratings of continuous impairment in both aspects of problem-solving behaviour, showed a significantly lower impairment after the training period.

Regarding single items, a significant decline for 10 out of 19 items was noted in the total group (Sign-Test). Even "apathy (abulia)", "unawareness of (cognitive) deficit" and "perseverations" were among the behavioural disturbances obviously reduced. For all items but two, the number of patients with continuous behavioural disturbances diminished.

In selecting the 15 patients with severe pretreatment problem-solving deficits, a substantially higher incidence of behavioural disturbances occurred

**Table 5.** Frequency of behavioural disturbances in patients with severe initial problem-solving deficit

| | PS− (with severe problem-solving deficit ($n$ = 15)) | | | | | | |
|---|---|---|---|---|---|---|---|
| | Pretreatment | | | Posttreatment | | | $p^a$ |
| | % | Occasional occurrence | Continuous occurrence | % | Occasional occurrence | Continuous occurrence | |
| Inflexibility | 100 | 2 | 13 | 100 | 4 | 11 | |
| Unawareness | 93 | 2 | 13 | 87 | 5 | 8 | |
| Apathy (abulia) | 93 | 3 | 11 | 73 | 3 | 8 | |
| Lack of ideas | 93 | 2 | 12 | 87 | 6 | 8 | |
| Concrete attitude | 93 | 5 | 9 | 93 | 9 | 5 | |
| Rule breaking | 80 | 4 | 8 | 47 | 2 | 5 | * |
| Lack of empathy | 73 | 2 | 9 | 67 | 1 | 9 | |
| Premature actions | 67 | 5 | 5 | 47 | 4 | 3 | |
| Perseverations | 67 | 3 | 7 | 47 | 1 | 6 | |
| Violent outbursts | 60 | 6 | 3 | 47 | 6 | 1 | |
| Emotional reactions | 53 | 2 | 6 | 47 | 3 | 4 | |
| Lack of mental effort | 47 | 1 | 6 | 47 | 3 | 4 | |
| Reduced speech | 47 | 1 | 6 | 40 | 2 | 4 | |
| Action slips | 40 | 1 | 5 | 40 | 3 | 3 | |
| Tactless behaviour | 40 | 3 | 3 | 33 | 2 | 3 | |
| Reduced exploration | 33 | 2 | 3 | 33 | 2 | 3 | |
| Logorrhea | 13 | 1 | 1 | 0 | – | – | |
| Utilization behaviour | 13 | 2 | – | 7 | 1 | – | |
| Euphoria | 0 | – | – | 0 | – | – | |

[a] Pre-/posttreatment comparison (Sign-Test); $^*p<0.05$.

than in the total group. With the exception of the item "rule breaking", no other single item had significantly declined after treatment in this subgroup (Table 5).

## Discussion

This contribution is meant to challenge other researchers to provide a still more refined and complete Rating Scale for behavioural disturbances in patients with frontal lobe dysfunction than we actually accomplished. We consider it a hindrance to further progress in this field that many authors seem content with a more or less intuitive understanding of these intricate aspects of disturbed behaviour instead of trying to find reasonable operational definitions which could gradually replace the vagueness of meaning and connotations we all have of these aspects of behaviour in brain-injured people. A clarification is especially needed for the clinicians who are forced to make repeated judgments on a patient's behavioural profile to decide on future rehabilitative measures.

As we would have expected, patients without problem-solving deficits showed a few behavioural disturbances.

It should be emphasized, however, that there are some patients, e.g., with "apathy (abulia)" and/or "lack of empathy", items considered to be rather specific for frontal lobe dysfunction, which had no obvious problem-solving deficit. This held true for the rating of their problem-solving behaviour and the psychometric findings as well. These dissociations of performance deficits which we observed in some patients with (proximal) anterior cerebral infarctions deserve further attention. Even after an intensive remediation programme over three months, patients with problem-solving deficits never reached the level of "good" problem solvers. A restitutio ad integrum regarding these behavioural disturbances did not take place in any of our chronic brain-injured patients.

As indicated in the introduction, we were primarily interested in learning whether a remediation programme, consisting of systematic and specific cognitive training (PST), has an impact on associated behavioural disturbances. We can answer this question with a cautious "yes". We found a significant global effect in the sense that, after the treatment period, the majority of items had declined in the group of patients with problem-solving deficits? This favourable effect could also be observed in chronic patients with a post-onset time of more than 9 months, which inclines us to accept that the reduction in behavioural disturbances was due to the remediation programme rather than to spontaneous recovery. Whether the PST alone or the entire remediation programme (cognitive training plus physical and recreational therapy) was responsible for the favourable effects cannot be determined on the basis of our study design.

As we have shown elsewhere (von Cramon et al. 1991), explicit PST seems to be superior to, for instance, memory training with respect to various behaviourally and psychometrically assessed aspects of problem solving. This study replicated these findings. Thus, it is not unreasonable to assume that the PST played a major though not the exclusive role in the changes observed.

Our data also revealed a significant overall reduction in behavioural impairment for 15 patients with severe problem-solving deficits, although the positive effect was smaller than for the total group of 46 patients. Pondering the consequences of this observation, we do not feel justified to exclude a priori patients with initially serious problem-solving deficits from a remediation programme including cognitive retraining.

With respect to single items, it is obvious that "inflexibility", "lack of ideas" and "concrete attitude" remained impaired in the majority of cases. However, the number of patients declined where such problems occurred continuously. It is our experience that even small ameliorations may be of considerable practical relevance to the patient's "significant others" in handling living with these patients.

## Conclusions

1. Brain-injured patients without problem-solving deficits showed only few associated behavioural disturbances as they have been defined in our rating scale.
   Nonetheless, there was a small number of good problem solvers with obvious behavioural abnormalities (e.g., "lack of ideas" or "apathy/abulia").
2. A 3 month remediation programme, consisting mainly of systematic cognitive retraining (problem solving training) significantly reduced the majority of those associated behavioural disturbances. This positive effect was observable even for highly chronic patients. The more severe the initial problem-solving deficit, the less the amelioration.
3. The study confirmed previous findings that our PST seems to be effective in the sense that both behavioural and psychometric measures indicated improved problem-solving abilities in a number of patients.

## References

Amthauer R (1973) I-S-T 70 Intelligenz-Struktur-Test. Handanweisung. Hogrefe, Göttingen

Arrow KJ (1966) Social choice and individual values, 2nd edn. Yale University Press, New York

Brems C (1989) Dimensionality of empathy and its correlates. J Psychol 123:329–337

Deutsch RD, Kling A, Steklis HD (1979) Influence of frontal lobe lesions on behavioral interactions in man. Res Commun Psychol Psychiatry Behav 4:415–431

D'Zurilla TJ, Goldfried MR (1971) Problem solving and behavior modification. J Abnorm Psychol 78:107–126

Goldstein K (1971) Abstract and concrete behavior. In: Gurwitsch A, Goldstein-Haudek EM, Haudek WE (eds) Selected papers/Ausgewählte Schriften. Nijhoff, The Hague, pp 365–399

Horn W (1983) Leistungsprüfsystem L-P-S. Handanweisung. Hogrefe, Göttingen

Jäger AO, Althoff K (1983) Der WILDE-Intelligenz-Test. Ein Strukturdiagnostikum. Handanweisung. Hogrefe, Göttingen

Kotovsky K, Hayes JR, Simon HA (1985) Why are some problems hard? Evidence from Tower of Hanoi. Cogn Psychol 17:248–294

Lhermitte F, Pillon B, Serdaru M (1986) Human autonomy and the frontal lobes. I. Imitation and utilization behavior. A neuropsychological study of 75 patients. Ann Neurol 19:326–334

Matthes-von Cramon G (1988) Der Einsatz des „Turm von Hanoi"-Computerprogramms zur Diagnostik von Störungen des problemlösenden Denkens bei Patienten mit erworbenen Hirnschädigungen. Biomed J 19:10–13

Mosey AC (1986) Psychosocial components of occupational therapy. Raven, New York, pp 274–293

Nelson HE (1976) A modified card sorting test sensitive to frontal lobe defects. Cortex 12:313–324

Norman DA (1981) Categorization of action slips. Psychol Rev 88:1–15

Rowe HAH (1985) Problem solving and intelligence. Erlbaum, Hillsdale

Sandson J, Albert M (1984) Varieties or perseverations. Neuropsychologia 22:715–732

Schwartz T (1970) On the possibility of rational policy evaluation. Theory Decision 1:89–106

Stoltze A (1991) Konstruktion eines neuropsychologischen Tests zur Messung von Planungsfähigkeiten nach Frontalhirnschädigung. Diplomarbeit Fachbereich Psychologie Universität Konstanz

Von Cramon D, Matthes-von Cramon G, Mai N (1991) Problem solving deficits in brain injured patients: a therapeutic approach. Neuropsych Rehabil 1(1):45–64

# Post-stroke Depression: Psychological and Biochemical Interpretations

*G. Gainotti*

## Introduction

Affective disturbances of different kinds (ranging from agitated depression to disinhibited attitude and from irritability with outbursts of anger to apathy with loss of motivation) are very frequent in brain-damaged patients. For the behavioral neurologist and the clinical neuropsychologist, these disturbances are of both theoretical and practical interest. On the one hand, they can supply previous information about the cerebral representation of emotions and affects, but, on the other hand, they generally have a very deleterious influence on rehabilitation.

Since it was impossible in this paper to survey all the facets of this complex set of behavioral modifications, we have decided to focus our attention on only one instance of affective disorder resulting from brain damage, namely post-stroke depression (PSD). This choice was made for three main reasons:

1. The incidence of this phenomenon, which is observed in a large number of stroke patients
2. The controversial meaning and the suggested multifactorial nature of this affective change, which allows us to take into account several biological, psychological, and psycho-social variables which probably also intervene in other kinds of affective disorders resulting from brain damage
3. The important implications that PSD has for rehabilitation.

## Clinical Aspects of the Post-Stroke Depression

### Prevalence

Despite the great number of problems concerning the criteria to be used for the diagnosis of PSD, several studies conducted with different methodologies in acute stroke units (Robinson et al. 1983; Ebrahim et al. 1987; Eastwood et al. 1989), rehabilitation hospitals (Sinyor et al. 1986b), out-patient clinics (Robinson and Price 1982; Feibel and Springer 1982) or in a community (Wade et al. 1987) have consistently shown that: (a) depression is very frequent in stroke patients, occurring in about 50% of those observed in the acute post-stroke stage and in about 30% of those seen in more chronic stages; and (b) about one half of these patients present a severe form of depression, whereas the other half show mild to moderate depressive symptoms.

## Clinical Phenomenology and Diagnostic Problems

The clinical phenomenology of PSD includes a large array of signs and symptoms, ranging from verbal reports of sadness and thoughts of death or suicide to objective phenomena, such as bursting into tears and vegetative signs of anxiety and to somatic signs, such as sleep or appetite disturbances. Different authors have given a different weight to these different signs and symptoms, both to make a diagnosis of PSD and to distinguish different subtypes of depression. Thus, Robinson and coworkers have consistently used DSM-III (American Psychiatric Association 1980) diagnostic criteria in their systematic series of investigations in this area (Robinson and Benson 1981; Robinson and Price 1982; Robinson et al. 1983, 1984a, b; Lipsey et al. 1984, 1985, 1986; Starkstein et al. 1987; Starkstein and Robinson 1988, 1989). Ross and co-workers (Ross and Rush 1981; Ross et al. 1986) have questioned an approach to diagnosis based mainly on DSM-III criteria, arguing that the presence of aphasia and of other signs of brain damage (such as verbal denial) may so distort the depressive syndrome as to render very questionable a standard detection with DSM-III-based criteria. The same criticism could be addressed to the distinction made by Robinson and co-workers between a major depression (considered as a form of "endogenous" biological depression) and a minor depression (considered as a form of "dysthymic", neurotic or reactive depression).

The equivalence between major PSD and "endogenous" psychosis is also hindered by the fact that some of the most typical symptoms of endogenous depression (namely self-reproach and feelings of guilt) are generally absent in PSD, whereas other patterns of behavior usually not observed in melancholy are often on the foreground in this form of depression. We refer here in particular to the "catastrophic reactions" (CR) first described by Goldstein (1948) and then studied in more detail by us (Gainotti 1969, 1972) in unselected groups of patients with right- and left-hemispheric brain injury, usually of vascular etiology. The CR can be considered as the disorganized, anxious, desperate reaction of a patient faced with a situation that he is actually unable to solve due to the consequences of brain damage.

Although a depressive state certainly increases the risk and the frequency of CR and the phenomenology of the latter often consists of bursting into tears and of other depressive signs, CR and PSD must be considered as partly distinguishable entities. The first is a phasic event, strictly related to the frustrations met in an interactive (generally communicative) situation, whereas the latter is a long-standing, not-event-related and relatively stable mood state. In spite of this, in PSD the lack of symptoms of endogenous psychosis strictly independent of the patient's actual condition (such a self-reproach or feelings of guilt) and, by contrast, the importance of the CR, seem to suggest that PSD is related more to psychological than to biological consequences of the brain lesion.

## Relationships Between Post-Stroke Depression and Severity of Functional Impairment

Several investigators have assumed that a study of the relations between severity of PSD and degree of functional impairment could be used to check the "psychological reaction" hypothesis that we have just advanced. Results of these investigations have been rather inconclusive, since some authors (e.g., Finklestein et al. 1982; Robinson and Price 1982; Robinson et al. 1983; Sinyor et al. 1986a) have found no relationship between depression and functional impairment, whereas other authors (e.g., Feibel et al. 1979; Ebrahim et al. 1987; Wade et al. 1987; Eastwood et al. 1989) have found a significant correlation between severity of depression and degree of functional impairment. This contrasting set of data can be explained by admitting that the correlation between functional impairment and PSD is not a simple and a direct one and that, therefore, an undifferentiated study of the relationships between physical disability and mood disorders is not a good test of the psychological reaction hypothesis. The above-mentioned hypothesis could, perhaps, be tested more appropriately by: (a) focusing attention on the correlations between PSD and some signs of brain injury which could a priori be considered as causing the greatest impact upon the mood of the patient; and (b) studying how the correlations between physical disability and affective change evolve in the post-stroke period.

As for the first point, the symptom of brain damage which could be more critically related with PSD is probably aphasia, owing to the importance that language disturbances can have in disrupting interpersonal relationships. However, the meaning of PSD is not really clarified by a study of the correlations between language and mood disorders, since a strong association exists between Broca's (non-fluent) aphasia and PSD, but a depressive state is less frequent in patients with global aphasia and definitely rare in those with Wernicke's aphasia (Benson 1973; Robinson and Benson 1981). The meaning of the association between PSD and Broca's aphasia is, therefore, controversial: Benson (1979) maintains that Broca's aphasics are the most depressed because of their greater awareness of the language disorder, whereas Starkstein and Robinson (1988, 1989) suggest that the lesion location within the left frontal region could explain both Broca's aphasia and the major PSD. The second point (i.e., a longitudinal study of the correlations between functional impairment and affective change) could be suggested by the fact that a psychological (depressive) response to the consequences of brain damage presupposes an appropriate cognitive appraisal of the implications that the disability will have for the quality of life of the patient. Since in the acute post-stroke period it is often difficult to properly evaluate the long-term consequences of brain damage, whereas these consequences are much more clear some months after the onset of the disability, it could be predicted that the correlations between functional impairment and PSD should increase with time. Results supporting this prediction have been recently obtained by several authors: Ebrahim et al. (1987), Robinson et al. (1984b), and Parikh et al. (1987) have, in fact, observed that severity of depression and degree of functional impairment are weakly related in the acute post-stroke period, but become strongly related 6 months after the stroke.

## Anatomical Correlates

In a series of investigations conducted at the end of the 1960s, we demonstrated that patients with left- and right-hemispheric lesions show different emotional reactions to the disabilities caused by brain damage (Gainotti 1969 and 1972). Left-brain-damaged patients showed frequent CR when confronted with difficulties in verbal expression, whereas right-hemispheric patients showed a strange "indifference reaction" when confronted with motor, visual-perceptual, and visuo-constructive disabilities (see Gainotti 1983, 1989 for discussions of these findings). In the following years, the notion of a prevalence of CR in patients with left-brain injury was interpreted as pointing to a greater incidence of depression after left-hemispheric lesions. A series of reports (e.g., Gasparrini et al. 1978; Finklestein et al. 1982; Robinson and Price 1982; Robinson et al. 1984a) seemed to confirm that depression is more frequent in left- than in right-brain-damaged patients.

In the same time, however, it became more and more clear that the equivalence between depression and CR is a misleading one and an increasing number of papers began to question the prevalence of depression in left- (as opposed to right-) brain-damaged patients (e.g., Black and Black 1982; Robinson et al. 1983; de Bonis et al. 1985; Gordon et al. 1985; Reding et al. 1985; Sinyor et al. 1986b; Ebrahim et al. 1987; Wade et al. 1987).

Even more recently, two (complementary, rather than antithetical) tendencies have emerged in this area: (a) the first assumes that qualitative rather than quantitative differences do exist between depression induced by left- and right-hemispheric lesions; and (b) the second maintains that only a subset of left-hemispheric lesions (namely those encroaching upon the frontal lobe and the related subcortical structures) provokes a "major" depression. According to the proponents of the first position (Ross and Rush 1981; Kinsbourne and Bemporad 1984; Finset 1988; Kinsbourne 1989), depression following left-hemispheric (and mainly left frontal-lobe) damage would be more overtly and dramatically expressed (often showing the typical features of the CR), whereas depression following right-hemispheric injury could often be masked by a flattened affect or by difficulty in overtly expressing emotions. According to the proponents of the second position (i.e., Robinson et al.), an important distinction should be made between major and minor PSD. The former, considered as indistinguishable from endogenous depression, would be significantly more frequent among patients with left-anterior lesions, involving either the cortical mantle or subcortical structures, such as the basal ganglia (Robinson and Szetela 1981; Robinson et al. 1983, 1984a; Starkstein et al. 1987; Starkstein and Robinson 1988, 1989).

The latter, considered as a form of dysthymic depression, would not have a similar, highly specific anatomic correlate, being observed both in right- and in left-hemispheric lesions with anterior and posterior localization.

Robinson et al. repeatedly claimed that in left-brain-damaged patients the proximity of the anterior border of the lesion to the frontal pole significantly correlates with severity of depression. Sinyor et al. (1986b) have only in part confirmed this observation. They found a negative correlation between severity of depression and distance of the lesion from the frontal pole in left-brain-damaged patients, but this association was weak and failed to reach the level of statistical significance.

## Biological Markers

The dexamethasone suppression test (DST) is a valuable neuroendocrine marker for endogenous depression (Carrol et al. 1981; Carrol 1982). Several authors (e.g., Ross and Rush 1981; Finklestein et al. 1982; Bauer et al. 1983; Lipsey et al. 1985; Reding et al. 1985) have, therefore, used this test in stroke patients, both to improve the diagnosis of PSD and to clarify the meaning of this kind of depressive disorder. The usefulness of the DST as a diagnostic criterion can be exemplified by case 4 of Ross and Rush's (1981) paper. This right-hemispheric stroke patient denied depression verbally but showed dependence, irritability, and vegetative signs (insomnia and weight loss) suggesting a post-stroke depression. This diagnosis was confirmed by a nonsuppressive DST response. A treatment with tricyclic medication led to a resolution of the symptomatology and to a normalization of the DST.

On the other hand, data relevant to clarify the meaning of PSD have been obtained by Finklestein et al. (1982), Bauer et al. (1983); Lipsey et al. (1985) and Reding et al. (1985). These authors have consistently shown that:

1. No difference is found between right and left hemisphere stroke patients as for the prevalence of abnormal DST responses.
2. Abnormal DST results correlate with moderate to severe levels of depression and with vegetative signs, such as appetite and sleep disturbances.
3. Nonsuppressory DST responses are not clearly related to lesion location within either hemisphere and tend in general to be associated with large lesion volumes (a fact which may lead to a sizeable number of false positive results).
4. The DST is an indicator of PSD, but not a predictor of rehabilitation outcome (Reding et al. 1985).

## Psycho-Social Factors

The long-term consequences of a stroke obviously concern the full range of the social activities of the patient (family relationships, occupational status, leisures and so on). Several authors have, therefore analyzed the relationships between psycho-social factors and PSD. Results of these investigations have consistently shown that a significant relationship exists between poor social functioning and PSD (Feibel et al. 1979; Feibel and Springer 1982; Robinson et al. 1984b). Furthermore, a number of studies which have investigated longitudinally the relationships between degree of social impairment and severity of PSD, have observed that this correlation is weak in the acute post-stroke period, but increases steadily in more chronic stages (Robinson et al. 1984b, 1985). This finding, which parallels results obtained studying longitudinally the correlations between functional impairment and PSD, can be explained in a very similar way. In the acute period patients can only in part predict how long and how much they will be deprived of significant social contacts. In the more chronic stages, on the contrary, the real extent of their social loss becomes clear and its consequences are more fully appreciated. The correlation between poor social functioning and severity of PSD will, therefore, show a very similar progression.

## Interpretations of Post-Stroke Depression

We have seen, in the first part of this survey, that several different biological, psychological, and psycho-social variables seem to play a role in PSD. In this second part we would like to focus attention on the main interpretations that can be advanced to explain this form of depression. The most thorough interpretation has been advanced by Robinson and co-workers, who, on the ground of their systematic investigations in this area, have come to the conclusion that the most typical form of post-stroke depression (namely the major depression observed in left-frontal patients) is indistinguishable from the "endogenous" depression. According to Robinson and co-workers, the clinical phenomenology (Lipsey et al. 1986), the length of the depressive episode (Robinson et al. 1987), and the presence of a non-suppressive response on the DST (Lipsey et al. 1985), render the major PSD very similar to the endogenous depression. The same authors also maintain that this set of clinical similarities stems from a common biochemical mechanism, namely from a defect in the noradrenergic and serotoninergic input to the neocortex. The association between left-frontal injury and major PSD plays a pivotal role in this interpretation, since, according to Robinson and co-workers, a lesion at this level could disrupt the noradrenergic and serotoninergic pathways directed to the cerebral cortex at their origin.

Although interesting and supported by a large body of empirical data, this interpretation can be criticized from several points of view. In the first part of this survey we discussed, for example, the clinical findings which, according to Robinson and co-workers, could contradict the "psychological reaction" hypothesis and those which could support the "identity with the endogenous depression" hypothesis. As for the first point, in our opinion, the weak correlation observed in the acute post-ictal stage between functional impairment, reduction of social activities, and severity of depression does not necessarily contrast with the psychological-reaction hypothesis, whereas the increased correlation obtained 6 months after the stroke supports the same hypothesis. As for the second point, we have cast some doubts on the assumed equivalence between the clinical phenomenology of the PSD and the endogenous depression. Furthermore, we have noticed that in studies conducted with the dexamethasone suppression test, no significant correlation has been found between abnormal DST response and localization of the lesion to the left-frontal lobe. If we pass now from the clinical findings to the hypothesized links between left-frontal lesions and disruption of the noradrenergic and serotoninergic pathways, we are faced with two further difficulties.

The first concerns the fact that, according to the hypothesis, the monoaminergic systems should be lateralized to the left hemisphere in the human brain, whereas the second concerns the overlap that should exist between frontal regions transversed by noradrenergic and serotoninergic pathways and frontal regions usually damaged in patients with major post-stroke depression. As for the first point, no independent evidence supports the existence of this lateralization. As for the second point, this overlap seems very limited. The main pathways providing noradrenergic and serotoninergic inputs to the neocortex actually enter the medial forebrain bundle up to the septal nuclei and then turn around the genu of the corpus callosum, running caudally in the cingulum (Johnsson et al. 1974; Smith and Sweet 1978; Moore and Bloom 1979; Moore and Card 1984). They are, therefore, located on the mesial part of the frontal lobes and are supplied by branches of the anterior cerebral artery. In contrast, the frontal regions usually damaged in stroke patients are located in the frontal convexity and are supplied by the upper branches of the middle cerebral artery (Gacs et al. 1982; Kertesz and Black 1985).

Thus, in spite of its biological appeal, the interpretation proposed by Robinson and co-workers meets important clinical and theoretical difficultes. An alternative (and more traditional) interpretation is that psychological rather than biochemical factors subserve the depressive disorders presented by stroke patients and that a pivotal role in the onset of PSD is played by a full awareness of the defect and of its personal and social implications. The stress put on the awareness of the disability proceeds from the fact that this kind of awareness is not a purely "mental" process, but is deeply rooted in neurophysiological mechanisms inherent to the various brain functions, so that different kinds of brain lesions can produce different levels of awareness. Although the mechanisms subserving these different levels of awareness are still poorly understood (see, for example the recent review of the problem by McGlynn and Schacter 1989), certain agreement still exists on some very general points. The first of these points is that an acute awareness of the disability is usually present in conditions where the defect concerns the motor level and requires from the patient a sustained, continuous effort to be surmounted. Prototypical of these conditions are, for example, the expressive language disorders observed in Broca's aphasia and the motor disturbances observed in Parkinson's disease. The second point is that a more or less complete unawareness of the disease can, on the contrary, be observed in conditions where the defect concerns the sensory rather than the motor level and where detection of the defect is probably prompted by mechanisms of automatic orienting of attention and of subsequent monitoring of performance. Instances of this condition are, for example, the unawareness of language disorders observed in Wernicke's aphasia, the unawareness of hemianopia presented by patients with unilateral neglect, and, perhaps, the unawareness of the cortical blindness observed in the so-called Anton's syndrome (Anton 1899).

Intermediate levels of awareness may be present in conditions where both the motor and the sensory levels are impaired and where an automatic orienting of attention is needed to detect the deficit, but we don't intend to dwell on these questions, which are at present purely speculative.

We only intend to suggest that the existence of neurobiological mechanisms subserving the acute awareness of expressive language disorders observed in Broca's aphasia could in part explain the prevalence of post-stroke depression in patients with left-frontal lesions. Apart from this anatomo-clinical correlation, which cannot be explained by an interpretation framed in generic psychologic terms, all the other aspects of the post-stroke depression (and in particular its evolutive aspects) are fully consistent with a psychological interpretation in which psychodynamic and psychosocial factors play an important role. From this point of view, we completely agree with Schuell et al. (1964) and with Tanner et al. (1988), who have rightly noted that aphasic patients (and brain-damaged patients in general) are not different from the rest of humanity and that the loss of something of value, such as language, functional integrity, or social activities, always produces depression in an aware patient when the loss can no longer be regained or compensated.

The therapeutic implications of this "psychological" interpretation will certainly not consist in neglecting in these patients the pharmacological approach with antidepressants, since at least two well-controlled double blind trials (Lipsey et al. 1984; Reding et al. 1986) have shown that these drugs are effective in post-stroke depression. They will rather consist in integrating the pharmacological treatment with a more individually-centered approach to the problems, needs, and main sources of distress for the patient and his family. It is interesting to note, from this point of view, that some authors (e.g., Isaacs et al. 1976; Anderson and Kottke 1978; House 1987) have recommended rehabilitation as the most effective treatment for PSD and that Hartman and Landau (1987) have shown that emotionally supportive counselling can produce as much improvement as formal language therapy among aphasics.

## Implications of Post-Stroke Depression for Rehabilitation

Several years ago, Adams and Hurwitz (1963) claimed that depression is an important barrier to recovery after stroke. This view has been repeatedly expressed since and is shared by many authors working in the field of neurorehabilitation. It must be acknowledged, however, that depression has been examined as an independent factor only in very few studies designed to identify variables influencing functional recovery after stroke. In one of these studies, Kotila et al. (1984) showed that depression and emotional lability exert a negative influence on recovery 3 and 12 months after stroke. More complex results were obtained in another study (Sinyor et al. 1986a), since depressed patients, although showing a lower level of participation in the rehabilitation process, did not differ from nondepressed patients in the degree of improvement over the course of a formal rehabilitation program. However, 6 weeks after discharge, depressed patients showed a significant impairment in their functional status. According to the authors, this could be due to the fact that, while in hospital, the patients' participation in the rehabilitation program was actively sought and reinforced, thus reducing the negative impact of depression on the rehabilitation process. Following discharge, in the absence of this external continuous support, depression exerted a greater interference with the patient's personal initiative to engage in the recommended therapeutic exercises and activities, and this reduced activity resulted in a loss of gains achieved while in hospital.

In conclusion, a complex set of interactions exists between the functional and the social consequences of brain damage, post-stroke depression, and the rehabilitation process. It is surprising, as Hachinski (1989) recently noted in a discussion of different stroke-rehabilitation programs, that, in spite of the high prevalence of this disorder and of its influence on rehabilitation, depression is often not discussed as a factor to always be taken into account in the rehabilitation of stroke patients.

## References

Adams GF, Hurwitz LJ (1963) Depression as a barrier to recovery after stroke. Lancet 1:533–537

American Psychiatric Association (1980) Diagnostic and statistical manual of mental disorders (DSM-III), 3rd edn. American Psychiatric Press, Washington

Anderson TP, Kottke FJ (1978) Stroke rehabilitation: a reconsideration of some common attitudes. Arch Phys Med Rehabil 59:175–181

Anton G (1899) Über die Selbstwahrnehmung der Herderkrankungen des Gehirns durch den Kranken bei Rindenblindheit und Rindentaubheit. Arch Psych Nervenkrank 32:86–127

Bauer M, Gans J, Harley J (1983) Dexamethasone suppression test and depression in a rehabilitation setting. Arch Phys Med Rehabil 64:421–422

Benson DF (1973) Psychiatric aspects of aphasia. Br J Psychiatry 123:555–566

Benson DF (1979) Aphasia, alexia, and agraphia. Livingstone, New York

Black FW, Black IL (1982) Anterior-posterior locus of lesion and personality: support for the caudality hypothesis. J Clin Psychol 38(3):468–477

Carrol BJ (1982) The dexamethasone suppression test for melancholia. Br J Psychiatry 140: 292–304

Carrol BJ, Feinberg M, Greden JF, Tarika J (1981) A specific laboratory test for the diagnosis of melancholia: standardization, validation and clinical utility. Arch Gen Psychiatry 38:15–22

De Bonis M, Dellatolas G, Rondot P (1985) Mood disorders in left and right brain damaged patients: comparison between ratings and self-rating on the same adjective mood scale: some methodological problems. Psychopathology 18:286–292

Eastwood MR, Rifat SL, Nobbs H, Ruderman J (1989) Mood disorder following cerebrovascular accident. Br J Psychiatry 154:195–200

Ebrahim S, Barer D, Nouri F (1987) Affective illness after stroke. Br J Psychiatry 151:52–56

Feibel JH, Springer CJ (1982) Depression and failure to resume social activities after stroke. Arch Phys Med Rehabil 63:276–278

Feibel JH, Berk S, Joynt RJ (1979) The unmet needs of stroke patients. Neurology (Minneap) 29:592

Finklestein S, Benowitz LJ, Baldessarini RG, Arana GW, Levine D, Woo E, Bear D, Moya K, Stoll AL (1982) Mood, vegetative disturbance and dexamethasone suppression test after stroke. Ann Neurol 12:463–468

Finset A (1988) Depressed mood and reduced emotionality after right hemisphere brain damage. In: Kinsbourne M (ed) Cerebral hemisphere function in depression. American Psychiatric Press, Washington, pp 51–64

Gacs G, Merei FR, Bodosi M (1982) Ballon catheter as a model of cerebral emboli in humans. Stroke 13:39–42

Gainotti G (1969) Réactions “catastrophiques” et manifestations d’indifférence au cours des atteintes cérébrales. Neuropsychologia 7:195–204

Gainotti G (1972) Emotional behavior amd hemispheric side of the lesion. Cortex 8:41–55

Gainotti G (1983) Laterality of affect: the emotional behavior of right- and left-brain-damaged patients. In: Mislobodski M (ed) Hemysindromes: psychobiology, neurology, psychiatry. Academic, New York, pp 175–192

Gainotti G (1989) The meaning of emotional disturbances resulting from unilateral brain injury. In: Gainotti G, Caltagirone C (eds) Emotions and the dual brain. Springer, Berlin Heidelberg New York, pp 149–170

Gasparrini WG, Satz P, Heilman KM, Coolidge FL (1978) Hemispheric asymmetries of affective processing as determined by the Minnesota Multiphasic Personality Inventory. J Neurol Neurosurg Psychiatry 41:470–473

Goldstein K (1948) Language and language disturbances. Grune and Stratton, New York

Gordon WA, Hibbard MR, Egelko S, Diller L (1985) The multifaceted nature of the cognitive deficits following stroke: unexpected findings. Arch Phys Med Rehabil 66:338

Hachinski V (1989) Stroke rehabilitation. Arch Neurol 46:703

Hartman J, Landau WM (1987) Comparison of formal language therapy with supportive counseling for aphasia due to acute vascular accident. Arch Neurol 44:646–649

House A (1987) Depression after stroke. Br Med J 294:76–78

Isaacs B, Neville Y, Rushford I (1976) The stricken: the social consequences of stroke. Age Ageing 5:188–192

Johnsson G, Einarsson P, Fuxe K, Hallman H (1974) Microspectrofluorimetric studies on central 5-hydroxytryptamine neurons. Adv Biochem Psychopharmacol 10:55–65

Kertesz A, Black SE (1985) Cerebrovascular disease and aphasia. In: Speech and language evaluation in neurology. Grune and Stratton, New York, pp 83–122

Kinsbourne M (1989) A model of adaptive behavior related to cerebral participation in emotional control. In: Gainotti G, Caltagirone C (eds) Emotions and the dual brain. Springer, Berlin Heidelberg New York, pp 248–259

Kinsbourne M, Bemporad B (1985) Lateralization of emotion: a model and the evidence. In: Fox NA, Davidson RJ (eds) The psychobiology of affective development. Erlbaum, Hillsdale

Kotila M, Waltimo O, Niemi ML, Laacsonen R, Lempinen M (1984) The profile of recovery from stroke and factors influencing outcome. Stroke 15:1039–1044

Lipsey JR, Robinson RG, Pearlson GD, Rao K, Price TR (1984) Nortriptyline treatment for post-stroke depression: a double-blind study. Lancet 1:297–300

Lipsey JR, Robinson RG, Pearlson GD, Rao K, Price TR (1985) Dexamethasone suppression test and mood following stroke. Am J Psychiatry 142:527–529

Lipsey JR, Spencer WC, Rabins PV, Robinson RG (1986) Phenomenological comparison of post-stroke depression and functional depression. Am J Psychiatry 143:527–529

McGlynn SM, Schacter DL (1989) Unawareness of deficit in neuropsychological syndromes. J Clin Exp Neuropsychol 11:143–205

Moore RY, Bloom FE (1979) Central catecholamine neuron system: anatomy and physiology. Annu Rev Neurosci 1:129–169

Moore RY, Card P (1984) Noradrenaline containing neurons systems. In: Bjorklund A, Hökfelt T (eds) Classical transmitters in the C.N.S. Elsevier, Amsterdam, pp 123–148 (Handbook of chemical neuroanatomy, vol 2)

Parsikh RM, Lipsey JR, Robinson RG et al. (1987) Two-year longitudinal study of post-stroke mood disorders: dynamic changes in correlates of depression at one and two years. Stroke 18:579–584

Reding MJ, Orto LA, Willenski P, Fortuna I, Day N, Steiner SF, Gehr L, McDowell F (1985) The dexamethasone suppression test is an indicator of depression in stroke but does not predict rehabilitation outcome. Arch Neurol 42:209–212

Reding MJ, Orto LA, Winter SW, Fortuna IM, Di Ponte P, McDowell FN (1986) Antidepressant therapy after stroke: a double-blind trial. Arch Neurol 43:763–765

Robinson RG, Benson DF (1981) Depression in aphasic patients: frequency, severity and clinical-pathological correlations. Brain Lang 14:282–291

Robinson RG, Price TR (1982) Post-stroke depressive disorders: a follow-up study of 103 patients. Stroke 13:635–641

Robinson RG, Szetela B (1981) Mood change following left hemispheric brain injury. Ann Neurol 3:447–453

Robinson RG, Kubos KL, Starr LB, Rao K, Price TR (1983) Mood changes in stroke patients: relationship to lesion location. Compr Psychiatry 24:555–566

Robinson RG, Kubos KL, Starr LB, Rao K, Price TR (1984a) Mood disorders in stroke patients: importance of location of lesion. Brain 107:81–93

Robinson RG, Starr LB, Lipsey JR, Rao K, Price TR (1984b) A two-year longitudinal study of post-stroke mood disorders: dynamic changes in associated variables over the first six months of follow-up. Stroke 15:510–517

Robinson RG, Starr LB, Lipsey JR et al. (1985) A two-year longitudinal study of post-stroke mood disorders: in-hospital prognostic factors associated with six-month outcome. J Nerv Ment Dis 173:221–226

Robinson RG, Bolduc PL, Price TR (1987) A two-year longitudinal study of post-stroke mood disorders: diagnosis and outcome at one and two-year follow-up. Stroke 18:837–843

Ross ED, Rush AJ (1981) Diagnosis and neuroanatomical correlates of depression in brain damaged patients. Arch Gen Psychiatry 38:1344–1354

Ross ED, Gordon WA, Hibbard M, Egelko S (1986) The dexamethasone suppression test, poststroke depression, and the validity of DSM-III-based diagnostic criteria. Am J Psychiatry 143:1200–1201

Schuell H, Jenkins J, Jimenez-Pabon E (1964) Aphasia in adult. Harper and Row, New York

Sinyor D, Amato P, Kaloupek D, Becker R, Goldenberg M, Coopersmith H (1986a) Post-stroke depression: relationship to functional impairment, coping strategies, and rehabilitation outcome. Stroke 17:1102–1107

Sinyor D, Jacques P, Kaloupek DB, Becker R, Goldenberg M, Coopersmith HM (1986b) Post-stroke depression and lesion location: an attempted replication. Brain 109:537–546

Smith BH, Sweet WH (1978) Monoaminergic regulation of the central nervous system function. II. Serotoninergic systems. Neurosurgery 3:257–272

Starkstein SE, Robinson RG (1988) Aphasia and depression. Aphasiology 2:1–20

Starkstein SE, Robinson RG (1989) Affective disorders and cerebral vascular disease. Br J Psychiatry 154:170–182

Starkstein SE, Robinson RG, Price TR (1987) Comparison of cortical and subcortical lesions in the production of post-stroke mood disorders. Brain 110:1045–1059

Tanner DC, Gerstenberger DL (1988) The grief response in neuropathologies of speech and language. Aphasiology 2(1):79–84

Wade DT, Legh-Smith J, Hewer RA (1987) Depressed mood after stroke: a community study of its frequency. Br J Psychiatry 151:200–205

# Spontaneous Remission Versus Rehabilitation of Aphasia

*A. Basso*

## Introduction

Most patients who have suffered acute onset of aphasia improve over the succeeding months. The precise course of recovery, its speed and duration, and reasons for this are still largely unknown. One question that has attracted much attention is whether the course of recovery from aphasia can be positively influenced by deliberate language intervention.

In this presentation I will review the prognostic factors related to recovery, the effects of treatment and the patterns of recovery in groups of patients and in individual patients.

## The Period of Spontaneous Recovery

In the early period after onset, spontaneous recovery is a reasonable expectation, and studies of changes in the language behavior of untreated aphasic patients have generally confirmed that some recovery occurs, although some patients have different degrees of recovery. Most investigators agree about the shape of the curve of spontaneous recovery but there is no general agreement about the exact time limits. The curve is a decelerating one, steepest in the first month post-onset, flattening out subsequently and finally reaching a plateau sometime between 6 and 12 months post-onset.

## Factors Influencing Recovery

The influence on recovery of some specific factors has been experimentally studied and results will be briefly reported below. These factors are not independent and often interact, making it more difficult to study their specific effects on recovery. Moreover, other factors that are not amenable to experimental investigation appear intuitively to be important: motivation is an example of these. An indirect proof of the importance of motivation for recovery comes from the observation that left-brain-damaged patients, who are in general aware of their handicap, recover better than right-brain-damaged patients, who often are unmoved by their illness (Denes et al. 1982). In the following, I will only consider those prognostic factors for which we have some experimental results. These can be grouped under two headings: anagraphical and neurological factors. Age, sex and handedness are the anagraphic factors that we will consider, etiology, site and size of lesion and severity and type of aphasia are the neurological ones. The effects of aphasia therapy will be considered separately. For a detailed review of factors influencing the natural course of aphasia and the effects of treatment, see Darley (1982).

## Anagraphic Factors

### Age

Age has often been considered an important determinant of degree of recovery but data for the effects of age on recovery are in some conflict. Some studies (Vignolo 1964; Sands et al. 1969; Gloning et al. 1976; Marshall et al. 1982) suggest that younger patients have a more favorable outcome than older ones, but other studies (Messerli et al. 1976; Basso et al. 1979; Sarno 1980) have not found age to have a significant effect on recovery. Recently, evidence that patients with fluent aphasia are older than patients with nonfluent aphasia has been obtained (Obler et al. 1978; Basso et al. 1980; De Renzi et al. 1980; Miceli et al. 1981). The effects of age in the above-mentioned studies have not been considered independently of the type of aphasia and this makes it difficult to interpret the results, as the type of aphasia could, itself, be a prognostic factor, even though no significant effect on outcome has been found when fluent and nonfluent patients were compared (Basso et al. 1979). All in all we can say that age is not a very important factor in recovery.

### Sex

Sex has been claimed to influence the presence and type of aphasia, with females less frequently and less severely aphasic than males (McGlone 1977, 1980). These results have not been reproduced in better controlled experiments with larger series of patients (De Renzi et al. 1980; Basso et al. 1980; Miceli et al. 1981), but two studies directly aimed at investigating the effects of sex on recovery from aphasia have shown a better prognosis for females than for males for oral expression (Basso et al. 1982a) or auditory comprehension (Pizzamiglio et al. 1985). In a previous study, where sex was but one of the factors considered, no significant difference was found (Kertesz and McKabe 1977).

### Handedness

Handedness is the last anagraphic factor studied. It has been considered important in determining the functional organization of the brain, since laterality of the lesion giving rise to language disturbances is much more heterogeneous among left-handers than among right-handers: some left-handers have right-hemisphere representation for language, the majority has left-hemisphere representation, and probably some have a more bilateral representation of language function (see Joanette 1989, for a review). Better recovery in left-handers is expected, at least for this last group. Both Subirana (1969) and Gloning et al. (1976) do, in fact, report a better prognosis for left-handed and ambidextrous patients than for right-handed patients. Moreover, according to Luria (1970), recovery from aphasia occurs more frequently in patients with familial sinistrality. In a retrospective study, we (Basso et al. 1990) compared recovery of oral and written production and comprehension in 15 non-right-handed rehabilitated patients with the recovery in a group of right-handed subjects and found no significant differences.

## Neurological Factors

These play a more important role in recovery from aphasia.

### Etiology

Traumatic aphasia has a better prognosis than vascular aphasia (Alajouanine et al. 1957; Luria 1970; Kertesz and McCabe 1977; Basso et al. 1980) but here again, as for age, the type of aphasia is a confounding factor, with fluent aphasia more frequent in traumatic patients than in vascular patients (Basso et al. 1980). Moreover, the different prognosis may not be directly due to etiology (traumatic vs vascular) but be a side-effect, since traumatic patients generally are neurologically healthy while patients who undergo strokes often are vasculopathic and not healthy neurologically. Cerebro-vascular disease is known to be the major cause of aphasia in adult patients. Different vascular etiologies, such as infarcts or hemorrhages, have generally been grouped together and only rarely has their effect on recovery been compared, with conflicting results. Anderson et al. (1970) studied predictors of recovery in complete stroke and concluded that hemorrhages are followed by the least recovery. Rubens (1977) considers that language recovery in patients with circumscribed intracerebral hemorrhage may begin late, even months after onset, but the deficit is often reversible. According to Nagata et al. (1986), the prognosis is good for patients with localized hematoma in CT.

We compared the recoveries from aphasia of 46 patients with intracerebral hematoma and 101 patients with ischaemic infarcts, comparable for CT lesion size. All patients were right-handed with a single left-hemisphere lesion, had a first neuropsychological examination performed no more than 6 months post-onset and a control examination at least 6 months after the first. More patients with intracerebral hematoma than patients with ischaemic lesions recovered all four language modalities considered (oral and written production and comprehension), but the difference was significant only for written production and comprehension. The better prognosis for hemorrhage, if it be confirmed by more data, may be ascribed to the fact that hemorrhage displaces the fiber bundles without completely destroying them, as is the case in infarcts.

## Extent and Location of the Lesion

As for the importance of extent and location of the lesion on recovery, it is difficult to disentangle their effects on *amount* of recovery from those on initial severity of aphasia which, in its turn, is directly associated with extent and location of lesion.

The negative effect of extent of lesion on initial severity of aphasia is unquestionable (see, for example, Kertesz 1979) but once initial severity has been taken into account, the effect of lesion size on rate of recovery is not clear-cut. Demeurisse et al. (1985) did not find any significant correlation between recovery 3 months post-onset and size of lesion in ten patients with subcortical lesion. They did, however, find a significant negative correlation between size of cortico-subcortical lesion and recovery of oral production, but not of comprehension. Selnes et al. (1983) studied the relationship between lesional volume and recovery of comprehension, as evaluated by the Token Test, in 39 vascular patients. There was a significant negative correlation for large but not for smaller lesions. A significant positive correlation – the larger the lesion the better the recovery – between size of lesion and recovery of auditory comprehension has been found (Kertesz et al. 1979), but this is probably due to a ceiling effect in moderate and mild aphasics with smaller lesions.

Lesions limited to Broca's area give rise to moderate and transient language disturbances (Mohr et al. 1978; Brunner et al. 1982) and lesions in Wernicke's area are accompanied by severe and long-lasting aphasia (Brunner et al. 1982). Recently, evidence in support of the importance of a posterior lesion on determining long-lasting aphasia has appeared (Ludlow et al. 1986; Naeser et al. 1987). In a group of 39 traumatic patients who had Broca's aphasia 15 years prior to the study (Ludlow et al. 1986), the only significant difference in the locations of the lesions between those patients who were no longer aphasic and those with clinical evidence of aphasia was in the posterior extension of the lesion: clinically aphasic patients had lesions that extended more posteriorly. Five Wernicke aphasics with sparing of at least half of Wernicke's area were found to have good comprehension 6 months post-onset; the five Wernicke aphasics with larger lesions in Wernicke's area still had poor comprehension (Naeser et al. 1987). The two groups, however, did not significantly differ in degree of recovery, showing that the lesion site has more influence on initial severity than on the degree of amelioration.

To summarize, a large or a posterior lesion initially causes severe aphasia but after removing the effect of initial severity, their effect on amount of recovery is not clearly demonstrated.

### Initial Severity of Aphasia

Level of impairment soon after onset is a significant indicator of the level of ultimate recovery: the lower the level of performance at onset, the more limited the amount of recovery. This result has been confirmed whenever the level of initial severity was included in studies evaluating recovery and it holds for whichever language performance was studied (Sands et al. 1969; Kenin and Swisher 1972; Gloning et al. 1976; Kertesz and McCabe 1977; Basso et al. 1979).

### Type of Aphasia

The type of aphasia cannot be studied independently of the severity since it is intrinsically related to it. Some syndromes are by definition more severe than others: A transcortical sensory aphasic, for example, is always more severely impaired than a Broca's, a conduction or a transcortical motor aphasic. When only fluent and nonfluent patients of approximately the same severity were compared, no differences in recovery were detected (Basso et al. 1979).

## Aphasia Therapy

Studies of the effect of aphasia therapy have used very different methodologies. We can roughly recognize a clinical approach, soon followed by a more methodologically correct approach, and lately by the single-case approach. In the earliest studies (Butfield and Zangwill 1946; Wepman 1951; Marks et al. 1957; Leischner and Linck 1967; Broida 1977) only treated aphasics were considered and recovery was evaluated subjectively after treatment. Moreover, the patients included did not have the same amount of therapy, which varied from 1 to 110 therapy sessions in one study (Marks et al. 1957) and from 5 to 290 in another (Butfield and Zangwill 1946). All these papers firmly stated that aphasia therapy is effectual, but the studies are, unfortunately, beset with methodological weaknesses. Probably the most important is the fact that effect of spontaneous recovery is not considered, and treated patients were not compared with untreated patients.

Later studies utilized a more experimentally correct approach and compared improvement of treated and untreated patients. At first sight the results of these studies are contradictory. Some of them report that aphasia therapy has a significant effect (Gloning et al. 1976; Basso et al. 1975, 1979; Hagen 1973); others did not find any significant difference between treated and untreated patients (Vignolo 1964; Sarno et al. 1970; Levita 1978). This approach to the study of efficacy of language therapy also has weak points: the treated and untreated patients are seldom properly comparable and the assignment to treatment or not was not random. Moreover, other factors known to influence recovery, such as site and extent of lesion, generally were not considered. However, the major objection that has been made to these studies is that the difference between rehabilitated and non-rehabilitated patients may be a consequence of showing interest and attention to the patient and not a specific effect of language therapy.

In the past few years, different treatments or speech-pathologists and volunteers have been compared in a certain number of studies. Patients rehabilitated by speech therapists or with formal language therapy do not recover significantly more than the other groups rehabilitated either by volunteers or with different therapeutic procedures (Meikle et al. 1979; Wertz et al. 1981; David et al. 1982; Lincoln et al. 1982, 1984). These studies suggest that treatment need not be specific and that recovery can be a nonspecific effect of receiving attention, but they, too, are not free from some methodological weaknesses. Their major limitation concerns the duration of therapy. In one study treatment lasted for 8 weeks (Lincoln et al. 1982) and in another patients received 30 therapy sessions over a period of 15–20 weeks (David et al. 1982). A careful reading of the literature shows that whenever untreated patients and patients treated for long periods were compared, the difference between the two groups was significant (Hagen 1973; Basso et al. 1979; Sarno and Levita 1981; Marshall et al. 1982), but no difference was found when rehabilitation was carried out for shorter periods of time (Vignolo 1964; Sarno et al. 1970; Levita 1978). In a retrospective study (Basso 1987), we investigated the effects of length of treatment on improvement of oral comprehension and expression. It was found that whether rehabilitation was for 3 months or 6 months caused significantly different effects on improvement of expression – but not on comprehension –, patients rehabilitated for 3 months faring less well.

Recently, the use of group-studies for evaluating the effect of therapy has been repeatedly criticized. Two general criticisms have been made: that the question is too broad and general for serious scientific investigation and that the treatments involved were widely different and underspecified, thus preventing replication (see Howard 1986). These criticisms are correct, but a methodologically valid clinical trial is certainly possible, even if beset with difficulties. Data from the group-studies reviewed vary in scientific merit. No single study provides by itself an unequivocal answer to questions about the efficacy of aphasia therapy. However, the question is too broad for a single unqualified yes-or-no answer. Taken together these results support the general notion that language treatment does positively influence the course of recovery from aphasia in a number of patients.

Lately the single case approach in studies aimed at evaluating efficacy of aphasia therapy has been preferred. Coltheart (1983), for example, claims that the methodological problems of group-studies can only be circumvented by longitudinal single-case studies, in which patients act as their own controls, which avoids the difficulty of matching one patient with another. An experimental design such as a cross-over treatment design, which allows comparison of two methods of treatment as well as providing ways of distinguishing between specific treatment effects, nonspecific treatment effects, and effects due to spontaneous recovery can be used. Multiple baseline designs can also be used. The more recent literature reports descriptions of a few individual patients rehabilitated according to principles of cognitive neuropsychology (Hatfield 1983; Byng and Coltheart 1986; de Partz 1986; Jones 1986; Byng 1988). Effects of therapy have generally been positive, but no negative cases have been published. Criticisms of the single-case approach have not been half as frequent as criticisms of the group-study approach. This, however, does not mean that single-case studies are above all criticism and I will mention two shortcomings of such an approach.

A serious objection that can be raised against the single-case study methodology is the fact that there is no possibility to find replications which would enable us to reject a previously reported result. Secondly, the performance of an individual patient may be *too* specific for meaningful generalization, it may simply be an idiosyncratic performance.

To summarize, while the effects of aphasia therapy have not been – and in such broad terms cannot be – unequivocally stated, clinical studies have satisfactorily demonstrated specific effects of treatment, and single-case studies have offered different therapeutic techniques that could be usefully utilized in larger samples.

## Pattern of Recovery

We have considered the time course of aphasia and what factors can affect it, but we have not yet specified the pattern of recovery, whether for example, all language modalities progress in parallel, or the most impaired first, or each independently of the others. Few longitudinal studies have addressed this problem or compared improvement in different language modalities by comparing the number of patients improving in one modality with the number of patients improving in another modality. In the few studies published all, or the same, modalities were not always compared, nor were the subjects studied always representative of the general aphasic population. Notwithstanding this, a common pattern emerges. A higher percentage of patients improve in comprehension than in production, and a higher percentage improve in oral than in written language (Kenin and Swisher 1972; Hanson and Cicciarelli 1978; Lomas and Kertesz 1978; Prins et al. 1978). These results are only valid for a group and do not say what happens in an individual patient. In a recent study, we (Basso et al. 1982b) found that in an individual rehabilitated patient, improvement of oral and written comprehension and production are always significantly associated. In nonrehabilitated patients, the recovery pattern is nearly the same, the only exception being that comprehension tends to be the only modality to improve in a consistent number of patients.

Considering the evolution from a qualitative point of view, characteristics of production – such as presence of apraxia of speech, semantic paraphasias and so on – are relatively constant, although they fade away with time. This means that many more patients are not classifiable into the classical aphasia syndromes if seen a long time post-onset. This pattern of evolution is the same for rehabilitated and nonrehabilitated patients, the only difference being a higher percentage of improvement within rehabilitated patients.

## Conclusion

As I have already said, none of the variables considered in relation to improvement exists in vacuo and we must understand how they interact if we want to be able to predict outcome. From data in the literature, it is now possible to draw certain group generalizations about recovery with some degree of accurateness, but it is much more difficult for the individual patient.

All factors must be taken into account, but it appears safe to say that anagraphic factors do in fact play only a minor role. The factors that really do influence outcome are initial severity of aphasia (which is inextricably associated with the extent and the location of the lesion) and rehabilitation. Rehabilitation does not alter the pattern of the natural course of restitution, but brings it about in a number of patients that would not show any improvement and accelerates it in some other patients.

## References


Alajouanine T, Castaigne P, Lhermitte F, Escourolle R, de Ribaucourt B (1957) Etude de 43 cas d'aphasie post-traumatique. Encephale 46:1–45

Anderson TP, Bourestom N, Greenberg FR (1970) Rehabilitation predictors in completed stroke: final report. American Rehabilitation Foundation, Minneapolis

Basso A (1987) Approaches to neuropsychological rehabilitation. Language disorders. In: Meier M, Benton A, Diller L (eds) Neuropsychological rehabilitation. Livingstone, London

Basso A, Faglioni P, Vignolo LA (1975) Etude controlée de la rééducation du langage dans l'aphasie: comparaison entre aphasiques traités et non-traités. Rev Neurol (Paris) 131:607–614

Basso A, Capitani E, Vignolo LA (1979) Influence of rehabilitation on language skills in aphasic patients. A controlled study. Arch Neurol 36:190–196

Basso A, Capitani E, Laiacona M, Luzzatti C (1980) Factors influencing type and severity of aphasia. Cortex 16:631–636

Basso A, Capitani E, Moraschini S (1982a) Sex differences in recovery from aphasia. Cortex 18:469–475

Basso A, Capitani E, Zanobio ME (1982b) Pattern of recovery of oral and written expression and comprehension in aphasic patients. Behav Brain Res 6:115–128

Basso A, Farabola M, Grassi MP, Laiacona M, Zanobio ME (1990) Aphasia in left-handers. Brain Lang 38:233–252

Broida H (1977) Language therapy effects in long term aphasia. Arch Phys Med Rehabil 58:248–253

Brunner RJ, Kornhuber HH, Seemuller S, Surger G, Wallesch CW (1982) Basal ganglia participation in language pathology. Brain Lang 16:281–299

Butfield E, Zangwill OL (1946) Re-education in aphasia: a review of 70 cases. J Neurol Neurosurg Psychiatry 9:75–79

Byng S (1988) Sentence processing deficits: theory and therapy. Cogn Neuropsychol 5:629–676

Byng S, Coltheart M (1986) Aphasia therapy research: methodological requirement and illustrative results. In: Hjelquist E, Nilsson LB (eds) Communication and handicap. North-Holland, Amsterdam

Coltheart M (1983) Aphasia therapy research: a single case study approach. In: Code C, Mueller D (eds) Aphasia therapy. Arnold, London

Darley F (1982) Aphasia. Saunders, Philadelphia

David R, Enderby P, Bainton D (1982) Treatment of acquired aphasia: speech therapists and volunteers compared. J Neurol Neurosurg Psychiatry 45:957–961

Demeurisse G, Capon A, Verhas M (1985) Prognostic value of computed tomography in aphasic stroke patients. Eur Neurol 24:134–139

Denes G, Semenza C, Stoppa E, Lis A (1982) Unilateral spatial neglect and recovery from hemiplegia. Brain 105:543–552

De Partz MP (1986) Reeducation of a deep dyslexic patient: rationale of the method and results. Cogn Neuropsychol 3:149–177

De Renzi E, Faglioni P, Ferrari P (1980) The influence of sex and age on the incidence and type of aphasia. Cortex 16:627–630

Gloning K, Trappl R, Heiss WD, Quatember R (1976) Prognosis and speech therapy in aphasia. In: Lebrun Y, Hoops R (eds) Recovery in aphasics. Swets and Zeitlinger, Amsterdam

Hagen C (1973) Communication abilities in hemiplegia: effect of speech therapy. Arch Phys Med Rehabil 54:454–463

Hanson WR, Cicciarelli AW (1978) The time, amount and pattern of language improvement in adult aphasics. Br J Dis Commun 13:59–63

Hatfield FM (1983) Aspects of acquired dysgraphia and implications for re-education. In: Code C, Muller DJ (eds) Aphasia therapy. Arnold, London

Howard D (1986) Beyond randomised controlled trials: the case for effective case studies on the effects of treatment. Br J Dis Commun 21:89–102

Joanette Y (1989) Aphasia in left-handers and crossed aphasia. In: Boller F, Grafman J (eds) Handbook of neuropsychology, vol 2. Elsevier, Amsterdam

Jones EV (1986) Building the foundations for sentence production in a non-fluent aphasic. Br J Dis Commun 21:63–82

Kenin M, Swisher L (1972) A study of pattern of recovery in aphasia. Cortex 8:56–68

Kertesz A (1979) Aphasia and associated disorders. Grune and Stratton, New York

Kertesz A, McCabe P (1977) Recovery patterns and prognosis in aphasia. Brain 100:1–18

Kertesz A, Harlock W, Coates R (1979) Computer tomographic localization, lesion size, and prognosis in aphasia and non-verbal impairment. Brain Lang 8:34–50

Leischner A, Linck HA (1967) Neuere Erfahrungen mit der Behandlung von Aphasien. Nervenarzt 38:199–205

Levita E (1978) Effects of speech therapy on aphasics' responses to the Functional Communication Profile. Percept Mot Skills 47:151–154

Lincoln NB, Pickersgill MJ, Hankey AI, Hilton CR (1982) An evaluation of operant training and speech therapy in the language rehabilitation of moderate aphasics. Behav Psychother 10:162–178

Lincoln NB et al. (1984) Effectiveness of speech therapy for aphasic stroke patients: a randomised controlled trials. Lancet 1:1197–1200

Lomas J, Kertesz A (1978) Patterns of spontaneous recovery in aphasic groups: a study of adult stroke patients. Brain Lang 5:388–401

Ludlow CL, Rosemberg J, Fair C, Buck DE, Schesselman S, Salazar A (1986) Brain lesions associated with nonfluent aphasia fifteen years following penetrating head injury. Brain 109:55–80

Luria AR (1970) Traumatic aphasia. Mouton, The Hague

Marks M, Taylor M, Rusk HA (1957) Rehabilitation of the aphasic patient: a survey of three years experience in a rehabilitation setting. Neurology (Minneap) 7:837–843

Marshall RC, Thompkins CA, Phillips DS (1982) Improvement in treated aphasia: examination of selected prognostic factors. Folia Phoniatr (Basel) 34:305–315

McGlone J (1977) Sex differences in the cerebral organization of verbal function and cognitive impairment in stroke. Age, sex, aphasia type and laterality differences. Brain 100:775–793

McGlone J (1980) Sex differences in human brain asymmetry: a critical survey. Behav Brain Sci 3:215–263

Meikle M, Wechsler E, Tupper E, Benenson J, Mulhall D, Stern G (1979) Comparative trial of volunteer and professional treatments of dysphasia after stroke. Br Med J 2:87–89

Messerli P, Tissot A, Rodriguez J (1976) Recovery from aphasia: some factors of prognosis. In: Lebrun Y, Hoops R (eds) Recovery in aphasics. Swets and Zeitlinger, Amsterdam

Miceli G, Caltagirone C, Gainotti G, Masullo C, Silveri C, Villa G (1981) Influence of age, sex, literacy and pathologic lesion on incidence, severity and type of aphasia. Acta Neurol Scand 64:370–382

Mohr JP, Pessin MS, Finkelstein S, Funkestein HH, Duncan GW, Davies KR (1978) Broca aphasia: pathology and clinical. Neurology (Minneap) 28:311–324

Naeser AM, Helm-Estabrooks N, Haas G, Auerbach S, Srinivasan M (1987) Relationship between lesion extent in Wernicke's area on computer tomographic scan and predicting recovery of comprehension in Wernicke's aphasia. Arch Neurol 44:73–82

Nagata K, Yunoki K, Kabe S, Suzuki A, Araki G (1986) Regional cerebral blood flow correlates of aphasia outcome in cerebral hemorrhage and cerebral infarction. Stroke 17:417–423

Obler LK, Albert M, Goodglass H, Benson DF (1978) Aphasia type and aging. Brain Lang 6:318–322

Pizzamiglio L, Mammucari A, Razzano C (1985) Evidence for sex differences in brain organization in recovery in aphasia. Brain Lang 25:213–223

Prins RS, Snow CE, Wagenaar E (1978) Recovery from aphasia: spontaneous speech versus language comprehension. Brain Lang 6:192–211

Rubens AB (1977) The role of changes within the central nervous system during recovery from aphasia. In: Sullivan MA, Kommers MS (eds) Rationale for adult aphasia therapy. University of Nebraska Medical Center, Omaha

Sands E, Sarno MT, Shankweiler D (1969) Long-term assessment of language function in aphasia due to stroke. Arch Phys Med Rehabil 50:202–206

Sarno MT (1980) Language rehabilitation outcome in the elderly aphasic patient. In: Obler LK, Albert ML (eds) Language and communication in the elderly: clinical therapeutic and experimental issues. Heath, Lexington

Sarno MT, Levita E (1981) Some observations on the nature of recovery in global aphasia. Brain Lang 13:1–12

Sarno MT, Silverman M, Sands E (1970) Speech therapy and language recovery in severe aphasia. J Speech Hear Res 13:607–623

Selnes OA, Knopman DS, Niccum N, Rubens AB, Larson D (1983) Computed tomographic scan correlates of auditory comprehension deficits in aphasia: a prospective recovery study. Ann Neurol 5:558–566

Subirana A (1969) Handedness and cerebral dominance. In: Vinken PJ, Bruyn GW (eds) Handbook of clinical neurology, vol 4. North-Holland, Amsterdam

Vignolo LA (1964) Evolution of aphasia and languge rehabilitation: a retrospective exploratory study. Cortex 1:344–367

Wepman JM (1951) Recovery from aphasia. Ronald, New York

Wertz RT et al. (1981) Veterans administration cooperative study on aphasia: a comparison of individual and group treatments. J Speech Hear Res 24:580–594

Wertz RT et al. (1986) Comparison of clinic, home, and deferred language treatment for aphasia. Arch Neurol 43:653–658

# Speech Disturbances of Organic and Functional Genesis and Their Therapy

*V. M. Shklovsky*

Speech disturbances usually appear as one of the syndromes or symptoms of a pathological process which, as a rule, occurs in a neurological or psychosomatic context. The problems of speech pathology, especially of organic genesis, can only be solved if the mechanism of the underlying illness is taken into account. This indicates a close connection between speech disturbances and other medical problems, which are topics in defectology, psychology, and neurolinguistics.

It is a known fact that the most severe and frequent speech disorders in adults are aphasia, dysarthria, and stuttering. In spite of the etiological and clinical differences between these speech disturbances, all of them are based on the disturbance of one of the most important psychological functions, the function of speech. This forces us to look upon speech disturbances as a scientific problem both from the organic and functional point of view.

Speech disturbances of organic genesis generally result from a stroke or neurotrauma, producing invalids quite often still young. The decreasing age of stroke patients is an international phenomenon; 23%–27% of stroke victims are younger than 50 years. The severest consequences of stroke are hemiparalysis and disturbances of speech function. About 75%–80% of stroke victims are completely unable to work, quite often as a result of speech disturbances.

Among the disturbances of basic psychological functions, aphasia is very frequent. People acquire not only neurological but also psychopathological symptoms, which result directly from the brain lesions and brain disturbances or occur in reaction to the deficient speech and motor functions and altered social and family status (Shklovsky 1985). Many of these people require extensive, long-term treatment and special forms of therapy and rehabilitation, including a wide range of biological and psychological measures radically different from those in cardiology, traumatology, surgery, etc.

The complex character of the rehabilitation of this patient collective has been confirmed (Basso et al. 1979; Sarno 1979; Beck 1983; Poeck 1982; Schmieder 1983; Busch 1983). Kabanov (1978), Gianotti and Lemmo (1983), and Shklovsky et al. (1982) view the rehabilitation process as a set of the state social, economic, medical, and pedagogic measures. Principles of rehabilitation have already been theoretically formulated and widely applied. Nevertheless, the theoretical and practical level of rehabilitation of aphasics, due to its very specific character, does not always meet the needs of the modern clinic. The latest achievements in neurology, psychiatry, psychology, psycholinguistic, and pedagogic sciences are not always taken into account. There is still no network of specialized clinics where the complex rehabilitation of people with aphasia could take place.

The Center of Speech Pathology was the first to work out a complete set of treatment modalities for people with aphasia as used now in Moscow clinics. The set includes pharmacological treatment, physical therapy, massage, restoration training, social rehabilitation, and psychotherapy (including family therapy). A special service has been established in Moscow to help people with speech disturbances. This has enabled us to organise the speech therapy and rehabilitation (in a broader sense of the word) at different stages of illness for people who have suffered a stroke or a brain trauma. There is a speech-therapy service for the early stages of the illness functioning in neurological stroke departments in Moscow hospitals and in regional polyclinics. Facilities also exist for people with speech pathology, where the complete range of rehabilitation measures is offered.

Most important for people with aphasia is the restoration therapy, aimed at the overcoming of disturbed psychological functions, primarily speech function. Due to the success of Soviet neuropsychology, a system of restoration treatment for victims of stroke or brain trauma has been worked out (Luria 1947, 1948; Kogan 1962; Bein 1964). The methodological platform has been established, as well as the principles of compensation for the disturbed functions, and a series of the treatment measures has been described. Recent scientific achievements, however, call for a further study of the disturbed psychological functioning and new forms of rehabilitation.

The All-Union Center for Speech Pathology conducts extensive scientific research in this field. Speech therapy plays the major role in determining the effective forms of restoration and rehabilitation. A series of studies have resulted in new methods of speech therapy to augment the traditional ones. The most important of these is the use of nonverbal communication, which is widely applied not only in communication between healthy people, but also in impaired verbal communication (Silverman 1980; Schindler 1984).

We revert to nonverbal, symbolic forms of communication when dealing with aphasics who have experienced a long-term lack of verbal communication despite extensive rehabilitation measures. The problem of "speechless" people goes beyond the limits of pure speech therapy and includes social adaptation. Deprived of the ability to speak, these people find themselves outcasts, which makes their hard life even harder. Nonverbal communication (pictograms and gestures) is meant to ensure communication at the elementary level at least.

Besides, the use of nonverbal communication is meant to produce an enlivening effect, which actually takes place in the majority of cases. Recent observations confirm that the use of the pictograms and gestures (if they are constantly followed by speaking) reinforces the nonverbal-verbal connection and the realization of words and simple phrases corresponding to the nonverbal signs in oral and written speech. These observations enable us to view nonverbal communication as a new, independent way to rehabilitate people with speech pathology (Shklovsky et al. 1982, 1985).

Another problem speech therapy faces is the use of work and everyday activity for the restoration of speech function. The close interrelation between work and speech, which can be assumed on the basis of phylogenetic or ontogenetic considerations, explains the stimulating influence of work on speech function. Today ergotherapy has gained a recognized position in the treatment regimens used for rehabilitation of invalids in various medical groups. It is based mainly on the patient's involvement in working activity and restitution of mobility. Ergotherapy plays an important role in social adaptation. Speech therapy is practically never used directly for the restoration of speech function, although there are authors who consider it appropriate. This approach is of principal importance and represents a new, independent branch of rehabilitation for aphasics. The collective work stimulates communication and enables people to realize one of the most important principles of rehabilitation, the principle of working with intact sense organs. Besides, work provides a generally enlivening stimulant (Kosheleva 1985). These branches of speech therapy are used both for individual and group therapy. The experience of group treatment confirms the importance of this kind of rehabilitation, which both teaches and provides social rehabilitation of patients.

As has been already mentioned, the modern concept of rehabilitation presupposes the integrative, systematic approach to the person, "the complete understanding of a sick person, his relation to the environment, to restoration of his personal and social status" (Kabanov 1978). Since we view aphasia not as a separate speech disturbance, but as a cause of desintegration of the whole psychological sphere, the aim of restoration treatment and the neuropsychological side of rehabilitation is not only the restoration of speech, but also the restoration of the personal qualities of the patient. It is necessary to define the interrelation between the neurological and the somatic states of the person on the one hand and the disturbances of the psychological functions on the other. Strengthening the individual's personality is necessary, as well as social and psychological adaptation of the person, which includes involving a person in communication activity of different kinds.

We study the methods of social and psychological rehabilitation in the following ways: (a) the study of personality change among aphasics; (b) the study of the subjective representation of the illness; and (c) the study of the character of the disturbed family relations and the influence of the illness on the family status in general, resulting in the adequate choice of family psychotherapy. Each of the above-mentioned points has its own scientific and practical importance and is closely connected with the others.

The results of diagnostic analysis on symptom production, the subjective representation of the illness, the patient's understanding of his illness, the motivation, and the spared sensory capacities form the basis of the psychological rehabilitation.

The significance of psychotherapy for victims of stroke or neurotrauma has not been fully researched. There is some work in this field (e.g., Sarno 1979), in which the relatives of an afflicted person are told about the illness and its consequences and also advised on how to treat the patient. Experience shows that psychotherapy is most important for this population. The reaction to the defect and also to the altered conditions may be very strong (especially among young people); it may even involve suicide attempts. In such cases, the psychiatrist's help is necessary, which can include both psychopharmacological treatment and/or special psychotherapy. Moreover, people with aphasia not only have disordered speech, but also disordered perception of verbal communication. Thus, immense difficulties arise in using the traditional forms of psychotherapy, in which speech provides the main source of psychological impact. This makes it necessary to look for further social methods of psychotherapy.

People with speech pathology of functional origin, primarily stuttering, also need complex medical and pedagogical treatment, which should include speech therapy, pharmacological treatment, psychotherapy, rhythmics, etc. None of these branches has been fully developed yet. This can be explained by: (a) the immense theoretical complexity of stuttering, in which the biological, psychological, and social aspects are closely interrelated; (b) the fact that new information on normal communication is not being fully integrated, i.e., concepts from theories of communication, results of research on individual or interpersonal psychology or the role of extralinguistic, paralinguistic and other factors for speech, and also results from lateralization studies; or (b) practical difficulties concerned with the absence of specialized clinics for stammerers.

Today the goal of perfecting every sphere of the complex therapy of stuttering is very important, but some of the spheres appear more urgent because solutions have already been found. One of these goals is the study and treatment of stuttering by means of group psychotherapy. In the last decades, there has been an increase in the interest in group psychotherapy in medicine and psychology, which has resulted in a series of publications (Petrovsky 1978; Shklovsky 1979; Shklovsky et al. 1988; Karvasarsky 1984, 1989; Kratochvil 1978), and also the use of psychotherapy in different fields of medical care.

Recently, the theoretical methods of the individual-based group psychotherapy of stutterers have been studied more extensively. One of the main tasks is the definition of the stammering group character and the corresponding form of treatment. Since stutterers not only have disturbed interpersonal relations, but also a disturbed communication, the group needs intense interrelations which would enable the communicative behavior to be analysed at the level of its separate parts. The improvement and development of nonverbal components of communication plays an important role in this type of group psychotherapy. It is important to note that the group psychotherapy study for this population is of theoretical interest as well, because it offers the opportunity to directly study different levels of disturbed communication in the process of communication among the patients. That is why group psychotherapy for stutterers may be viewed as a natural experiment in the field of communicative psychology.

Personality-oriented group psychotherapy is an important part of the complex medical and pedagogical system of treatment for stuttering, and it is naturally linked with its other components, which are also being developed and perfected. The complex diagnostic study of a patient, establishment of different individual treatment regimens, and the development of methods of speech therapy are aimed at increasing therapeutic efficacy. The study of communication, self-consciousness, and attitudes toward people who stutter presents a prominent way to understand the nature of this speech disturbance.

## References

Basso A, Capitani E, Vignolo L (1979) Influence of rehabilitation language skills in aphasic patients. Arch Neurol 36:190–196

Beck M (1983) Medizinische und berufliche Rehabilitation im Spannungsfeld zwischen Leistungsgesellschaft und Wirtschaftskrise. In: Leistungsdiagnostik und Rehabilitation von organischen Hirnschädigungsfolgen. Karlsruhe, pp 15–19

Bein ES (1964) Aphasia i puti ejo preodolenija (Aphasia and its treatment). Medgiz, Moscow

Bein ES (1970) Klinika ilechenije aphasij (Clinics and treatment of aphasia). Meditsina i Fizkultura, Sophia

Bloodstein O (1987) A handbook of stuttering. Easter Seals

Busch G (1983) Neuroradiologische Diagnostik organischer Hirnschädigungsfolgen in der Rehabilitationsphase. In: Leistungsdiagnostik und Rehabilitation von organischen Hirnschädigungsfolgen. Karlsruhe, pp 49–68

Gianotti G, Lemmo M (1983) Comprehension of symbolic gestures in aphasia clinic. In: Nervous and mental diseases. Rome

Kabanov MM (1978) Reabilitacija psikhicheski bolnykh (Rehabilitation of mentally ill). Meditsina, Leningrad

Karvasarsky BD (1984) Meditsinskaja psikhologija (Medical psychology). Meditsina, Leningrad

Karvasarsky BD (ed) (1989) Gruppevaja psikhoterapija (Group psychotherapy). Meditsina, Leningrad

Kogan VM (1962) Vosstanovlenije rechi parli insulta (Rehabilitation of speech after an attack). Meditsina, Moscow

Kosheleva NV (1985) Stimulating the capacity for speech by processes of practical-objective activities (in Russian). In: Kovaljov VV (ed) Patologija rechi organicheskogo i funktsionalnogo geneza. Collection of papers of the Moscow Institute of Psychiatry, Moscow, pp 100–106

Kratochvil S (1966) Skupinova psychotherapie neuroz. Prague

Luria AR (1947) Trouwaticheskaja aphasia (Traumatical aphasia). Academy of Medical Sciences, Moscow

Luria AR (1948) Vosstanovlenije funktsij mozga posle vojennoj trawny (Rehabilitation of brain function after war injuries). Academy of Medical Sciences, Moscow

Petrovsky AV (1978) Istorija sovetskoj psikhologii (History of psychology in the Soviet Union). Moscow

Poeck K (1982) Modern methods of phasia therapy. 7th Annual Meeting of the CVD-Society, Hirosaki

Sarno MT (1979) Rehabilitation of the client with communicational impairment.

Schindler O (1984) Immediate logopedical treatment global acute rehabilitation system. 1st International Aphasia Rehabilitation Congress, Cracow

Schmieder F (1983) Was macht die Rehabilitation von Hirngeschädigten so schwierig? In: Leistungsdiagnostik und Rehabilitation von organischen Hirnschädigungsfolgen. Karlsruhe, pp 30–33

Shkovsky VM (1979) Psychotherapy in the complex system of stutter therapy (in Russian). In: Rozhnov VE (ed) Rukovodstwo po psykhoterapii. Meditsin Uzb. SSR, Tashkent, pp 400–420

Shklovsky VM (1985) Stutter. Several theoretical and clinical problems (in Russian). In: Kovaljev VV (ed) Patologija rechi organichoskogoi funktsionalnogo geneza. Collection of papers of the Moscow Institute of Psychiatry, Moscow, pp 12–21

Shklovsky VM, Vizel TG, Borovenko TG (1982) Possible applications of nonverbal symbolic communication standards in aphasia patients (in Russian). Defectologija 2:3–10

Shklovsky VM, Kroll LM, Mikhajlova EL (1988) The psychotherapy of stuttering: on the model of stuttering patients' group. Sov J Psychiatry Psychol Today 1(1):130–142

Silverman F (1980) Communication of the speechless. New York

# Therapy of Aphasia – Comparison of Various Approaches

*W. Huber**

## Introduction

Aphasia therapy is an ambiguous term, meaning either "therapy of aphasia" or "therapy of the aphasic patient". Of course, the two aspects cannot and should not be separated in clinical practice. First of all, there is always the individual person with her or his specific history of illness and handicap. Patients differ greatly in how they deal with their being aphasic, which, in most cases, has changed their lives drastically. The degree to which a new personal perspective can be built up and social integration be achieved depends on numerous factors, such as etiology and prognosis of the basic illness, premorbid personality, family support, friends and self-help groups, social status and profession, financial resources, etc.

The degree and kind of language impairment itself may also have an impact. However, the possible relationships between the patient's aphasia and his or her way of psychosocial adaptation and reintegration are largely unknown. In several studies, interviews of patients and their relatives were undertaken (e.g., Kinsella and Duffy 1979; Joussen and Pascher 1984; Herrmann and Wallesch 1989). The findings are inconsistent, and there were several methodological shortcomings.

Regarding emotional changes due to aphasia, one particularly simplistic claim was that patients with nonfluent language output are depressive as opposed to fluent aphasics being euphoric (Bay 1962). This claim was refuted by several authors, but nevertheless led to a still ongoing debate on possible causes for emotional changes in aphasic patients (cf. Poeck 1972; Gainotti 1972; Benson 1973; Robinson and Benson 1981).

Given no clear correspondence between patient's psychological conditions and their aphasic behavior, it remains unclear whether and to what extent aphasic patients may improve their specific language problems when they are generally encouraged by councelling or referred to general behavior therapy or

* This paper is dedicated to Professor Klaus Poeck on the occasion of his 65th birthday. I would like to thank him, Luise Springer and Klaus Willmes for many discussions on the topic of this paper. Several of the studies reviewed have been supported by the Deutsche Forschungsgemeinschaft.

psychotherapy (cf. Währborg and Borenstein 1989, and the succeeding discussion).

Theoretically, any approach to aphasia therapy that relies primarily on general encouragement and behavioral modification is in conflict with the classical neuropsychological view, according to which language is a highly specialized capacity of the human brain localized in the perisylvian area of the left hemisphere. Brain damage in this area leads to temporary or permanent loss of language functions, which either have to be reactivated or relearned (cf. e.g., Geschwind 1974). This does not occur automatically, but must be supported by aphasia therapy, which specifically aims at the linguistic impairment of the patient. According to this view, a general behavioral approach to the therapy of aphasic patients is useful but not sufficient for the remediation of the linguistic deficits themselves.

Since the Second World War, the field of aphasia therapy (in the strict neuropsychological sense) has developed rapidly, resulting in a variety of theories and methods, which, when taken together, make rather conflicting assumptions on the nature of aphasia and its consequence for therapy planning (cf. Chapey 1986b; Code and Müller 1989). In the 1950s and 1960s, theoretical work was mainly concerned with global goals and methodology (cf. Schuell et al. 1955; Wepman 1953). Activation of any verbal behavior was thought to be essential. The standard procedure was auditory stimulation. Given enough motivation of the individual patient, this would suffice to reactivate impaired language functions. Overall severity and time post onset were seen as important intervening factors. But neither a specific pattern of aphasic symptoms nor the possible underlying mechanisms in terms of linguistic structures, processing routines or strategies were systematically considered for therapy planning.

An outstanding exception is Luria's approach, which anticipated many later developments in cognitive neuropsychology. However, in Luria's view, too, facilitation and reactivation were the main goals for language rehabilitation. He postulated that multiple facilitation will eventually result in a functional reorganization of the impaired language system (cf. Luria et al. 1969).

Under the influence of behavioristic learning theory, the stimulation approach gradually changed into a methodological framework for behavior modification in aphasic patients. This is usually referred to as the programmed instruction approach (e.g., Holland 1970; cf. also the review by Seron 1987). Several standards were set for therapy procedures. Each therapy program should contain defined success criteria, which must be related to the baseline performance of the patient. The course of therapy has to be planned and conducted in small steps. For each step, intervention techniques are specified as well as mastery criteria for the patient's performance. Furthermore, a hierarchy of difficulties is introduced, which is defined for task demands and/or training material.

It was not before the 1970s that specific linguistic contents and communicative goals became important for therapy planning. This went hand in hand with the neoclassical revival of syndromes and symptoms.

## Syndrome Approach

In present clinical practice, therapy planning commonly starts from the aphasia syndrome given in an individual patient (Albert et al. 1981; La Pointe 1990; Springer 1986). There are two main reasons for doing that, one practical and one theoretical. First, syndromes are widely used as abbreviations for general performance characteristics to be expected in an individual patient. Second, syndromes stand for combination of symptoms that may have common underlying pathological mechanisms at which therapy should aim.

Syndrome classification requires systematic clinical observation of the patient's verbal behavior across several linguistic modalities and with respect to units and regularities in different linguistic levels of description (phonology, lexicon, morphology, syntax). Aphasic disturbances are associative and systematic in nature (Huber et al. 1989). They are multimodal. In general more than one linguistic modality is affected, namely oral production *and* comprehension, reading *and* writing. They are also supramodal in the sense that the same type of systematic failure may occur across several tasks (modalities), e.g., confusion of phonemes or of word meanings, inability to process low-frequency words, grammatical morphemes, complex sentence structures, etc.

Aphasic syndromes are described as characteristic combinations of symptoms. By symptoms, either quantifications of level of performance are meant, such as poor or good comprehension, or qualifications of erroneous utterances in production, such as recurring utterances, automatized elements, stereotypes, word-finding difficulties, semantic or phonemic paraphasias, neologisms, agrammatism, paragrammatism, etc. It is true that clinical practice is often vague in clustering symptoms into syndromes, which leads to considerable overlap between syndromes (Caramazza 1984; Schwartz 1984). Such "polytypical" syndromes cannot be unambiguously delineated from one another. In such a situation, it would be worthless and only time consuming to base initial therapy planning on syndromes. It would be much more informative to take the individual symptom as a starting point. The probability of symptoms to cluster together could be disregarded if syndromes were truly polytypical.

However, there are two arguments against this criticism of the clinical syndrome approach:

1. Syndromes can be classified by means of psychometric methods (Huber et al. 1984).
2. Syndromes can be described as prototypical rather than polytypical (Poeck 1983). Many clinical researchers agree that each of the four standard syndromes exhibits one or two cardinal symptoms that are typically observed in spontaneous language production. These cardinal symptoms are:
   - Automatized repetitive elements (recurring utterances, stereotypical words and phrases) in global aphasia
   - Paraphasias and paragrammatism in Wernicke's aphasia
   - Agrammatism with or without apraxia of speech in Broca's aphasia
   - Word-finding difficulties in amnesic (or anomic) aphasia.

These symptoms reflect specific disturbances either in access to or knowledge of phonological, lexical and syntactic units/regularities of the language system.

For initial therapy planning, the syndrome approach is indispensable. It identifies cardinal symptomes and modality-specific characteristics. With a valid, reliable and fully standardized test instrument at hand, the performance profile of an individual patient will allow conclusions on the severity and heterogeneity of impairments to be expected during early treatment, as well as the identification of outstanding language symptoms (cf. Willmes 1990). Thus, the syndrome approach enables satisfactory pretreatment evaluation. However, for planning the specific therapy contents, standard aphasia examinations are very often too gross. More specific supplementary examinations are required to determine the pathological mechanisms underlying the various symptoms and performance patterns across modalities (Poeck and Göddenhenrich 1988). Ultimately, therapeutic intervention has to aim at the underlying mechanism and not at superficial symptoms and/or performance profiles.

## Language-Oriented Approaches

Under this heading, several approaches are addressed which all start from descriptions and theories of normal language processing. This provides a framework in which aphasic symptoms and syndromes can be specified and consequences for therapeutic interventions can be formulated.

### Structure

Beginning in the late 1960s, research on aphasia increasingly made use of methods taken from descriptive linguistics, and aphasic symptoms were interpreted in terms of grammatical theories (e.g., Goodglass 1968). Studies of linguistic behavior in aphasia were conducted to determine which linguistic structures were affected and which preserved. Based on clinical and experimental findings, hierarchies of inherent linguistic difficulties were proposed.

This structural approach soon influenced principles and methods of aphasia therapy, especially in Europe (cf. Howard and Hatfield 1987; Peuser 1979). Aphasia therapists developed training materials that bore resemblence to grammatical exercises used in textbooks for second-language learning (e.g., Engl et al. 1982). Some authors call this approach didactic. And, indeed, the patient is typically presented with training material that exemplifies basic units and regularities of each component of the language system. Examples are phonemes and syllables with articulatory contrasts, words with minimal phonemic contrast, with classificatory- versus associative-meaning relations, or sentences with specific grammatical contrasts, such as intransitive vs transitive, active vs passive, coordination vs subordination, etc.

Simultaneously, metalinguistic tasks began to be used widely in aphasia therapy (cf. Springer and Weniger 1980), such as phonologic and orthographic spelling, sorting words to a given semantic criterion, rearrangement of word or sentence anagrams, sentence completion from multiple-choice sets of content or function words, etc. These tasks require the patients to make conscious decisions on phonemic and graphemic, lexical and grammatical structure, thereby activating what is left of their linguistic knowledge. Stimuli are often presented in several modalities simultaneously, mostly as pictures together with written and/or spoken words or phrases. Besides a target item, there are several distractors with varying degrees of linguistic similarity to the target. When the patient fails, systematic cues are given by the therapist contrasting stepwise correct and incorrect possibilities for finding a resolution to the linguistic problem given.

The therapeutic goal is to make the patient indirectly (without telling him) aware of linguistic units and regularities that are specifically lost in the patient or are available for one item but not for the next. By doing so, one hopes to induce relearning processes in the patient (cf. Poeck et al. 1977; Kotten 1981). These techniques are mainly based on exemplary selection of linguistic problems and material to be practiced. If necessary, they are supplemented by telling the patient explicit grammatical rules. For stabilizing the performance, most patients have to be asked to perform the same or similar items over and over again (so-called pattern drill).

The efficacy of the linguistic-structure approach to aphasia therapy was demonstrated in numerous single-case studies (cf. reviews in Howard and Hatfield 1987; Lang and von Stockert 1986). There is also evidence that specific linguistic training can be expected to be superior to general communicative stimulation (Wiegel-Crump and Koenigsknecht 1973). Weniger et al. (1980) pointed out that for the structure approach to be efficacious, it has to be demonstrated that there is not only a trivial training effect but also (a) stabilization, i.e., improved performance after a period of no therapy, and (b) generalization, i.e., transfer of improvement to nontrained problems and material of similar linguistic structures.

These strict methodological requirements were fully met in only a few studies reporting favorable results. In present therapy research, the methodology of the linguistic-structure approach together with principles of programmed instructions is used for the development of computer-assisted therapy of aphasia (cf. Katz 1986; Stachowiak 1987).

## Modality

As an alternative to focusing on linguistic structures, therapy may primarily aim at activating linguistic modalities. Even if aphasic disturbances are multimodal in nature, the severity of impairment usually differs from one modality to another. In therapy, one tries to make systematic use of these differences.

Linguistic modalities can be analyzed into input and output components, each of which has modality-specific codes for processing linguistic information. There are two primary ones, the accoustic-phonetic and the articulatory code and two secondary ones, the visual-orthographic and the graphomotor code.

The modality approach to therapy presupposes a detailed analysis of task demands in terms of output and input as well as central processing components. Depending on how many and which components are involved, tasks can be ranked according to their inherent difficulties. The more and the deeper the central processing that has to take place is, the more difficult the task for aphasic patients becomes. Shewan and Bandur (1986) developed a therapy program in which task hierarchies are introduced separately for several input and output modalities, namely for auditory, visual, gestural, oral and graphic processing.

It should be clear that, for each aphasic syndrome and possibly even for each individual patient, significant deviations from the general hierarchy of inherent task difficulties may be expected. Some task components can be more impaired than others. Some input or output routes may even appear to be blocked. Weigl (1961) suggested systematic deblocking as a therapy method. When a patient performs very badly on one particular task, the therapist tries to find related tasks in which the patient performs substantially better. The therapist then arranges the tasks into a deblocking chain with the relatively preserved tasks preceding the impaired one. This leads to facilitation, i.e., the patient now performs well on what he could not do before.

For example, there are aphasic patients who are unable to name objects. However, naming becomes possible after the patient has successfully activated the target name in some other task, such as reading the written name or comprehending the spoken name by pointing to the corresponding object. But how does the therapist exclude that the deblocking effect is not brought about by mere retention and verbal imitation? Deblocking effects can also be obtained when the training includes not just one, but several words from the same semantic field with randomized order from task to task. Facilitation is, however, less likely to occur when semantically unrelated words are used (Springer 1979; Weigl 1979). Parallel similarity effects were reported for deblocking syntactic and morphological structures (Weigl and Bierwisch 1970). From the perspective of modern cognitive neurolinguistics, it appears that these effects are based on preactivation of units/regularities of central processing components rather than on "deblocking" of impaired output or input routes.

## Strategy

The strategy approach offers an alternative to conscious structural relearning in aphasia. Instead of setting the goal in terms of linguistic units and regularities that are lost or only inconsistently available, the therapist tries to optimize those linguistic processing routines of which the patient still is capable (cf.

Seron 1982). In other words, the positive rather than the negative aspects of the aphasic symptoms are taken as a starting point.

The difference between the structure and the strategy approach can perhaps be best illustrated with respect to agrammatism (cf. Kearns 1990). Under the structure approach, the patient is instructed stepwise to practice morpho-syntactic units and regularities of increasing inherent difficulties (e.g., Helm-Estabrooks and Ramsberger 1986). Under the strategy approach, the therapist assumes that even in severe agrammatism, basic thematic relations can still be conveyed despite the lack of function words and inflectional endings. The content words used still refer to agents, actions, objects, goals of an action, instruments, locations, etc. Word order still indicates a logical or temporal sequence or a gradation of thematic importance. These positive functions of agrammatism can be systematically enhanced in therapy (cf. Jones 1986; Kearns 1990). The patients are told to ignore their grammatical and syntactic difficulties during sentence planning and to concentrate on a thematically consistent selection of content words. The therapist may introduce a thematic scheme which supports thematic sentence planning. The patient is instructed to consider WHO/IS DOING WHAT/TO WHOM/WHERE/WHEN/WITH/etc. This scheme is stepwise expanded. Only inappropriate selection of content words is corrected by the therapist. Morphological or syntactic errors are ignored.

Another symptom where the strategy approach works quite well is word-finding difficulties. The patient is systematically guided to produce circumlocations that specify the functional and/or situational characteristics of the object or person which cannot be named (Greitemann, personal communication). Several authors have described how they helped patients find strategies for compensating reading and writing disorders (e.g., Beauvois and Derouesné 1982; Hatfield 1989).

## Processing Models

Planning of aphasia therapy often lacks a coherent theoretical framework allowing the therapist to postulate underlying mechanisms of aphasic symptoms and to predict how impaired linguistic functions interconnect with others and whether unimpaired functions can possibly serve as a compensation. Such a framework, when demonstrated to have observational and explanatory adequacy, can guide the therapist to investigate step by step the pattern of impairments of an individual patient during the course of therapy (cf. Lesser 1987; Sasanuma 1986; Kotten 1989).

Since the late 1970s, frameworks of this kind have become increasingly available within the rapidly growing field of cognitive neuropsychology and neurolinguistics. Most processing models available so far specify information flow, i.e., they provide a system of components and routes which linguistic information runs through from input to output and vice versa. It was pointed out several times that these models bear some similarity to the classical diagram-maker's approach (cf. e.g., de Bleser 1987). However, the modern models do not aim at functional anatomy; instead they are designed to specify the functional architecture of language without claiming localization of function.

Most successful was the development of an information-flow model that specifies two processing routes for reading words, one being holistic and one segmental. Originally, this model was called the logogen model (Coltheart et al. 1980; Patterson et al. 1985). Many of its features were justified by observations made during therapy of patients. This is also true for expansions of the model and its application to other task demands, such as writing, repetition and naming.

In many respects, the processing-model approach combines aspects of the other language-oriented approaches. As in the modality approach, dissociations between task performances are of crucial importance. There are always three main possibilities for intervention:

1. Optimizing the preserved route: In deep dyslexia, for example, semantic word confusion may indicate general difficulties in access to word meanings and/or in degraded semantic knowledge. Consequently, the therapist engages the patient in general training of lexical semantics by metalinguistic classification and sorting tasks, naming and description exercises, etc. If the patient improves on these tasks, it can be expected that whole-word reading via the semantic route will improve likewise.
2. Enforcing the impaired route: Naturally, this can only be done by making it harder to process along the better preserved alternative route. For example, a patient with deep dyslexia is forced to read via the surface route when the stimuli are non-words. The therapist must then systematically try to build up skills for grapheme-to-phoneme conversions, e.g., by introducing spelling strategies, by making the patient aware of phonotactic analogies between non-words and real words, etc.
3. Provoking compensatory strategies: Very often the patients come up with them spontaneously. For example, a patient with surface dyslexia found out that he was able to make lexical decisions after he laboriously sounded out each string of letters (Klingenberg 1990). He spoke aloud the obtained sound pattern several times to himself with increasing speed. Thereby, via the acoustic-phonetic route, he was able to activate his knowledge of phonological word forms and discriminated correctly between words and non-words. Of course, his decisions were considerably delayed.

Processing routes start and end at components in which linguistic knowledge is stored. In an explicit model, these components have to be specified in terms of entries and principles of organization. Two main types of aphasic impairments can be expected: Either stored linguistic knowledge is degraded or the access to the knowledge is impaired. Shallice (1988) suggested distinguishing these disorders in the following way:

1. Knowledge deficits are more likely to result in consistent error patterns over testing and therapy sessions, i.e., the same or similar items are affected in the same or in similar ways. In contrast, fluctuation of errors across items and sessions is typical for access disorders.

2. Access disorders often have surprisingly little impact on metalinguistic operations, such as grammatical judgements, lexical categorization and semantic specification. In knowledge disorders, these operations are outstandingly difficult to perform.
3. Priming of targets by structurally or semantically similar items works better for access than knowledge disorders. Many logopedic cuing techniques make systematic use of similarity relations between stored units. If the knowledge is degraded, these cuing techniques are of little help.
4. Access disorders are sensitive to frequency and familiarity of stored units, whereas knowledge disorders vary as a function of the linguistic complexity of the items to be processed.
5. Time intervals between training may improve the performance of patients with access disorders, but not with knowledge disorders.

This list of expectations provides the therapist with criteria for differential diagnosis and points out possible interventions and stimulation techniques (cf. e.g., Howard et al. 1985).

## Working Memory

So far, I have discussed processing components that are taken to provide automatic activation of stored units, i.e., the retrieved information becomes immediately integrated into formulation or comprehension. However, there are also components that function as a working space for controlled processing (cf. Shallice 1988). Activated units have to be assembled and compared with alternative units, and a decision has to be made to select those units that best fulfill the given goal or purpose of the task. Processing components of this kind do not function as long-term stores, and, therefore, are neither vulnerable to access nor to knowledge deficits. However, the processing capacity of these control components may be limited either by reduced memory span or by deficits of attention and/or problem solving. As these deficits are frequently associated with aphasia (cf. von Cramon and Zihl 1988; Poeck 1989), limited capacity for controlled linguistic processing must be expected.

There are two areas where limitations in processing capacity become immediately relevant for therapy planning: selection of tasks and improvement of the patients' capacities to monitor and self-correct linguistic errors. Especially under the language structure approach to therapy, metalinguistic tasks are frequently used, many of which require controlled linguistic processing. Failure in these tasks does not necessarily reflect primary deficits of access or knowledge. When the therapist reduces the nonlinguistic demands, the patients will more often come up with appropriate responses than when specific linguistic cues or contrasts are provided. There may also be trade-off effects, depending on task demands. For example, dysgrammatic patients may be able to handle morphological structures quite well as long as they practice isolated sentences. However, when processing of texts is required, their previous difficulties show up again.

Findings of this kind are not fully understood (cf. the discussion of related issues in Kolk 1987; Huber et al. 1988). One possibility is that multiple activation of automatic processing components, such as semantics, syntax, morphology, and lexicon, is limited. When it is required, as in text processing, the central executive system of the whole processing apparatus may give priority to the most needed one, e.g., to processing the semantics of words and phrases at the cost of syntax and morphology. Another possibility is that the temporal aspects of the originally impaired processing component are still more affected than those of unimpaired components. For example, in dysgrammatic patients, it might take much longer to process morphology than lexical semantics. Given the overall time constraints of the text-processing task, it would take too long for morphology, and, therefore, morphological processing is neglected. Finally, as a third possibility, one may hypothesize that the originally impaired capacity was not restored as a set of automatic language functions, but was relearned as a consciously controlled mode of processing. Consequently, the patient fails whenever the overall processing load is increased.

It is not clear how these possibilities of limited working-memory capacity can be dealt with in language therapy (cf. Chapey 1986a). Simply increasing the task demands step by step may be too unspecific, especially when the underlying disorder is a pathological delay with respect to one particular component. Similarly, general neuropsychological training of attention, psychomotor speed and problem solving may be of little help if the impairment is restricted to components of the language system.

As a rule, aphasic patients monitor failure of access better than overt errors. Prepairs are most frequent than repairs (Schlenck et al. 1987). An obvious consequence for therapy is focusing on treatment of comprehension. But success may be limited, even when comprehension itself improves substantially. The reason again is a limitation in working-memory capacity, which makes it difficult for the patient to plan and execute the language output and, at the same time, to monitor for possible errors.

## Natural Course of Aphasia

From a neurophysiological point of view, there are three basic mechanisms of functional recovery in the brain: restitution, substitution and compensation (Singer 1982). Each one appears to correlate in different ways with changes in linguistic behavior at different time periods post onset (cf. Rothi and Horner 1983). Consequently, principles and methods of aphasia therapy vary depending on the phase of recovery the patient is in. In our clinical regimen, we distinguish three phases of aphasia therapy: activation, symptom-specific training and consolidation (Springer and Weniger 1980; Huber et al. 1991).

Restitution of impaired language functions occurs typically during the first 4 weeks and leads to full recovery in about a third of the patients. These are patients in whom the lesion affects regions of the brain in the neighborhood of the perisylvian language areas. Transitory aphasia arises due to edema or bleeding into brain tissues of the language areas. While resorption takes place, the impaired language functions normalize. Initially, it is language comprehension which improves rapidly. Expressive language changes more gradually from mutism to short passages of paraphasic and jargon-like speech with long interruptions characterized by strained and often unsuccessful attempts to formulate the intended message. From day to day, the language output becomes more fluent, with word-finding difficulties remaining as a residual symptom. The goal of aphasia therapy in these patients is to enhance the evolution of temporarily impaired language functions. The classical stimulation approach as well as modality-oriented facilitation techniques seem to be best suited. In some patients with severely reduced speech output, melodic-intonation therapy works surprisingly well (Sparks et al. 1974).

Stimulation is not the only therapeutic method during the acute phase. In patients with evolving global or severe Wernicke's aphasia, the therapist attempts to block automatisms, perseverations, jargon and logorrhoic speech from the very beginning. The overall therapeutic goal during the acute phase is to activate the patient by all available means to respond communicatively as appropriately as possible.

The next phase of aphasia therapy starts when stable physical conditions have been attained and when an extensive clinical examination of the aphasic syndrome is possible. Now symptom-specific training is provided, aiming primarily at relearning of degraded linguistic knowledge, at reactivation of impaired linguistic modalities, and at learning of compensatory linguistic strategies. In other words, methods of the language-oriented approaches are applied.

During the phase of linguistic relearning, a gradual functional reorganization of the impaired language system is assumed (cf. Luria et al. 1969). This may be brought about by both substitution and compensation of impaired brain functions. It is not clear to what extent functional reorganization presupposes some intact language functions of the left dominant hemisphere and/or carry over to right-hemispheric functions (cf. e.g., Moore 1989).

Conscious linguistic relearning during aphasia therapy is not an absolute prerequisite for language improvement. Up to 12 months post onset, there is also spontaneous recovery (Kertesz 1984; Reinvang 1984), i.e., the severity of the aphasic disturbances decreases even if there is no professional language therapy. Of course, there is always some amount of communicative stimulation by families, friends, physical therapists, etc. In a follow-up study, Willmes and Poeck (1984) examined 96 patients who did not receive professional therapy between 1 and 7 months post onset. Nineteen percent were fully recovered at 4 months, and another 8% at 7 months post onset. Not only did the number of patients decrease during the course of recovery, but also the amount of improvement among those patients who did not reach full spontaneous recovery. From these figures, it can be concluded that restitution of function may continuously play a role during the early phase of recovery up to 4 months post onset. Later on, unspecific stimulation in everyday situations may suffice to induce some reactivation and/or relearning in aphasic patients.

The consequences for professional therapy are clear. Any demonstration of treatment success has to be corrected by the amount of improvement that can be expected from spontaneous recovery alone. Poeck et al. (1989) were able to meet this strict methodological requirement and still reported favorable outcome of language-oriented therapy. Treatment was intensively provided for 7 weeks with nine full-hour sessions per week.

The phase of symptom-specific training is continued as long as comparisons of post- and pretreatment testing demonstrate substantial improvement. In many patients, treatment can be extended well into the chronic course of recovery beyond 12 months post onset until a learning plateau is reached (cf. also Hanson et al. 1989).

The symptom-specific training must be complemented by a phase of consolidation. Consolidation aims at enhancing the transfer of practiced linguistic skills to everyday communicative situations (cf. Davis 1986; Prutting 1982). Standard techniques are linguistic role playing (Schlanger and Schlanger 1970; De Bleser and Weismann 1981) and PACE-therapy (Davis and Wilcox 1985). Present therapy research is intended to specify contents, scope and efficacy of these pragmatic approaches to aphasia therapy (cf. e.g., Glindemann and Springer 1989; Springer et al. 1991).

Of course, each phase of aphasia therapy has to be accompanied by family councelling and psychosocial support of the patient. As stated at the beginning of this review, the clinical regimen should always comprise both, therapy of aphasia and therapy of the aphasic patient.

## References


Albert ML, Goodglass H, Helm NA, Rubens AB, Alexander MP (1981) Clinical aspects of dysphasia. Springer, Vienna

Bay E (1962) Aphasia and non-verbal disorders of language. Brain 85:411–426

Beauvois MF, Derouesné J (1982) Recherche en neuropsychologie cognitive et rééducation: quels rapports? In: Seron X, Laterre C (eds) Rééduquer le cerveau. Logopédie, psychologie, neurologie. Mardaga, Bruxelles

Benson FD (1973) Psychiatric aspects of aphasia. Br J Psychiatry 123:555–566

Caramazza A (1984) The logic of neuropsychological research and the problem of patient classification in aphasia. Brain Lang 21:9–20

Chapey R (1986a) Cognitive intervention: stimulation of cognition, memory, convergent thinking, devergent thinking and evaluative thinking. In: Chapey R (ed) Language intervention strategies in adult aphasia, 2nd edn. Williams and Wilkins, Baltimore

Chapey R (ed) (1986b) Language intervention strategies in adult aphasia, 2nd edn. Williams and Wilkins, Baltimore

Code C, Müller DJ (eds) (1989) Aphasia therapy. Studies in disorders of communication, 2nd edn. Whurr, London

Coltheart M, Patterson JC, Marshall RC (eds) (1980) Deep dyslexia. Routledge and Kegan Paul, London

Davis GA (1986) Pragmatics and treatment. In: Chapey R (ed) Language intervention strategies in adult aphasia, 2nd edn. Williams and Wilkins, Baltimore

Davis GA, Wilcox MJ (1985) Adult aphasia rehabilitation: applied pragmatics. College-Hill, San Diego

De Bleser R (1987) From agrammatism to paragrammatism. German aphasiological traditions and grammatical disturbances. Cogn Neuropsychol 4:187–250

De Bleser R, Weismann H (1981) Übergang von Strukturübungen zum spontanen Dialog in der Therapie von Aphasikern mit nichtflüssiger Sprachproduktion. Sprache Stimme Gehör 5:74–79

Engl E, Kotten A, Ohlendorf I, Poser E (1982) Sprachübungen zur Aphasiebehandlung: Ein linguistisches Übungsprogramm mit Bildern. Marhold, Berlin

Gainotti G (1972) Emotional behavior and hemispheric side of lesion. Cortex 8:41–55

Geschwind N (1974) Late changes in the nervous system: an overview. In: Stein DG, Rosen J, Butters N (eds) Plasticity and recovery of function in the central nervous system. Academic, New York

Glindemann R, Springer L (1989) PACE-Therapie und sprachsystematische Übungen – Ein integrativer Vorschlag zur Aphasietherapie. Sprache Stimme Gehör 13:188–192

Goodglass H (1968) Studies on the grammar of aphasics. In: Rosenberg S, Koplin J (eds) Developments in applied psycholinguistic research. Macmillan, New York

Hanson WR, Metter EJ, Riege WH (1989) The course of chronic aphasia. Aphasiology 3:19–29

Hatfield F (1989) Aspects of acquired dysgraphia and implications for reeducation. In: Code C, Müller DJ (eds) Aphasia therapy. Studies in disorders of communication, 2nd edn. Whurr, London

Helm-Estabrooks N, Ramsberger G (1986) Treatment of agrammatism in long-term Broca's aphasia. Br J Dis Commun 21:39–45

Herrmann M, Wallesch C-W (1989) Psychosocial changes and psychosocial adjustment with chronic and severe nonfluent aphasia. Aphasiology 3:513–526

Holland A (1970) Case studies in aphasia rehabilitation using programmed instruction. J Speech Hear Dis 35:377–390

Howard D, Patterson K, Franklin S, Orchard-Lisle V, Morton J (1985) Treatment of word retrieval deficits in aphasia. Brain 108:817–829

Howard D, Hatfield FM (1987) Aphasia therapy: historical and contemporary issues. Erlbaum, Hove

Huber W, Poeck K, Willmes K (1984) The Aachen Aphasia Test. In: Rose FC (ed) Progress in aphasiology. Raven, New York

Huber W, Lüer G, Lass U (1988) Eye movement behavior in aphasia. In: Johnston CW, Pirozzolo FJ (eds) Neuropsychology of eye movements. Erlbaum, New York

Huber W, Poeck K, Weniger D (1989) Aphasie. In: Poeck K (ed) Klinische Neuropsychologie, 2nd edn. Thieme, Stuttgart

Huber W, Poeck K, Springer L (1991) Sprachstörungen. Trias, Stuttgart

Jones EV (1986) Building the foundations for sentence production in a non-fluent aphasic. Br J Dis Commun 21:63–82

Joussen K, Pascher W (1984) Empirische Untersuchungen der sozialen Situation von Aphasikern. Folia Phoniatr, Basel 36:66–73

Katz RC (1986) Aphasia treatment and microcomputers. Taylor and Francis, London

Kearns KP (1990) Broca's aphasia. In: La Pointe LL (ed) Aphasia and related neurogenic language disorders. Thieme, Stuttgart

Kertesz A (1984) Recovery from aphasia. In: Rose FC (ed) Progress in aphasiology. Raven, New York

Kinsella G, Duffy FD (1979) Psychosocial readjustment in the response of aphasic patients. Scand J Rehabil Med 11:129–132

Klingenberg G (1990) Zur Erfassung von Oberflächendyslexie mit Hilfe des AAT-Supplements 'Dyslexie'. In: Mellies R, Ostermann F, Winnecken A (eds) Beiträge zur interdisziplinären Aphasieforschung. Narr, Tübingen

Kolk HHJ (1987) A theory of grammatical impairment in aphasia. In: Kempen G (ed) Natural language generation: new results in artificial intelligence, psychology and linguistics. Nijhoff, Dordrecht

Kotten A (1981) Aphasietherapie: Linguistisch gesteuerter Wiedererwerb der Muttersprache. In: Peuser G (ed) Methoden der angewandten Sprachwissenschaft. Bouvier, Bonn

Kotten A (1989) Evaluation von Aphasietherapie. Neurolinguistik 3:83–106

Lang C, von Stockert TR (1986) Zum gegenwärtigen Stand der Aphasietherapie. Fortschr Neurol Psychiatr 54:119–137

La Pointe LL (ed) (1990) Aphasia and related neurogenic language disorders. Thieme, Stuttgart

Lesser R (1987) Cognitive neuropsychological influences on aphasia therapy. Aphasiology 1:189–200

Luria AR, Naydin VL, Testvetkova LS, Vinarskaya EN (1969) Restoration of higher cortical function following local brain damage. In: Vinken PJ, Bruyn GW (eds) Handbook of clinical neurology, vol 3. North-Holland, Amsterdam, pp 368–433

Moore WH (1989) Language recovery in aphasia: a right hemisphere perspective. Aphasiology 3:101–110

Patterson KE, Marshall JC, Coltheart M (eds) (1985) Surface dyslesia. Erlbaum, London

Peuser G (1979) Studien zur Sprachtherapie. Fink, Munich

Poeck K (1972) Stimmung und Krankheitseinsicht bei Aphasien. Arch Psychiatr Nervenkr 216:246–254

Poeck K (1983) What do we mean by "aphasic syndromes"? A neurologist's view. Brain Lang 20:79–89

Poeck K (ed) (1989) Klinische Neuropsychologie, 2nd edn. Thieme, Stuttgart

Poeck K, Göddenhenrich S (1988) Standardized tests for the detection of dissociation in aphasic language performance. Aphasiology 2:375–380

Poeck K, Huber W, Stachowiak F-J, Weniger D (1977) Therapie der Aphasien. Nervenarzt 48:119–126

Poeck K, Huber W, Willmes K (1989) Outcome of intensive language treatment in aphasia. J Speech Hear Dis 54:471–479

Prutting CA (1982) Pragmatics as social competence. J Speech Hear Dis 47:123–134

Reinvang I (1984) The natural history of aphasia. In: Rose FC (ed) Progress in aphasiology. Raven, New York

Robinson RG, Benson DF (1981) Depression in aphasic patients: frequency, severity and clinical-pathological correlations. Brain Lang 14:610–614

Rothi LJ, Horner J (1983) Restitution and substitution: two theories of recovery with application to neurobehavioral treatment. J Clin Neuropsychol 5:73–81

Sasanuma S (1986) Universal and language-specific symptomatology and treatment of aphasia. Folia Phoniatr (Basel) 38:121–175

Schlanger PH, Schlanger BB (1970) Adapting role-playing activities with aphasic patients. J Speech Hear Dis 35:229–235

Schlenck KJ, Huber W, Willmes K (1987) "Prepairs" and repairs: different monitoring functions in aphasic language production. Brain Lang 30:226–244

Schuell HM, Carrol V, Street BS (1955) Clinical treatment of aphasia. J Speech Hear Dis 20:43–53

Schwartz MF (1984) What the classical aphasia categories can't do for us, and why? Brain Lang 21:3–8

Seron X (1982) Les choix de stratégies: rétablir, réorganiser ou aménager l'environnement? In: Seron X, Laterre C (eds) Rééduquer le cerveau. Logopédie, psychologie, neurologie. Mardaga, Bruxelles

Seron X (1987) Operant procedures and neuropsychological rehabilitation. In: Meier MJ, Benton AL, Diller L (eds) Neuropsychological rehabilitation. Livingstone, Edinburgh

Shallice T (1988) From neuropsychology to mental structure. Cambridge University Press, Cambridge

Shewan CM, Bandur DL (1986) Treatment of aphasia. College-Hill, San Diego

Singer W (1982) Recovery mechanisms in the mammalian brain. In: Nicholls JG (ed) Repair and regeneration of the nervous system. Springer, Berlin Heidelberg New York

Sparks R, Helm N, Albert M (1974) Aphasia rehabilitation resulting from melodic intonation therapy. Cortex 10:303–316

Springer L (1979) Zur Anwendung der Deblockierungsmethode in der Sprachtherapie. In: Peuser G (ed) Studien zur Sprachtherapie. Fink, Munich

Springer L (1986) Behandlungsphasen einer syndromspezifischen Aphasietherapie. Sprache Stimme Gehör 10:22–29

Springer L, Weniger D (1980) Aphasietherapie aus logopädisch-linguistischer Sicht. In: Böhme G (ed) Therapie der Sprach-, Sprech- und Stimmstörungen. Fischer, Stuttgart

Springer L, Glindemann R, Huber W, Willmes K (1991) How efficacious is PACE-therapy when language systematic training is incorporated? Aphasiology 5:391–399

Stachowiak F-J (1987) Computer als Werkzeug der Sprachtherapie. Neurolinguistik 1:57–94

Von Cramon D, Zihl J (eds) (1988) Neuropsychologische Rehabilitation. Grundlagen – Diagnostik – Behandlungsverfahren. Springer, Berlin Heidelberg New York

Währborg P, Borenstein P (1989) Family therapy in families with an aphasic member. Aphasiology 3:93–98

Weigl E (1961) The phenomenon of temporary deblocking in aphasia. Z Phonetik Sprachwiss Kommunikationsforsch 14:337–364

Weigl E, Bierwisch M (1970) Neuropsychology and linguistics: topics of common research. Found Lang 6:1–18

Weigl I (1979) Neuropsychologische und neurolinguistische Grundlagen eines Programms zur Rehabilitation aphasischer Störungen. In: Peuser G (ed) Studien zur Sprachtherapie. Fink, Munich

Weniger D, Huber W, Stachowiak F-J, Poeck K (1980) Treatment of aphasia on a linguistic basis. In: Sarno MT, Höök O (eds) Aphasia. Assessment and treatment. Almqvist and Wiksell, Stockholm

Wepman JM (1953) A conceptual model for the processes involved in recovery from aphasia. J Speech Hear Dis 18:4–13

Wiegel-Crump C, Koenigsknecht R (1973) Tapping the lexical store of the adult aphasic: analysis of the improvement made in word retrieval skills. Cortex 9:411–418

Willmes K (1990) Statistical methods for a single case study approach to aphasia therapy research. Aphasiology 4:415–436

Willmes K, Poeck K (1984) Ergebnisse einer multizentrischen Untersuchung über die Spontansprache von Aphasien vaskulärer Ätiologie. Nervenarzt 55:62–71

# Discussion: Treatment of Specific Deficits

*A. Kertesz*

The task of discussing today's papers is an enjoyable one because of their high quality. Previously it has been suggested that therapists should concentrate on devising new therapies, rather than trying to prove existing ones, mainly because of the lack of available ones that are reliable. It seems to me that the papers we have heard today show that reliable therapies do exist in certain areas but not in others, and that there are also methodologies to evaluate them.

The most difficult areas of rehabilitation it seems, and the least proven methodologically, is the treatment of attention problems and the speed of mental processing, as reviewed so ably by Ed van Zomeren. The levels of attentional mechanisms of the CNS are multiple and complex. Dr. van Zomeren stayed mainly at the clinical level, although he touched upon psychophysiology as well. The usefulness of psychophysiological approaches to rehabilitation may become evident in the future. Event-related potentials (ERP) appear to be useful to monitor attentional or central processing. These techniques show promise to follow spontaneous recovery and to find some theoretical explanation for the physiologial changes that take place. The concepts of focused and divided attention seem to be important and testable. Reaction time paradigms continue to enjoy a degree of popularity in psychological research. Their clinical relevance is yet to be demonstrated convincingly, but they may help to quantitate the slowness to respond and to think. Sensitive tests of processing capacity, such as the "Paced Auditory Serial Addition Test" (PASAT), will detect mild damage but cannot be performed by significantly brain-damaged patients. Similarily, demanding tests excel in sensitivity, they lack in specificity. Dr. van Zomeren recommended the "Digit symbol task", which is a test to measure divided attention and the continuous performance test for sustained attention. Most of these are applicable only to the high level patient and have a certain amount of variance that decrease their discriminative value.

"Supervisory Attentional Control" (SAC) is a difficult concept, somewhat remote from clinical symptoms, although it seems that the "Tower of Hanoi" is being built in London, Munich, Groningen, Toronto, and even in London, Ontario. Puzzles, games, and their computerized versions are endless and there is a good chance that many more will be introduced into neuropsychological testing on the basis of one theoretical explanation or another. Clinicians will be asking which one should we use? This question can be further developed: Which one tells us about brain processing or which one can be a useful marker of deficit or recovery? Which one is going to uncover rehabilitation potential or quantitate a functionally relevant deficit? This areas needs more clinical data. The relative expense of computerized testing confines them to the research domain. Their future utility, quite apart from their theoretical importance, will become evident after a period of clinical research that needs to be supported.

On the more practical side, behaviour therapy and cognitive therapy are in their infancy. Stimulation therapy to achieve improvement of general attentional function seems logical but so far rather non-specific. Efforts to treat hemiattention by moving stimuli in the neglected field are largely uncontrolled. The "Orientation Remedial Module" is more comprehensive, but it was still uncontrolled at the time this was written. The most rigorously controlled studies of computer therapy of head injured patients seem to be negative. Therefore, the continuing enthusiasm for computer training of patients is hardly justifiable.

Therapeutic efforts, that utilize an independent measure to indicate recovery, may actually measure spontaneous recovery rather than generalizations as their promoters (not quite disinterestedly) claim. Anecdotes of verbal mediation of visuospatial problems, such as the report about the radiologist who improved his reading of x-rays after describing movies are entertaining examples of what various investigators in the past called deblocking or facilitation, and what is now renamed as "strategy substitution". Behaviour modification is as old as mankind. The common man on the street calls it bribery. Franz, 70 years ago, described an anecdotal case of an amnesic who could not remember to say the alphabet, but after being offered a carton of cigarettes he learned it faultlessly until the reward was paid.

According to Barbara Wilson, memory rehabilitation is probably a misnomer not so much that memory recovers, but in reality compensatory strategies are learned. These strategies consist mainly of memory aids, such as restructuring the environment, placing reminders of internally stored information, as well as externally recorded information in the shape of labels, sign posts, colour, coding of special places and asking others to remind the patient of appointments, etc.

The description of memory therapy is a mixed affair, but Dr. Wilson brings order and sense into a difficult area. She reviewed computer rehabilitation of memory and concluded that so far this has not been controlled appropriately. Studies that evaluated computer rehabilitation carefully reported negative results recently. Other rehabilitation techniques include mnemonics and songs, but there is no guarantee that the patient will use them and generalization cannot be expected to occur automatically. Dr. Wilson also described other memory games, exercises and the technique of expanding rehearsal, backward and forward chaining, and the method of vanishing cues. We also heard about the fractionation of memory, such as the distinction between visual and semantic memories, and between episodic and procedural learning, which have different therapeutic implications. The loss of autobiographical memory is linked with damage to the limbic system and is often associated with severe anxiety.

Memory therapy is most seriously being investigated in Britain. Dr. Wilson indicated that one of the significant achievements was that most of the patients are using external aids. Evaluating outcome with the "Rivermead Behavioural Memory Test" (RBMT) indicated that this test distinguished those who eventually were able to return to gainful occupation and to live independently. On the hand, Wechsler Memory Test could not predict this. This kind of ecologically valid test of memory appears to be very promising in the evaluation of memory therapy.

One of the most interesting and scientifically satisfactory evaluation of problem-solving therapy in frontal lobe deficit came from the Munich group of von Cramon and Matthes-von Cramon. This is a most difficult field, yet they managed to define and measure problem solving, and describe a domain-specific therapy for it and contrast it with memory training. They matched patients in comparable groups and measured the effect of therapy. The results of their relatively brief but intense and well-defined intervention is impressive, and deserves confirmation in a larger group of patients or by another centre.

Dr. Gainotti considered a range of behaviour from agitated depression to disinhibited attitude as affective disturbance and he focused on post-stroke depression, and on the so-called catastrophic reaction. The hemispheric differences in the causation of post-stroke depression are interesting and Guido Gainotti suggested that they may be related to loss of language being so important to man rather than to the postulated asymmetries of serotoninergic and adrenergic systems. Gainotti has also made the point that different kinds of brain mechanisms produce different levels of awareness. Lack of awareness occurs more often with sensory deficit, such as in Wernicke's aphasia, neglect or in Anton's syndrome. Broca's aphasics, on the other hand, are more aware of their deficits and are more prone to depression. The psychological factors or interpretations should not preclude the pharmacological approach with tricyclic antidepressants as there are well controlled clinical trials to show their efficacy in post-stroke depression.

Anna Basso reviewed the rather mature field of recovery from aphasia and aphasia therapy. Biological and neurological factors, such as initial severity and etiology, appear to represent a major portion of variance. Lesion location and severity are difficult to evaluate because they interact with initial severity and aphasia type, but they also contribute significantly. This suggests that in other areas of rehabilitation, such as in diffuse brain damage, biological factors may also be important and should be carefully considered besides the psychological ones. "Anagraphic" factors, such as age, sex, and handedness, were less important in most of the studies. The evaluation of therapy results remains controversial, but Dr. Basso concluded that aphasia therapy bring about improvement in some and accelerates normal recovery in others. Just what kind of therapy and how long remains to be settled.

Walter Huber's summary of therapies is quite comprehensive. The Aachen unit considers the reactivation of temporarily impaired linguistic function in the early phase of spontaneous recovery in the first four months different from specific linguistic training in the chronic phase. Therapy included specific training of semantic fields, phonemic contrasts, sentence constructions, question particles, modal words, reflecting the linguistic orientation of the Aachen unit. In their comparison, the treated and untreated patients were from different populations. In the single case analysis the progression of each treated individual was compared to the average of a multi-centre control group. The conclusions were in favour of therapy (extra recovery in 78% in the early group and in 46% of the late group). The statistics were complex, but Klaus Willmes' methodological paper provided a good argument in their favour. Dr. Huber finally called for the integration of specific linguistic and more general cognitive aspects of therapy.

## Conclusion

Aphasia therapy has evolved to be a standard form of rehabilitation with reasonable evidence of efficacy, although the best forms of therapy and the duration and the suitability of patients are yet to be agreed upon. Cognitive rehabilitation of head injury and amnesia is relatively in its infancy, but we have seen impressive results indicating that research and existing therapies, particularly problem-solving therapy, need to be supported, and some forms of memory aids seem promising. I take a somewhat different view from Norbert Mai and suggest that before everyone puts forth a new innovative method of therapy, efforts to evaluate existing therapies need to be fully supported before new therapy clinics are established. If I were to rank the priorities for funding, research would stay on the top and existing services to patients would follow closely. This does not mean that therapists should not generate new ideas how to deal with the large number of brain-damaged patients with rehabilitation potential. Keep on innovating, but do not publish it as a panacea until some reasonable proof exists towards its efficacy or superiority over existing methods. It is just that we should not run off in every unproven direction with a waste of resources. There is time to inject a healthy dose of science into the honourable therapeutic efforts.

# Subject Index